Ward Sister's Survival Guide

Second Edition

Edited by Elizabeth M. Horne and Tracy Cowan

A collection of articles first published in *Professional Nurse* and here revised and updated for inclusion

Wolfe Publishing Ltd

Published by
Mosby–Year Book Europe Ltd.
Lynton House
7–12 Tavistock Square
London WC1H 9LB
England

Printed and bound in Great Britain by
BPCC Hazells Ltd

Member of BPCC Ltd

© 1992 Wolfe Publishing Ltd

Reprinted 1993

Wolfe is an imprint of Mosby–Year Book Europe Ltd.

ISBN 0 7234 18071

For full details of all Wolfe and Mosby Nursing titles please
write to Mosby–Year Book Europe Ltd, Lynton House,
7–12 Tavistock Square, London WC1H 9LB, England.

The Professional Developments Series

These eight books provide you with a wealth of insight into all aspects of nursing practice. The series is essential reading for qualified, practising nurses who need to keep up-to-date with new developments, evaluate their clinical practice, and develop and extend their clinical management and teaching skills. Through reading these books, students of nursing will gain an insight into what the essence of nursing is and the wide range of skills which are daily employed in improving patient care. Up-to-date, referenced and appropriately illustrated, The Professional Developments Series brings together the work of well over 200 nurses.

Other titles in The Professional Developments Series:

Contents

Managing Stress and Handling Aggression

Primary Nursing

Legal and Ethical Issues

Introduction

Since the first edition of the *Ward Sister's Survival Guide* was published, quality assurance, resource management and standard setting have become firmly established in nursing practice. The ward sister's role has, as a result, become firmly management orientated, and it is now the sister's key responsibility to ensure that available resources are matched to patients' needs and that optimum quality is achieved in all clinical circumstances. Managers in industry and commerce would easily recognise and identify with such a demanding role.

Basic management training often has to be supplemented with instinct and common sense. This book offers a constructive analysis of the key areas of the ward sister's role, showing how effective management can achieve optimum clinical results. Chapters on professional development, resource management, quality assurance, recruiting and managing staff, your teaching role and product appraisal cover the essential components of the ward sister's role, and present first hand examples of how good management can be put into practice. All articles were first published in *Professional Nurse* magazine, and have been updated and revised for this new edition. I hope you and your colleagues will find them useful in your own practice and professional development.

Tracy Cowan
Assistant Editor, *Professional Nurse*
London, March 1992

Your Professional Development

1

Can continuing education ease the nursing shortage?

Janet D. Duberley, MSc, SRN, RSCN, RCNT, Dip. Adv. Nurs. Stud.
Regional Nurse, Education and Practice, South West Thames Regional Health Authority

Nursing is facing major problems as the shortage of nurses begins to bite, and since there is no single reason for the shortage, there can be no single solution. It seems, however, that continuing professional education (CPE) is currently being used as the panacea to cure all the ills of staff recruitment and retention. I would suggest that at best it could serve as 'First Aid', at worst it could exacerbate the problem unless structural and organisational changes are also made.

What is continuing education?

Generally considered to be a 'good thing' CPE has an aura of common knowledge. However, common knowledge, like common sense, is remarkably uncommon, so I would like to explore the concept of CPE.

Houle (1980) says it relates to a dynamic concept of professionalisation with the ultimate aim "to convey a complex attitude made up of a readiness to use the best ideas and techniques of the moment, but also to expect that they will be modified or replaced. Everyone must expect constant change and with it new goals to be achieved and new understanding and skill to be mastered". This preparation for change is rather nebulous, so what does it mean in real terms? The American Nurses Association (ANA) defines CPE as "learning activities intended to build upon the educational and experimental basis of the professional nurse for the advancement of practice, education, administration, research or theory development to the end of improving the health of the public."

This definition contains a sense of what Houle calls the dynamic concept of professionalisation – the major focus builds on what has gone before to improve the public's health. However, what the learning activities might be is open to interpretation – the definition focuses on the different activities of nursing practice, education, administration and research. There is no mention of the *what* or *how* the public's health might be improved. In comparison, the American Medical Association (AMA, 1979) says "continuing medical education is composed of any education and training which serves to maintain, develop or increase the knowledge, interpretive and reasoning proficiencies, appropriate technical skills, professional performance standards or ability for interpersonal relationships that a physician uses to provide the service needed by patients or the public."

This comprehensive and thought provoking definition does not relate solely to 'keeping up-to-date', nor does it focus on how medicine is practised, but to maintaining, developing and increasing intellectual and cognitive skills as well as psychosocial and psychomotor skills. The definition's goals relate to the ideals of professionalism – the possession of a unique body of knowledge – but also, and especially, to the expert application of that knowledge through the development of the intellectual skills of interpretation and reasoning.

How do employers see CPE?

How do these definitions compare with the way employers might view CPE? The type of CPE supported and promoted by employing organisations give us a clear idea of their perspective. In 1985 Rogers conducted a national review of CPE in nursing, and found a tremendous amount fell primarily into three categories:

- In-service training. Staff orientation/introduction, policy dissemination.
- Clinical updating. Issues and trends in clinical practice and practical skills training.
- Post registration clinical role preparation. Six to 12 month courses in clinical nursing.

The activities most heavily supported and prevalent in all organisations were in-service training. These were well planned, with records of attendance kept in many cases, especially for those on fire and safety policies. Clinical updating activities were also present in most organisations, but tended to be less well planned and coordinated. Post registration clinical role preparation was provided where appropriate experience was available, but not all experience supported clinical courses.

These findings suggest that employees value the activities they see as contributing to the achievement of their organisational goals – providing a high quality, effective service. To fulfill these goals, staff must be aware of the environment, geography, personnel, operational and safety policies. Surely nurses' clinical knowledge and skills should have at least equal standing?

How do practitioners see CPE?

From the practitioner's point of view, the meaning of CPE may be determined by her or his age, previous experience of preregistration and continuing education and career goals. Cervero (1981) identified four major factors motivating doctors to participate in CPE:

- To maintain and improve professional competence and service to patients.

- To understand oneself as a professional.
- To interact with colleagues.
- To enhance personal and professional position.

The practitioner's view of CPE is different to those of the profession and the employers. It retains the service ideal but focuses more on the individual – CPE has a personal meaning as well as a professional one.

Potential areas of conflict

It is generally believed that responsibility for the continuing high quality of professional practice is equally shared by the profession, the employer and the practitioner, but their priorities may differ. The profession wants to advance its position in service to the public, and the employer wants to provide a high quality and cost-effective service to the public. The practitioner is pulled four ways – serving the public; fulfilling professional ideals; serving the employer, and meeting (or not meeting) personal goals.

This fourth component can cause real conflict. In undertaking CPE and acquiring more knowledge and skills, the practitioner may come to expect more of professional practice and of its financial remuneration. However, while enhancement of the individual's position featured in practitioners' goals, it did not feature in those of the profession or the employer, so the practitioner may not have a forum in which to practise these newly acquired skills or to be recompensed for them.

This conflict, I would suggest, is reflected in current nurse staffing problems. Nurses are expressing frustration, they have a poor self-image, and this contributes to high staff turnover and wastage. Obviously, pay levels and the high cost of living in the south of England have an effect, but I believe that even if the problems over pay were to be rectified tomorrow, the frustration would be evident again in a very short time. Why? Because pay is not the whole problem.

Over the last three years, the nursing shortage has assumed considerable political significance. People are anxious to know why nurses are leaving the profession. Analysis of the 1981 census data in two regional health authorities demonstrates that only 20 per cent of people holding nursing qualifications are currently employed in the profession. This suggests there is not a shortage of nurses, but a shortage of nurses employed in the profession. This in turn suggests there is something about the workplace or practice of nursing that makes people leave.

In 1986, Oxford District Health Authority, concerned about high staff turnover among clinical nurses conducted an extensive study to find the cause of nurses' dissatisfaction. The overwhelming response was that nurses felt unable to provide the care they believed their patients deserved. This was partly due to low staffing levels, but also due to frustration. Having trained in the profession, nurses were increasingly less able to practise nursing – their time was spent doing other things.

Waite (1986) undertook a national survey for the RCN, which came up with similar findings. Nurses who had left the health service or who had seriously considered doing so reported not feeling they were doing a worthwhile job; being unable to use their initiative; poor promotion prospects; not being valued. These sentiments indicate a restricted framework which does not allow nurses to practise nursing. Their expertise is not valued either in monetary terms or in years of professional practice, and they do not have a structure in which they can function as expert practitioners.

When nurses feel frustrated in their profession, they have a number of options. Many simply continue in their frustration – they have a poor image of both themselves and their profession, and take no action 'because it wouldn't make any difference'. Others use their frustration as an impetus for change. These nurses may seek greater challenge by changing jobs within clinical nursing, thus contributing to the high staff turnover in the profession. Others may pursue further education.

Since Rogers' survey of CPE opportunities in 1985, and the recognition of the nursing shortage there has been a great deal of investment in CPE. In some cases it has been used as a carrot to attract and retain nurses, but unfortunately it often only works for the duration of the course. On completion of the course, many nurses either change jobs or leave the profession altogether. I believe this is because employing authorities do not consider how to use the newly acquired skills, which means the nurses remain in their state of frustration and have no alternative but to consider a job change. While by no means all job changes within nursing can be attributed to this, the reality is that with few exceptions, employers have no structure for recognition or acceptance of clinical nurses who pursue education for advanced clinical practice.

Could a structure be created?

In the USA, clinical career structures have developed in a different way than in this country. Using a theoretical model of skill acquisition, Benner (1984) identified distinguishable differences in the competence of nurses with different levels of expertise. This has provided a rationale for the development of a career ladder within clinical nursing. Benner describes five stages of clinical development: novice; advanced beginner; competent; proficient and expert. The latter three are relevant here.

The competent practitioner   This practitioner is typified by the nurse who has been doing the same or a similar job for two or three years. She demonstrates a mastery of and ability to cope with the many contingencies of clinical nursing. Nursing care is conscious, deliberately planned and effective.

The proficient practitioner   This practitioner perceives situations as wholes rather than as aspects of the whole. Previous experience enables the proficient practitioner to recognise when the expected normal picture does not materialise. Decision making is improved because the nurse has a perspective on which of the many aspects are the important ones. Proficient performance is usually found in nurses who have worked in similar clinical settings for three to five years.

The expert practitioner This practitioner has an intuitive grasp of clinical situations. Her enormous background of experience enables her to home in on the accurate region of the problem without time consuming consideration of a wide range of alternative problems and solutions. While the expert practitioner appears not to rely on analytical principles, highly skilled analytical ability is necessary for those situations in which the nurse has no previous experience.

Implications for staff development

In describing levels of clinical expertise, Benner has provided the basis for a clinical career structure based on clinical competence, rather than managerial criteria as we have at present. But such defined career rungs have implications for staff development and continuing education in general. We must re-examine the goals and practice of CPE. It is the possession of cognitive, intellectual and interpretive skills that distinguishes the expert from the competent practitioner. CPE must address how it will facilitate the development of these skills.

However, as stated earlier, education and the acquisition of skills may not assist the retention of qualified nurses. These skills must be valued and recognised by employers. The current review of nursing manpower in terms of demand, supply and skill mix must take on a broader meaning than simply qualified:unqualified ratios. An examination of the level of skill requirements in clinical areas lends itself to the concept of clinical career ladders, to the proper use of scarce nursing resources and to proper levels of remuneration for clinical expertise. Unless this happens, CPE will only serve as First Aid. CPE should support the development of professional practice, but in association with the aims and goals of employing authorities.

References
AMA (1979) Proceedings of the 128th Annual Convention of the Council of Medical Education. July 22-26. Council on Medical Education, Report C.
Benner, R. (1984) *From Novice to Expert*. Addison Wesley, Mento Park, California.
Cervero, R. (1981) A factor analytical study of physicians' reasons for participating in continuing education. *Medical Education,* **56**, July, 29-34.
Houle, C.O. (1980) *Continuing Learning in the Professions*. Jossey-Bess, San Francisco.
Oxford District Health Authority (1986) DHA Member Report (Unpublished).
Rogers, J. (1987) *Continuing Professional Education for Qualified Nurses*. Austen Cornish Publishers and Ashdale Press, London. (Research carried out in 1985.)
Waite, R. and Hutt, R. (1987) *Attitudes, Jobs and Mobility of Qualified Nurses*. A report for the RCN. Institute of Manpower Studies, Brighton.

2
Will the minumum become an optimum? PREPP: mandatory study leave for nurses

Ann Shuttleworth, BA
Editor, Professional Nurse

You could be forgiven for heaving a big sigh at the prospect of yet more change in the nursing professions when the document PREPP and You (UKCC, 1991) landed on your doormat. Sent to all practitioners registered with the Council, it solicits your opinions about the recommendations made in Post Registration Education and Practice Project (PREPP: UKCC, 1990). The implications are far reaching and will affect how every practitioner keeps up-to-date, so it is important that people let Council know their opinions. This chapter will raise some of the many issues you will need to think about when making your response, starting with the recommendation that all practitioners complete a minimum of five days study leave every three years.

Ensuring effective practice
There are a number of reasons why you may welcome this recommendation in principle. Most fundamentally, you may think it is essential that nurses keep up-to-date if they are to practise effectively and efficiently and offer their patients the standard of care to which they are entitled. In the past, it has been perfectly possible (at least in theory) for nurses to sail through 40 year careers without undertaking any professional development or updating. While it is unlikely that there have been many instances of this, imagine the effect on patient care if such a nurse was involved in dressing wounds, or in any other field which has developed radically in the past few years? It doesn't bear thinking about, does it?

However, most nurses already see it as essential that they keep up-to-date with developments in their profession in general and their specialty in particular - the wellbeing and even the lives of their patients are at stake. Is this not enough? Do the small proportion of nurses who do not wish to update cause unnecessary stress or suffering to patients as a result? Is that enough to justify a mandatory requirement to update being imposed on everyone? What effect does it have on people when things are made compulsory? Those nurses who do not wish to update may resent being forced to do so. How well can they be expected to learn under those circumstances? And what about nurses who did update before it became mandatory? Will they resent being 'told', and will this affect the quality of their learning?

What about the managers?

Mandatory updating may, on the other hand, equally be directed at those responsible for sanctioning nurses' attendance at continuing professional education events. Many nurses who have been keen to update themselves have found it far from easy. Delegates to *Professional Nurse* National Study Days, to take one example with which I am familiar, testify to the fact that nurses all too often have to pay their own fees and travel for courses and study days *and* take the day as holiday! While these cases are by no means a majority, they do constitute a significant number of nurses, whose managers appear to to regard clinical updating as a low priority for their staff. Perhaps the introduction of mandatory updating will make these managers more amenable to the idea of supporting their nurses in maintaining and improving their competence.

Why five days?

If nurses are to be compelled to update, should we be talking in terms of days - why not hours? And why specifically five? Surely, as individuals, working in a wide range of fields, some will need more time than others to do the same amount of updating. What about those who need more than five days to maintain their practice at an acceptable standard, either because they work in a rapidly developing specialty or because they simply lose their 'edge' more quickly than others? Should they still be allowed to re-register, simply because they have completed a prescribed number of days? The problem with setting fixed numbers is that, while it makes for ease of administration, it does not take individuality into account. Also, with money as tight as it is currently, could the minimum become the optimum, the prescribed amount of updating employers require their nurses to undertake? Will nurses wishing to undertake more than the five days in three years find it difficult to obtain funds or time away from clinical practice? While it is currently unclear who will be responsible for funding these five days, if the bill has to be picked up by the health authorities, how keen will they be to add to their education costs for qualified staff by paying for extra days study leave? Will nurses too begin to see five days as the target beyond which they need not go?

A diverse enough range?

Since nursing is such a diverse profession, there will need to be a diverse range of updating opportunities to take account of individual, local and specialist needs. Unless this is made clear in the final PREPP legislation, there is a danger that the continuing education opportunities available, rather than growing, will shrink. Would it not be an attractive, cost-effective option for health authorities, if they are expected to fund this, to simply run a standard five day course and compel all nurses to attend? Easy to administer and cheap to run, could it become virtually the only updating available to some nurses?

Whatever final form PREPP's legislation and recommendations take, it is bound to cause difficulties for someone, in terms of cost and administration. It is important, however, that this prospect does not lead to them taking the simplest possible form, because although this may improve the minority of nurses who do not currently take any interest in maintaining their competence, and the minority of employers who see continuing professional education as a low priority for their nurses, it could also have dire consequences for the rest of the profession. Education budgets are all too easy to cut - they don't make the same waves as special care baby units, and if they exceed a minimum standard laid down in law, all the easier to justify cutting them. Nurses are human, and humans are also notoriously adept at seeing the minimum requirement as their goal. Will the setting of a five day rule demotivate nurses who would previously have undertaken much more professional education, once they reach the magic number?

Until PREPP is fully implemented, we cannot answer the questions raised in this chapter. However, none could be described as going into the realms of fantasy. We must hope legislation will take account of such possibilities, and ensure, as far as is feasible, that implementation of PREPP contributes to development , not to stagnation. Perhaps extending individual performance review to cover all nurses, and tying PREPP into this system is a way ahead? It would certainly allow individual needs to be accounted for.

References
UKCC (1990) Post Registration Education and Practice Project, UKCC, London.
UKCC (1991) PREPP and You, UKCC, London.

3

Who pays for PREPP?

Ruth Paton, BA(Hons), RGN, DN Cert
District Nurse, Bath

The report of the Post-Registration Education and Practice Project's (PREPP; UKCC, 1991) aims are twofold: to meet the needs of patients and the health service and to maintain and develop existing standards of nurse education and practice. For the nursing profession as a whole, it heralds widespread change. Indeed, in the words of the chairman of the project, Professor Margaret Green: "The Council does not underestimate the scale and importance of the recommendations contained within this report and how critical they are to the professions and to the future."

The report highlighted nine major recommendations, devised to: "maintain and enhance standards in order to meet the needs of patients, clients and the health services" (UKCC, 1991). Briefly, these recommendations centre on the key issues of providing:
- support for newly qualified staff;
- a written record of maintenance and development of professional skills and knowledge;
- guidelines as to the minimum attendance at study days required to facilitate three yearly re-registration;
- specification for advanced practice;
- guidelines as to eligibility to practice.

For nursing to be regarded as a profession, it is vital that standards of practice are maintained and enhanced. It is also imperative that each practitioner has the implicit knowledge base which patients and clients consider essential for the provision of care. The PREPP proposals will enable nurses to present explicit evidence of their eligibility to practice; indeed, the introduction highlights: "The Council is confident that the final recommendations offer an exciting, workable and cost-effective framework for maintaining and enhancing standards in post-registration education and practice" (UKCC, 1991).

The PREPP document has been offered to the profession for debate, and the nine major recommendations approved for implementation. One central issue was not discussed in the document – that of funding for nurse education, and it is this issue which this article aims to discuss.

Funding
It is clear that post-basic nurse education is under considerable review. As we move into the business orientated health service, characterised by purchasers and providers, the future of nurse education is unclear within

this framework. Various options are available, and funding will come from either:

- the providers of care ie, the health trusts;
- nurses themselves, in the guise of self-funding;
- a combination of the two;
- from possible external sources such as drug companies.

No clear answers have yet emerged as to which of these are the favoured funding option. It is interesting, however, to speculate on the possible implications were one of these options to be adopted.

Funding from the providers of care

If funding were to come from the providers (the health trusts and health authorities), in an effort to keep costs low and to compete with other areas, would this mean that the minimum of five days study in each three year period will become the maximum offered to nurses, and that courses longer than five days will be rendered redundant? If the employers determine that five days study in each three year period is a maximum, what place will there be for provision of courses requiring longer periods of study, such as degree courses, sponsoring for diploma and masters places and the continuing impetus to align nurse training with universities and other centres for higher education? The impetus to promote professional development and enhance nurse status is clearly gaining momentum, but if we allow the links developed with centres for higher education to wither, what effect will this have for the standard and quality of nurse development? Concern over funding is also raised due to the fact that PREPP is competing for finance against other educational changes, such as Project 2000; the projected increase in educational costs facilitated by the introduction of Project 2000 has been calculated by York University to be £140 million (based on 1982-83 prices). In view of this, where will additional finance be found for PREPP?

If employers do finance nurse education, what effect will this have on course provision? At present, it is not uncommon for each area to provide similar or duplicated courses to meet local nursing needs, but as the new health trusts will undoubtedly demand value for money, it can reasonably be assumed that this will cease. As a more cost-effective alternative, course provision may instead be rationalised with regional centres, thus streamlining educational provision. This will have considerable implications for course attendance: if, for example, only one centre provides a particular course which necessitates the participating nurse finding accommodation, who will pay for this? Furthermore as the 'demographic time bomb' increases its impact on nurse recruitment, how will this affect recruitment of mature personnel, who may already have domestic commitments, which preclude either residential courses or self-financing of education? The PREPP report indicates that: "...the professions are already targeting more mature entrants as part of their recruitment drive" (UKCC, 1991), adding that they will bring "...greater expectations of themselves and the organisation they work for". These hidden implications may serve only to dash such expectations and create a new wave of frustration and resentment.

On a positive note, however, if nurses adopt a business orientated approach, health trusts may well have to compete for increasingly scarce and valuable nursing expertise. Why, therefore, work for one health trust, which offers only the minimum period of study leave, when another may fund one for longer periods of study? Similarly, in terms of residential courses, nurses may well use demographic trends to their advantage. In an effort to recruit personnel, funding provision for attendance on courses at regional centres may become important parts of salary and renumeration packages. At present, no clear answer has emerged, but nurses themselves have the power to determine which outcome prevails.

Self-funding

If it is accepted that the financial implications for PREPP are considerable, does this mean we are moving into the area of nurses funding their own professional update? Sylvester (1990) claims: "...it is possible that part of the cost would be met by the employer and part met by the practitioner."

Precedents for this have already been established, the Open Learning Programme being one example. Aimed primarily at enrolled nurses who wish to convert to first level registration, it is also considered suitable for nurses returning to practice and "registered nurses who have had no time to devote to study since they qualified" (Robinson, 1990). Initially, this may seem an ideal way to satisfy recommendations five and six of PREPP pertaining to study leave and return to practice. The cost of the Open Learning Programme, however, is £975 per year, and it is only "hoped that health authorities will help to support students" (Robinson, 1990); for nurses, particularly those at D and E grades, this is not an inconsequential sum. Although most would agree that it is their professional responsibility to ensure their continuing development, will every nurse see that: "putting time and money into study which can move them forward in their careers and ultimately enable them to earn more money can be a good investment?" What will happen to those who cannot afford this? The cost of preparation for first level registration per NHS entrant was £13,090 in 1988 (Bosanquet, 1988). If we rely on staff supplementing their own post-basic education, then the recruit and retrain programme may be seriously affected by the PREPP proposals.

External sources

Drug companies are increasingly realising the influence nurses have in product choice, especially within the community setting. The advent of nurse prescribing, however limited initially, is within sight; the pharmaceutical companies are increasingly promoting their products to nurses, and regional district nurse exhibitions, lunches and lectures are now common. Taking this a step further, what better way of establishing brand awareness than to sponsor educational courses for nurses? As a profession nursing would have to question the ethics of such developments, but it is a scenario with which we may find ourselves dealing.

Professional comparisons

As nursing strives to become recognised as a profession, are we wrong to express concern regarding this new concept of self-funding for post-registration education? How do we answer critics who argue that as individuals nurses should invest in their own future? In an endeavour to answer this question, it is useful to compare the PREPP proposals with systems already in place in the other main professional groups. Having contacted the professional bodies for chartered accountants, solicitors and teachers, it appears that there is no hard and fast rule. The Institute for Chartered Accountants for England and Wales has developed obligatory requirements known as continual professional education (CPE), and to meet these objectives, the Institute recommends "an appropriate mix of structured and unstructured CPE". Meeting these requirements is the individual's own responsibility, but accountants employed by the major practising firms are subsidised by their employers to do this. Accountants in Scotland have voluntary guidelines for continuing education, which amount to a minimum of 100 hours of structured learning, but again, course enrolments come from firms, as opposed to individuals. In the case of solicitors, the Law Society indicates that although responsibility to comply with the society's regulations on updating lies with the individual, most employers fund courses to meet these individuals' training needs.

It is, however, interesting to discuss the position of teachers, perhaps the professional group with which nurses have been most closely identified. In the case of teachers employed in further and higher education, until recently they have had their in-service training paid for by their employing institution, but this situation is now under threat. At present, the situation varies between institutions and individual authorities.

It appears, therefore, with the exception of teachers in further and higher education, that although funding for post-basic education is discretionary, it is unusual for employees to be expected to finance their own education. Although it would not be advisable for nursing to adhere *carte blanche* to the practices of other professional bodies, we should not ignore their example when debating and reviewing the PREPP proposals.

The underlying principle of PREPP is that of maintaining and enhancing standards "in order to meet the needs of patients, clients and the health services" (UKCC, 1991). It has given us an ideal opportunity to enhance our profession by potentially aligning ourselves with institutions of higher education, particularly under the credit accumulation and transfer scheme (CATS). In a purchaser/provider arena, we must be cautious that we do not price ourselves and our skills out of the market. Conversely, it would be a sad indictment of the system, if the positive aspects of PREPP were to be sacrificed as a result of financial insufficiency. As a profession, these are issues we need to be highlighting as we continue to debate the PREPP proposals.

References
Bosanquet, N. (1988) What will it cost? *Nursing Times*, **84**, 31, 34.
Millar, B. (1991) Investing in the future. *Nursing Times*, **87**, 8, 29.
Robinson, K. (1990) Open learning. *Nursing Times*, **86**, 43, 27.
Sylvester, J. (1990) Taking the road ahead. *Nursing Standard*, **4**, 25, 16.
UKCC (1991) The Report of the Post-Registration Education and Practice Project, UKCC, London.

4

A gap which must be bridged: nurses' attitudes to theory and practice

Sue Hawkett, MSc, RGN, RSCN, RM, DipN, CertEd, RNT
Senior Nurse, Palliative Care Co-ordinator, South West Thames Regional Health Authority

"It's all right in theory, but have you tried to actually do this in practice? What is the use of nursing models and curriculum planning when it has no relevance to what I do in practice?". These are no doubt familiar words to many, and they are often justified. This chapter traces the background of why some of these attitudes exist in nursing and suggests ways in which the practice-theory gap can be bridged.

Attitudes to theory

Our society sees nursing as a practical, vocational activity, and nurses themselves as a dependable and reliable workforce (Judge, 1985). Although today's nurses are increasingly concerned with ethical, political and economic questions which directly affect patient care, the notion that nursing is essentially practical and paternalistic still exists - nursing practice often consists of tasks designed to enable nurses to be in control of dependent patients.

Theoretical assumptions are often viewed with suspicion by nurses, and described as 'woolly', 'impractical' and 'airy-fairy', but as Chapman (1985) states, nursing cannot only be a practical activity, a viewpoint supported by McFarlane (1986) who points out that practice without theoretical basis becomes a ritualised performance, unrelated to the health needs of individuals and society. It is important, however, that innovative ideas spring from practice.

So why do nurses resist theory? One reason may be that nursing has suffered from the assumption that it has no unique function, that it borrows relevant theories from other disciplines, and consequently never identifies its own unique body of knowledge. If this were so, it would be difficult to identify the nature of nursing (Hawkett, 1989).

In considering the functions played by nurses as described by Hoy (1986), however, it is hard to understand why the profession's uniqueness is not more universally recognised and accepted. Nurses are described as the carers who are in contact with patients, often communicating at times of extreme human need, who help them attain independence according to their ability and condition. To maximise individuals' health potential, nurses require knowledge of environmental factors and the educative process. They value patients as individuals and act in accordance with this belief, and recognise that their role cannot be carried out in isolation, and so coordinate other services for their patients' welfare. Nursing, therefore, has a unique function, and needs to be encouraged to own and develop this.

Bridging the gap

How can theory and practice be brought together? The first step in achieving compatibility between theoretical frameworks and what is done in practice is to explore with practitioners the meaning of the nature, philosophy and practice of nursing. In an attempt to address this issue, a survey was conducted among nurses working in a hospice, to discover what they saw as the nature of the dying patient, and the role of the nurse. The survey was based on the belief that if nursing is a practice discipline, practitioners should be able to state their beliefs, which should then be translated into a working philosophy. From this position it should be possible to develop a nursing theory which is owned, understood and therefore accepted by nurses; practice should constantly challenge and stimulate theory.

The research question behind the survey was, "How does the educationalist, working in a multidisciplinary context caring for dying patients, prepare a curriculum which is congruent with the philosophy of practitioners?" (Hawkett, 1986). However, any defined philosophy needs to be considered against the background of the prevailing ethos of the organisation which is going to set standards and have certain expectations of staff. This raises fundamental questions: to what extent should the curriculum be based on the ethos of the organisation, which through years of experience has learnt what is needed and expected of carers? Should the curriculum grow out of the needs of the carers, meeting, matching and encouraging their development? To what extent are new recruits constrained by the organisation, and to what extent are they able to grow and contribute to the organisation?

To understand these issues, it is helpful to reflect on the kind of background many nurses have had. Some nurses will have followed a strong medical model, being directed and monitored by doctors, while others will have grappled with professional accountability. All, however, will have felt the conflict between education and service needs, and this debate will not disappear with Project 2000.

When nurses enter training, usually at 18 years, they are at a vulnerable stage of development - idealistic, energetic, with high hopes and expectations. This is inconsistent with what is observed at the end of training or in continuing education, when nurses' outlook is less positive.

Reconciling experience and theory

So what has been happening? The caring role is so often seen as innate, a virtue which is 'just there'. Both clinical nurses/managers and educators have adhered to the notion that to learn nursing you must do nursing. Many nurses have experienced the 'trial by fire', when they have found themselves vulnerable, defensive and ill-equipped to cope on a ward in the face of human tragedy. Professionals are often still expected to leave their emotions at home, which causes some nurses to feel guilty if they become sad, angry or despairing at work. Nurses exchange what they actually feel for what they 'ought' to feel, and in doing this they suppress real feelings, and with them their own self-awareness. As a result their personal growth and that of others is stunted.

The results of this process are familiar: absenteeism, frequent job changes, doing courses, and finally leaving nursing. Here lies some of the theory-practice gap - our treatment of each other.

Kitson (1985) describes a concept of care which aims to combine the emotional (experience) and cognitive (theory) dimension of a task. The concept is familiar; that of knowing oneself, being cared for, and having respect for others. She asserts that where this exists it leads to increased commitment to the job, eagerness to acquire skills and knowledge, and a growing respect for patients and colleagues. Only when people care about themselves and are cared for by colleagues are they free to care for others (Rogers, 1967). This poses a challenge to create a learning environment where such skills as compassion, empathy and imagination can be practised, and given equal importance with clinical objectives.

The philosophy of practice should also be the curriculum philosophy. An individual is not seen as a set of symptoms arising from a disease, but as a human being with rights, needs and wants, which will change and develop daily. Implicit in this statement is the belief that individuals need to grow and use their experiences in a positive way, seeking meaning and purpose within sometimes meaningless situations. Surely the role of the educator is to foster continued growth, recognising the uniqueness of each individual.

The link

Here is the link between practice and theory. In caring it is recognised that there is a need to provide a safe environment in which patients can explore their feelings, have control and choice over treatment, receive individualised care and be encouraged in personal growth. This can only be achieved if the carer is prepared to shift from the traditional custodian role to a partnership and facilitative role. The thrust of this model of care is that it is patient-centered, so the logical progression is that the curriculum model should be student-centred. The emphasis in both is the respect of, and the importance attributed to, individuals. The curriculum model which best fits is a process model (Stenhouse, 1975), whose elements stress the importance of learner participation and responsibility, recognising the partnership between learner and teacher.

Hoy (1986) describes eight elements of care which can be transferred from the clinical environment into the 'classroom', which serve as a useful basis for discussion when considering the process approach based on humanistic principles:

Knowing - the person, their needs and growth needs.

Alternating rhythms - doing and then reflecting, analysing, understanding and modifying the doing, so that the process recommences.

Patience - allowing another space, time, to think, feel and live.

Honesty - seeing the other person as they actually are, not as they ideally are.

Trusting - appreciating independent existence.

Humility - being responsive to the growth of another and continuing to learn about and from the other.

Hope - the other will grow through caring.

Courage - to move into the unknown.

Implementing a philosophy of practice

In pursuing a holistic and humanistic approach to nursing, practice models and curriculum models must embrace the same philosophy and understanding about the nature of nursing, which seems to be an activity based on humanistic principles, responding to individuals' needs on a continuum from total independence and health to dependence and death. This philosophy needs to be reflected in the curriculum, which could come about through pursuing the basic belief of negotiation and partnership between practitioner and educationalist.

The physical environments of hospital and college of nursing are often as separate as is the intellectual understanding of the philosophy of nursing from which they have designed a curriculum; but to what extent has the philosophy been understood and curriculum fitted into practice?

This was recently illustrated when a small group of educationalists met with the surgical directorate of a hospital to discuss the development of the Diploma of Higher Education in Nursing Adult Branch. The educationalists went with a carefully formulated theoretical framework and wished to explain to their clinical colleagues how they expected the theory that the students would receive in college to be enhanced and reinforced in the pratice setting. This approach was met with blank looks and frowns. What relevance would the theory have in helping the student care for the patient recovering from a hysterectomy? Would they be able to recognise if the patient was bleeding, developing an infection or deep vein thrombosis? Would they have the basic practical skills and confidence in order to develop further clinical expertise?

The problem was that the theoretical underpinning of all these clinical skills had been developed and described away from the wards in the college of nursing and midwifery. It had then been brought to the ward staff as an 'educational package'. The ward staff had had no input and because of this there was little understanding of the terms used and no ownership.

As a result of this experience the group decided that the starting point in the process must be to ask the question, 'what knowledge, skills, and attitudes do you expect a student to develop while gaining experience looking after patients undergoing surgery?' In this way the emphasis is put where it belongs, on practice. In becoming a competent surgical nurse he/she will require a body of knowledge and nursing skills based on nursing research.

These problems can be contrasted with a specialised unit such as a hospice, whose staff share an agreed philosophy. Here the physical environment means that education and teaching take place near or within the clinical area. There is an intellectual acceptance of the philosophy of 'total pain', which considers physical, emotional, social and spiritual pain experienced by patients and their families, and there is a commitment to a team approach in caring for patients and families.

The accepted philosophy of practice is translated into curriculum content. At St Christopher's Hospice, multidisciplinary courses have been developed which reflect this principle. Nurses, doctors, social workers and clergy join together for one or two week courses, spending approximately 75 per cent of their time following common components of the curriculum. The rest of the time is divided into sessions for doctors and nurses looking at specific aspects of symptom control together, and for social workers and clergy at other specific areas. This emphasises two points: first, each discipline works from a specialist knowledge base and has a unique role and function which must be acknowledged, owned and respected by others; second, there are many common areas as we work together as a healthcare team which need to be explored and recognised. The courses illustrate that it is possible to learn together and work together. Perhaps this is a brave attempt to break across guarded professional boundaries, but it is a challenge to allow our working philosophy to influence and drive our teaching, linking theory with practice on a number of levels and creating a realistic experience which makes sense to the healthcare team.

References
Chapman, C. (1985) Theory of Nursing. Practical Application. Harper and Row, London.
Hawkett, S. (1989) Model marriage? *Nursing Times*, **85**; 1, 61-62.
Hawkett, S. (1988) The Philosophy of Terminal Care - Towards a Common Philosophy and Curriculum. MSc Dissertation, University of Surrey.
Hoy, R. A. (1986) Balancing the Nurse Curriculum. Costello, Tunbridge Wells.
Judge Report. (1985) The Education of Nurses: a New Dispensation. Commission on Nursing Education, Royal College of Nursing.
Kitson, A. (1985) Educating for Quality. Paper presented at Annual Director of Nurse Education conference. Robinson Hall, Cambridge.
McFarlane. (1986) Models for Nursing. In: Kershaw B. (Ed) John Wiley, Chichester.
Rogers, C. (1967) On Becoming a Person. Constable, London.
Stenhouse, L. (1985) An Introduction to Curriculum Research and Development. Heinemann, London.

5

Coming down from the ivory tower: putting research into practice

Stephen G. Wright, RGN, RCNT, DipN, RNT, MSc
Consultant Nurse, Nursing Development Unit, Tameside General Hospital

Mark Dolan, RGN
Charge Nurse/Senior Primary Nurse, Nursing Development Unit, Tameside General Hospital

Nursing is renowned for the gaps it endures between theory and practice, and such a gap, it seems, applies as much to nursing research as to any other sector of nursing. Bergman (1986) has argued that "some researchers live in ivory towers, divorced from the reality of daily practice". The researcher, separated in this way, is seen as pursuing esoteric theory which has no bearing on the day-to-day world of nursing practice, instead working for or speaking to fellow like-minded academics. Preaching thus to the converted, the findings of nursing research reach a limited audience and fail to affect the huge mass of nurses engaged at the hard edge of practice.

"Practice can only be as sound as the knowledge on which it is based" (Jacox, 1974).

Some writers have suggested the term 'research' itself alienates many nurses because it is surrounded by mystique, and: "Because nursing is essentially a pragmatic discipline, the usefulness of research endeavours is sometimes equated with practical applicability. Hence, research which is not seen to have an immediate use is often dismissed as a waste of resources with which it is not worth bothering" (Luker, 1986).

Luker goes on to suggest that research may illuminate or bring new insight to what nurses do. It may help to test out and refine methodologies appropriate to nurses, discovering new knowledge which can directly affect practice, such as the work of Norton *et al*, (1962) and their work on pressure sore risk assessment. Given that there are such clear benefits to nursing research, why is it so often ignored and little applied? It is perhaps too simplistic to blame the 'ivory tower' researcher, though this is, no doubt, a contributing factor. Sometimes the language in which a research report is couched is itself counterproductive, simply because it is not described or expressed in such a way that most clinical nurses can comprehend. Sometimes nurses see themselves as too busy with patients to have time for research, and this is reinforced if they regard research as a theoretical issue which has no relevance to practitioners. They are, futhermore: "often unwilling to carry out research through shortage of funds, or lack of awareness of how to go about it, and are put off by the seeming complexities of the ethical issues. On top of this, nurses may simply feel that the 'bosses' (who may not be research minded) would be unsupportive and even hostile" (Wright, 1986).

Bond (1978) believes that nursing research must be 'proletarianised' if it is to have any meaning and relevance to the greatest number of nurses. In other words, thinking about, carrying out, and analysing research need to be commonplace activities accepted by all nurses in their day-to-day practice. The number of research courses available and the trend towards including research awareness in both statutory and continuing education programmes means that, to some extent, this is already underway. A great deal more can be done in the service side of nursing to proletarianise nursing research, and this has been one of the main aims of the Nursing Development Unit (NDU) at Tameside.

Promoting research awareness
Motivated experts at clinical level Benner (1984) argues cogently that clinical experts need to act as role models in promoting research-based practice. While all nursing staff on the NDU have research elements written into their job descriptions, there is no guarantee that this will happen in practice. Other key individuals are needed to be experts in their field, acting as good examples to others, helping them to carry out research and apply findings. A research nurse post was specifically created, and a team of clinical specialists and a consultant nurse also included research in their remit. These nurses can also use informal networks to guide colleagues to others who will assist with information or act as supervisors. This is also seen as a key role for the 'G' grade sister and charge nurse who are the key clinical leaders and innovators. Nurses who have conducted research through research appreciation on graduate courses are in an excellent position to facilitate awareness among others, especially if they work alongside them.

Staff development All the NDU's courses are research-based, and many contain specific education in areas such as research awareness and methodologies. Including research projects as part of course objectives stimulates a spirit of enquiry, while reinforcing the idea that research is 'ordinary'. Staff can be encouraged to attend research courses off site with similar research components or pursue open learning programmes.

Scale Making research 'ordinary' is a key feature in demystifying it. Nurses can be helped to realise that nursing research is simply 'finding out' and choosing the best methods with which to do so. Simple, practical projects related directly to nurses' working experiences (such as the effects of going out of uniform, costing of incontinence devices, evaluating the introduction of pet therapy) were found to be most helpful. Nurses do not need to feel that research should be highly complex in order to discover the meaning of life; setting research projects which are fairly simple, relevant to nurses' day-to-day work and which can be pursued within the time and resources available are good starting points for promoting an acceptance of the relevance of research.

Literature   This includes books, journals and articles on research reports as well as research methods, which need to be made available at ward level and accessible to all staff, day or night. The NDU has set up a small library on site which is open 24 hours a day, and which clearly makes access to literature much easier than relying on the more limited availability in, for example, a more distant school of nursing. Stocks of books and journals can also be kept at ward level. Additional access to literature can be gained by setting up arrangements with local colleges, polytechnics and universities – most will willingly permit external students entry to their libraries. Organisations such as the RCN have extensive library facilities, including assistance with literature searches.

Informal approaches   Introducing a research item to the agenda of a meeting, setting up a research appreciation forum, a journal, club or discussion groups are various methods in which groups of nurses can get together informally and treat research as part of the topic of the day. Nurses at ward level, for example, can introduce a topic of relevance to each ward meeting, while colleagues at all levels can read and précis research reports for discussion, and circulate written summaries to others. Peer group support is essential to successful research awareness. A research interest group can be set up, a quality circle developed or nurses can join in many research interest and development opportunities provided by such professional bodies as the RCN.

Funding and resources   How can we afford to promote research awareness? The real question is how can we afford not to? Nurses, like other professionals, are now being judged in cost-effective terms – a knowledgeable, expert nurse, whose practice is based on sound research, is required to make the best use of resources. Above all, however, patients have a right to a nurse who knows what he or she is doing, and is interested and well-motivated enough to offer skilled, expert care.

Whenever possible, funds and resources have been put to maximum use, for example by using staff training monies on secretarial or word-processing time. In addition a bursary has been set up, derived from various methods of fund raising (Purdy *et al*, 1988), to provide money to support nursing research and staff development which is independent of the limited health authority funds available. Staff can also be encouraged to apply for other sources of funding such as local industry, scholarships, the Nightingale Fund or the Department of Health.

Senior staff need to be prepared to actively support nurses making applications for funding and seeking resources – the latter including not just money, but time. Committed managers will find that releasing staff for study and research, however difficult this might seem in the short term in a hard-pressed service, will be more than rewarded in the long term by the greater energy, motivation and skill of those staff.

The above points have proved helpful to us in developing research awareness in the NDU. One final point is also worth considering: nurses are notorious for not valuing what they do, and much valuable research is lost because no-one is able to read it. The staff's research reports are kept in the NDU library, and summaries can be discussed at meetings or circulated to wards. Letters of appreciation for research projects reinforce researchers' morale and motivation. However small a project, it always provides difficulties which deserve recognition when they are overcome and good work is produced. On a wider scale, the project can be prepared for publication, and many journals will give advice on this. It is a real pleasure for researchers to see their work in print and to know that it has reached a wider audience than their immediate colleagues.

The effects
If research awareness and activity are encouraged, the question has to be asked – is it worth it? The value of nursing research is that it directly benefits both patients and staff. Staff who feel they are learning, trying out new things and improving practice feel better about themselves and

---

- **Uniforms** – trials of going out of uniform were conducted. Some areas remained out of uniform as a result of patient response.

- **Sharing mealtimes** to produce a more therapeutic environment – staff on rehabilitation wards carried out a trial of sharing mealtimes which has now been implemented.

- **Pet therapy** – a research project was completed in the light of earlier evidence of the benefits of pet therapy. A dog is now resident on one ward.

- **Quality circles** – these have been set up and are used as forums to produce change. For example, the night staff formed their own quality circle and examined various problems which affected them. This led to re-examining and changing the way that deceased are removed from the ward.

- **Primary nursing** – the staff have implemented primary nursing throughout the unit, and conducted various surveys to examine patients' and other responses.

- **Self-medication** – evidence of poor compliance with drugs by elderly people after discharge led to designing, implementing and evaluating a patient self-medication programme.

Table 1. Application of research.

more motivated at work, thus contributing to an improved staff morale (with consequent reduction in the costs of high sickness or leaving rates). It cannot be a coincidence that the NDU, with its aroused spirit of enquiry, has a waiting list of staff, while sickness and leaving rates are well below the national average (less than 1 per cent, compared with 18 per cent). Several projects completed in the unit also testify to a further feedback – that 'finding out' stimulates innovation, which in turn stimulates further 'finding out' (Table 1).

Encouraging staff to enquire, innovate and see research as a normal part of nursing practice can change and improve it in many ways. Nursing research achieves its true value in this way, not as an esoteric notion, but a tool to improve the lives of patients and nurses.

References
Benner, P. (1984) From Novice to Expert. Addison Wesley, London
Bergman, R. (1986) Escaping from the ivory tower. *Nursing Times*, **82**, 41, 58-60.
Bond, S. (1978) Dilemmas in Clinical Research. Unpublished paper presented at Northern Regional Health Authority Seminar on Developments in Nursing.
Jacox, A. (1974) Nursing research and the clinician. *Nursing Outlook*, **22**, 82, 16-18.
Luker, K. (1986) Who's for research? *Nursing Times*, **82**, 52, 55-56.
Norton, D., McLaren, R. Exton-Smith, A.N. (1962) An Investigation of Geriatric Nursing Problems in Hospital. National Corporation for the Care of Old People, London.
Purdy, E. and Wright, S.G. (1988) If I were a rich nurse. *Nursing Times*, **84**, 41, 36-38.
Treece, E.W. and Treece, J.W. (1977) Elements of Research in Nursing. Mosby, St Louis.
Wright, S.G. (1986) Building and Using a Model of Nursing. Edward Arnold, London.

6

Who needs nursing philosophies?

Dominic Mawdsley, BA, RGN

Charge Nurse, Urology, Hammersmith Hospital, London

Much has been said about philosophies for care, but little literature on the subject has been written for guidance. Most nurses know they are expected to have philosophies of care for their areas, but few know their purpose and how to go about writing them. The English National Board (ENB, 1988) states that all areas involved in nurse training must have a philosophy, while the other national boards also have similar requirements. The mention of national board directives makes most nurses roll their eyes upwards and start muttering profanities under their breath. However, if the boards say so, then that word tends to become law. Everyone rushes off, hurriedly writes a philosophy for care, breathes a sigh of relief when the visit is over and then puts the philosophy in the top drawer of sister's desk until the next visit.

The inclination is, therefore, to mention such directives as an afterthought in order to discourage the view that this is a time-wasting exercise devised to keep nurses busy. Encouragement and motivation are far more likely to get a philosophy written.

A philosophy is an invaluable tool which directs and influences patient care. It is a series of beliefs, feelings, values and outlooks that can be developed in any area concerned with patient care, with the purpose of demonstrating what nurses feel their particular specialty should be achieving both for patients and nursing staff. This will only be the case, however, if nurses have a true understanding of what a philosophy is and how to go about developing one.

How to write a philosophy

Various methods have been used for developing philosophies, such as being presented with one from management and asked to comment on it (the 'top down' approach), questionnaires, or a 'cascade' method. The disadvantage of these methods is that philosophies generated in these ways will all ultimately reflect the preconceived ideas of the initiator. More successful, however, is a 'bottom-up' approach, involving all the staff of the relevant area (Figure 1).

Time should be allocated for study days and fact finding so that all staff become familiar with the process of writing a philosophy and can obtain any relevant research or information required. A nurse specialist or facilitator should be included if one is available, to act as an objective party who can support and advise from the outside. However, if no nurse specialist is available, a facilitator usually emerges from within the group.

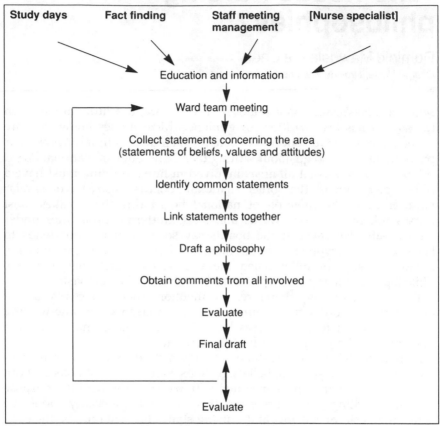

Figure 1. The process for writing a philosophy at a local level.

This initial ground work and organisation means there is a wealth of information and education which is pooled at the ward team meeting. By 'brainstorming', and sharing ideas, common beliefs and values will emerge which ultimately reflect philosophy, purpose and objectives. There are no strict rules and no set length, although a philosophy of three lines will provide little direction, and one several pages long will deter potential readers. What is desirable, however, is that nursing jargon and clichés are avoided. Moore (1971) wrote: "This tendency to make use of pot-boiler statements culled from the folklore of nursing does serve a purpose of sorts: it protects nurses from looking at the realities of their jobs and evaluating their own activities." This can also make a philosophy incomprehensible and indigestible to non-nurses.

Why bother?

Are there any benefits to be gained from having a philosophy, or is it yet another piece of paper produced by nurses who have nothing better to do with their time? If a philosophy is truly a statement of belief and intent, then it must have practical applications (Romhanyi, 1990). A written philosophy provides a chance to reflect on practice: the process of writing it necessitates examining and justifying nursing practice. This leads practitioners to question whether practices are carried out on a traditional basis "because we've always done it this way", or whether they truly benefit patient care, so not only will individual practice be questioned, but also the beliefs and practices of the team.

Philosophies translate practice into writing. Nurses as a group are good at 'feeling and intuition', but are sometimes hard-pushed to clarify these in black and white. This may be one of the most difficult aspects of formulating a philosophy, but once practice is committed to writing, it will direct a group in the achievement of a purpose and therefore promote continuity of care. This must be preferable to a situation where nurses deliver erratic care because they are following a 'gut feeling'.

This continuity will go on to develop a team and promote a harmonious relationship with clinicians from other disciplines. Philosophies need not be solely for nursing; if members of the multidisciplinary team are involved in writing them, a truly holistic approach can be adopted. For instance, physiotherapists in intensive care units play a crucial role in the care of critically ill patients and should therefore have their values and beliefs reflected in their unit's philosophy. It must also be remembered that a philosophy serves to clarify the nurse's role to other members of the team.

A philosophy can also be used as a justification of quality of service. Proof can be given to managers that quality care is being delivered – an extremely important aspect in the light of the proposals contained within Working for Patients (DoH, 1989). Leading on from this, it can also provide a base for the development of standards of care. Either problem areas will be identified when writing the philosophy, or standards will be developed as measuring tools for the quality service being guaranteed in the philosophy.

An appropriate model of nursing may also be developed from a philosophy; once beliefs and practices have been questioned, it may become apparent that care delivery is inappropriate. This, in turn, will lead nurses to question whether the framework being used within the nursing process for delivering care is meeting patients' needs, or whether it can be improved upon. Would the application of an alternative nursing model or the development of one's own enhance nursing care?

Patient expectations

A philosophy can increase the awareness of patients/clients about what they can expect during their period under care if it is displayed in a prominent position. In many ways this is a brave thing to do, as nurses are laying themselves open to potential criticism and complaint, but patients would be quite within their rights to challenge staff and ask why they are not doing what is laid down within the philosophy. However, it has been observed that patients have read philosophies and commented to staff that their care truly reflects them. Medical staff may also find it interesting to read a ward philosophy, as it may clarify the aims and objectives of nursing practices in the clinical area and help them understand the need for the nursing process and individualised patient care at a time when nurses are moving away from the traditional image of 'ministering angels'.

Ward philosophies can also provide invaluable information for student nurses, particularly if they are sent out in an orientation package prior to the start of their allocation. How many of us started on a ward as students and spent the first week hiding in the sluice room trying to work out sister's likes and dislikes – a phenomenon supported by research by Fretwell (1982) and Pembrey (1980)? The ward philosophy can provide insight into the workings and the personalities of the ward.

By the same token, philosophies can be used for recruitment purposes when sent out with job descriptions and application forms. Candidates can then decide whether the unit is compatible with their particular ethos or whether it would be a waste of time for both parties to continue with the application. Should they decide to continue with the application, philosophies can be useful at interview; candidates may question the philosophy and ask for elaboration, and interviewers may be able to ascertain if the candidate is right for the environment.

Taking this one step further, philosophies may then be used to aid nurse appraisal on both sides. If care appears inconsistent and of a poor quality, managers can use the philosophy to redirect care and serve the nurse a reminder of what has previously been guaranteed. On the other hand, nurses may actually use it to demonstrate that the objectives outlined are not being achieved, possibly due to lack of staff or equipment, and that patient care is being compromised.

Finally, philosophies provide tools for teaching. The process of writing a philosophy means all those concerned will have to have access to relevant education and information. This may well involve fact finding and study days, and thus lead on to other areas of interest. Should the need to examine standards of care or nursing models become apparent, that in itself is a different aspect of the trained nurse's education, so philosophies can play a significant part in continuing education.

Evaluation

A philosophy, therefore, is a useful tool with a variety of applications. Table 1 is an extract from one of the ward philosophies at Westminster Hospital, which demonstrates the values and intentions of the nursing staff on a dermatology ward.

It is important, however, to evaluate the philosophy of care regularly, and this should take into account staff changes or change of the clinical specialty; otherwise it should be done at least yearly. Even if the philosophy remains unchanged, the process will serve as a reminder and ensure that it continues to reflect the beliefs of the clinical area.

> "We feel that it is important to welcome patients warmly to the ward. We recognise that hospital is not home, but by being friendly and approachable we hope to portray a relaxed environment and also reduce some of the patients' fears and anxieties.
>
> "Any disfiguring disease can cause a distorted body image and also lower a person's morale and confidence. Therefore, it is important for us to promote patients' self-confidence in their appearance and in their personal value, and to be particularly sensitive to their needs and feelings.
>
> "An important part of our work is the education of patients and their relatives. We encourage them to participate in their care and we teach them how to apply any treatments that are to be continued at home. By educating patients and relatives we hope to increase their understanding and awareness of their conditions and also help to maximise the potential of individuals to adapt and to cope with any physical/psychological disorder."

Table 1. Extract from a dermatology ward philosophy.

Nursing philosophies, as well as providing nurses with an opportunity to reflect on ward practice, may also help them harmonise their working relationships; provide written proof that quality of care is being given; and lead to development of an appropriate model of nursing for their clinical environment. As such, they are a resource not to be underused.

References

DoH (1989) Working for Patients. HMSO, London.
ENB (1988) Institution and Course Approval/Reapproval Process: Information required, criteria and guidelines (1983/39/APS). ENB, London.
Fretwell, J.G. (1982) Ward Teaching and Learning. Royal College of Nursing, London.
Moore, M. (1971) Philosophy, purpose and objectives: why do we need them? *Journal of Nursing Administration,* **1**, 3, 9-14.
Pembrey, S. (1980) The Ward Sister: Key to Nursing. Royal College of Nursing, London.
Romhanyi, A. (1990) A time to reflect. *Nursing Times,* **86**, 21, 33-34.

Taking Charge of the Ward

7

What is management?

Gillian E. Chapman, SRN, RSCN, BSc, MSc, PhD

Gillian Chapman was Lecturer in Nursing, King's College, University of London when this chapter was written

Every day, clinical practitioners, at staff nurse and sister level, manage. With varying degrees of skill, they manage staff and the use of their time and skills. They control, predict and coordinate a series of complex events in the context of the human dramas of illness, recovery or death. This impressive achievement remains scarcely recognised by their colleagues, who may perceive management as being a restricted set of administrative practices such as writing the off-duty. While mastery of administrative techniques facilitates good management, it is not the essence of management. This chapter discusses the nature of management and those elements of nursing that might be described as managerial. A brief outline of the literature relevant to ward management is followed by a guide to the practical, short-term managerial goals which face the clinical practitioner in charge of a ward during one period of duty. Finally, the long-term managerial goals of the ward sister, and the skills required to sustain them, will be identified.

What is management?

In organisational theory the manager is portrayed as being somewhat like an orchestra conductor – at the centre, controlling parts of the organisation in order to produce a harmonious whole. She is advised to plan, direct, coordinate and control events by exercising leadership and decision-making skills and by using formal administrative techniques of budgeting, record-keeping and so-on. Clinical practitioners observing the sometimes haphazard and confused nature of ward life might be relieved to discover that this view is challenged by some organisational theorists.

Mintzberg (1975), for example, suggests that the orchestra leader view of managers is more folklore than fact. Reviewing research studies in organisational behaviour he notes first, that this view of a manager is not supported by research. In fact, managers work at an unrelenting pace and their tasks are characterised by discontinuity, brevity and variety. Further, managers are action-oriented rather than reflective. The idea that managers have no regular daily duties seems unsupported by the research evidence. Managers not only handle crises, but are regularly involved in negotiations and interactions related to the larger organisation. The idea that managers work with formal communications is also challenged by the evidence which suggests that they prefer verbal exchanges, telephone calls and meetings. The view that management has become a scientific profession backed up by systematic analytical procedures is a powerful one, but neglects the fact that management remains concerned with intuitive judgements about people and situations.

Research studies of ward sisters as managers (Lelean, 1973; Pembrey, 1980; Runciman, 1983) have demonstrated how complex and varied their role is, with discontinuity, fragmentation and brevity characterising their tasks, communications and interactions with others. Indeed, Walton (1984), in a useful text on management techniques contrasts the principles of management described in the literature with the practice of managing in the NHS. He argues that far from rationally planning and coordinating resources and activities of the day, nurses tend to 'get along' with the resources they have; coping and reacting to situations as they arise, rather than anticipating difficulties and planning for them. Further research would be required to see the extent to which the introduction of computer based clinical budgetting and resource management techniques have altered this picture. Despite these reservations, a means is found in hospitals across the country to manage ward and departmental life in a coherent and sustained way.

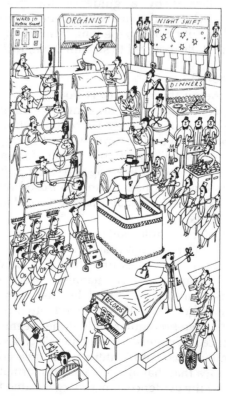

Managing a ward
— Ward management involves the attempt to identify needs and problems, set objectives and plan, implement and evaluate actions. The difference between this and individual patient care is that the whole ward, its environment, equipment and the groups of people within it, is the focus of attention rather than the individual patient.

What are the 'needs and problems' of a ward or unit? Each one will differ, of course, according to the priorities of care and the nursing and medical philosophy. It is vital for each clinical practitioner to make it clear what these might be. For example, nurses on a short-stay, five-day surgical ward might have the overall objective of ensuring safe pre- and postoperative care of patients in the context of a hospital policy or philosophy committed to efficiency and rapid turnover of patients. On the other hand, nurses on a long-term psychiatric ward might stress the development of a secure and consistent relationship with the patient, in order that rehabilitation to the community can be achieved. The important thing is that reasonable and achievable overall nursing objectives are set in keeping with unit quality assurance programmes and the contracts agreed between the purchasing health authority and the provider unit of which the ward is a part. This is largely a task for the ward sister, together with the nurse manager in liaison with the nursing, medical and administrative teams.

All clinical practitioners in the ward or department should be aware of what these goals are. Once known, the daily organisation of the ward, the priority of problems and the allocation of resources becomes a simpler exercise. For example, the allocation of one nurse to develop a long-term relationship with a patient admitted for day surgery is less important than allocating a skilled nurse to ensure his safe recovery from anaesthetic.

Like the nursing process, the process of management has both short- and long-term goals. For the purposes of this article, a short-term managerial goal will be related to running the ward during one period of duty; long-term goals will be those associated with maintenance of the ward over longer periods of time. Each will be discussed separately.

Managing a shift
What follows is one method of managing a shift while in charge of a ward, based on a judgement of the ward priorities as they relate to the needs of the group of patients under the clinical practitioner's care, and is sequential in nature. In other words, it describes the sequence a nurse in charge of a ward might follow when arriving on duty. Clearly, given the scope of this article, not all the possible problems and actions have been included.

Nurse's prior knowledge   Prior knowledge of the type of ward (medical, surgical or psychiatric) together with the number of patients and range of clinical conditions met on the ward will enhance the practitioner's capacity to prepare and think through her management plans. Similarly, knowledge of the ward layout and location of key facilities is essential; for example, clinical rooms, telephones, resuscitation equipment, fire doors and so on. Additionally, when arriving on duty, she should provide herself with an overview of the ward and its work before taking actions or making decisions. The most direct way of doing this is to tour the ward making observations.

Estimate of patient needs/dependency   Direct observation of patients during a brief tour of the ward enhances information on the patient's dependency needs gained from care plans during the handover report. While patient dependency is difficult to measure scientifically, professional judgement about the amount and quality of nursing time required has proved effective (Waite, 1986). Thus, the nurse in charge should assess the number of patients requiring constant nursing, the number requiring frequent nursing (for example, time-consuming treatments or observations) and the number of patients requiring only selective attention. It is important to remember that patients without life-threatening conditions can, at times, require as much attention as those more profoundly ill. For example, a patient requiring dressings for leg ulcers may need more time spent on this procedure than the patient recovering from a myocardial infarction. Once patient needs are known, the next step is to match them with available staff resources.

Establishing staff resources   The nurse in charge next establishes the staff resources available to care for patients. She needs to establish who is on duty, who is off sick, on annual leave, or on a study day, and the skill mix of trained staff to learners, experienced staff to newcomers.

Allocating staff to patients   Using her professional judgement, and based on her estimate of patient dependency, the available staff are allocated to patients, ensuring a balanced caseload for each primary nurse, and matching skills and experience of nurses to patient needs. At this early stage she should inform the nursing administration should she require extra staff.

Inform staff   Clarity of communication about the nurse's delegated duties and responsibilities with respect to the patients she is caring for is essential. The care plan and update received during the report should be enhanced by the nurse in charge checking that the nurse concerned understands and is familiar with the procedures required. Appropriate attachment of learner nurses to trained staff enables trained staff to supervise, monitor and teach learners as required. The fact that less experienced nurses have recourse to senior staff frees the nurse in charge to undertake other managerial duties.

Review organisational components of day As already noted, once management action has been taken to ensure the continuing care of patients (always the first priority), the nurse in charge is able to review other aspects of the day which require attention. This can take the form of a checklist with which to anticipate problems and delegate tasks. An example of what such a checklist might look like for a general ward is found in Table 1.

Number of empty beds?
Number of admissions: routine or emergency?
Number of transfers: Other wards or hospital? Transport? Time?
Number of discharges:
    Outpatient appointment: Booked?
    Drugs to take home: Ordered?
    District nurse: Arranged? Letter written?
    General practitioner's letter: Written?
    Health education information/advice on recovery: Given?
Number of theatre lists:
    Times?
    Preoperative preparations: Completed? Consent form signed?
    Preoperative medication: Written up? Time?
Drug rounds: Frequency?
Other investigations/treatments: X-rays? Scans?
Special equipment: Needed? Functioning?
Ward round: Nursing recommendations/observations available?
Doctors on call?
Medical teams on take?
Specific tasks: Ordering stores? Meals?
Teaching: Time available?
Liaison with other disciplines: Physio? OT? Dietitian? Ward clerk?
Coffee/lunch/supper breaks: Arranged? Trained staff cover?

Table 1. Organisational checklist.

Decide own priorities/delegate appropriately Once the clinical practitioner has informed herself of the likely predictable events of the day she can select her own priorities, allocate tasks to herself and delegate others. She is then in the position of being in command of her time and will be better able to respond to unusual or untoward events (like patient complaints, accidents or incidents), or to attend to long-term managerial tasks.

Ending the shift At the end of each shift information about the ward is collected and communicated to oncoming staff verbally in report and in written form on the patient's care plan. This exchange of information also provides an opportunity to review and evaluate care.

Managing long-term
There are a range of texts available which deal with long-term management issues (Matthews, 1982; Raybould, 1977; Rowden, 1984). It will not be possible to explain these in detail here; however, many of

the topics covered are concerned with techniques and activities aimed at maintaining the ward environment as a place in which patients' conditions improve, and staff and learners achieve job satisfaction (Ogier, 1982). Central to the maintenance of the work environment are the leadership skills of the ward sister. The capacity to motivate and lead a team of nurses depends, in turn, on quite specific managerial skills: first, the capacity to recruit and select staff via the mechanism of effective interviewing; second, the capacity to retain staff both in terms of skills in professional development, appraisal and performance review, and the sensitive planning and allocation of off-duty rotas; third, the demonstration of competence in relation to a range of management techniques, from ward budgeting to quality assurance to research appreciation (Pembrey and Fitzgerald, 1987). Finally, it seems, the perceived integrity and fairness of the manager is of fundamental importance.

References
Lelean, S.R. (1973) Ready for Report Nurse? RCN, London
Matthews, A. (1982) In Charge of the Ward. Blackwell Scientific Publications, Oxford.
Mintzberg, H. (1975) The Manager's Job: Folklore and Fact. Harvard Business Review No. 75409 July/August, 49-62.
Ogier, M.E. (1982) An Ideal Sister? RCN, London
Pembrey, S.E. (1980) The Ward Sister – Key To Nursing. RCN, London.
Pembrey, S. and Fitzgerald, M. (1987) Developing the potential of sisters. *Nursing Times,* 25 March, 27.
Raybould, E. (ed.) (1977) A Guide for Nurse Managers. Blackwell, Oxford.
Rowden, R. (ed.) (1984) Managing Nursing. Ballière Tindall, London.
Runciman, P. (1983) Ward Sister at Work. Churchill Livingstone, Edinburgh.
Waite, R. (1986) Nursing by numbers. *Nursing Times,* 19 February.
Walton, M. (1984) Management and Managing: A dynamic approach. Lippincott Nursing Series, Harper and Row, London.

8

Objectives for care: replacing procedures with guidelines

Gillian Snowley, M.Ed, BSc, RGN, DN,
District Education Manager, Mid Trent College of Nursing and Midwifery

Peter J. Nicklin, M.Ed, RGN, RMN, RNT,
Director of Nurse Education, York Health Authority

Since the inception of the NHS, demands upon the service and its employees have increased. Medical technology, demographic change, consumer expectation and managerial concerns for improved productivity, have all conspired to increase the workload of the caring professions. As these demands have intensified, there has been a tendency to forget the importance of the consumer's identity and personal needs. The nursing profession has recognised and acknowledged this neglect, and attempted to provide a solution by adopting the nursing process as a broad philosophy for the planning and delivery of healthcare.

Definitions of the 'nursing process' vary, but common to all are the assumptions that it is goal-directed, systematic, rational and problem-solving. The registered nurse is accountable for delivery of care, based on an assessment of the individual's needs, and for subsequent measurement of the effectiveness (evaluation) of that care. Implementing the nursing process continues to pose significant problems for the profession. The Nurse Education Research Unit (1986) has provided valuable insights into the difficulties experienced by nurses.

A significant barrier

In 1983, the North Lincolnshire Health Authority acknowledged that the 'nursing procedure manual' was a significant barrier to the successful implementation of the nursing process, as it gave no scope for an individualised and prescriptive approach to care. With its rampant and unbending concentration on task, the perfect completion of which would follow the same format on every occasion, the patient's individual needs seemed insignificant. All patients were expected to respond equally, and all nurses to behave with almost military precision on every occasion, despite any special circumstances which could prevail. The procedure manual restricted professional clinical freedom and became a recipe book for nursing. It also encouraged disregard for the psychosocial aspects of care delivery.

This was not to say that procedures were inaccurate, or that accuracy in performing procedures was and is unimportant or unnecessary. But they omitted extra dimensions of care which allow total consideration of the patient. The procedure manual tended to dictate specific technical and highly visible nursing actions in a ritualistic manner, with no concern for assessment, planning and evaluation of nursing care. It did not recognise the individual nurse's role in the process of care delivery – except perhaps for the favourite opening instruction: "Tell the patient what you are going to do". Even that became a regulation!

In 1983, North Lincolnshire's chief nursing officer recommended that "guidelines for nursing practice, which reflect acceptable standards of care" be formulated. Membership of the nursing guidelines committee was drawn from all the health units within the district, including the nurse education unit, so all nurses, midwives and health visitors were represented. The authors were members of this group.

Conceptual differences

During the early stages, we experienced some difficulty in grasping the conceptual differences between 'procedure' and 'guideline', and had little idea what the latter would look like. The prospect of reinventing the wheel did not inspire much enthusiasm, so we undertook the obligatory literature search to determine what had been published in this area. There was little or no information from UK sources, but American literature, while describing a guidelines approach, did not seem to offer anything very different, and was not always consistent with Lincolnshire nursing culture. However, we acknowledged that what we were calling 'guidelines' may not have been so defined by the rest of the nursing profession. Informal discussions with colleagues both regionally and nationally did not reveal any formal work of a similar nature, although it may well have existed. Work subsequently published by the Royal Marsden Hospital (Pritchard and Walker, 1984) while sharing some of the characteristics of our guidelines, was not entirely consistent with our philosophy. This meant we could not rely on precedents for guidance, but we were not going to distort someone else's structure to fit our own circumstances. In short, we started from scratch.

Although we did not realise it for some time, we needed to ask the question "what does nursing seek to achieve?" Certainly the procedure manual does not answer this. Once we had recognised the importance of the question, we needed to examine models of nursing to identify the structure of nursing guidelines. We considered Orem's (self-care), Roper et al's (activities of living) and Roy's (adaptation model), but eventually returned to basics – to Virginia Henderson's Basic Principles of Nursing Care (1969), which fulfilled our need for a comprehensive and readily understood model. The committee then began composing guidelines under the headings originally described by Henderson.

To say this was difficult would be an understatement. Our first attempts were either too long, too short, too esoteric, too academic, too trivial, too general or too detailed – and sometimes several of these combined! We had problems with semantics and grammar, and our morale sometimes slumped, but by a process of trial and error, consultation and cooperation, we agreed a style of describing nursing intention which had the potential for improving patient care.

Early guidelines

Our early guidelines were expressed as the aims and objectives of nursing on psychosocial, physiological and educational dimensions. Each had an evaluation component, but their most important feature was that each was generated from available literature and published research, and supported by a bibliography.

By late 1985, the committee had developed and disseminated 17 guidelines to all care points in the district. In addition to Henderson's 14 components of basic nursing care, we acknowledged the need to provide guidance on expressing sexuality; helping patients in pain and the care of the dying and bereaved.

Guidelines were intended to be used by trained nurses who can responsibly and reasonably interpret them with discretion and with the authority which the research base provides. We believed they should encourage thoughtful and individual delivery of care by nurses who are accountable for their own actions. The guidelines were recognised as the basis for teaching nurses in training, and for the use of nursing assistants with trained supervision.

Mixed reception

Not surprisingly, our guidelines had a mixed reception in the clinical areas where they were intended to be used. Their appearance coincided with many other recent changes in the philosophy and implementation of healthcare delivery, both nationally and locally directed. Many nurses regarded them as "just another new idea thrust upon us by nurse managers and nurse educators" – despite the fact that clinical nurses from all specialties were members of the committee, and joint authors of the guidelines. One specific problem was that they were seen as isolated documents, and not as an integral part of a systematic and prescriptive approach to individual care. Suddenly, the procedure manual became a highly valued lifeline, even though in many areas it gathered dust and its whereabouts remained unknown. In considering this dilemma, the committee suggested that guidelines were an important aid to the implementation of the nursing process, and that every opportunity to present them as such be pursued. The Open University's Distance Learning Course P553 – A Systematic Approach to Nursing Care (1984) was widely used within the district, both in the continuing education department and within individual units, where courses were being led by nurse managers. The guidelines were therefore introduced to staff undertaking this course as a tool for goal setting and care planning within whichever nursing model was being used in the clinical area. In fact, they provided suitably phrased goals and objectives which would not disgrace any care plan. Although the committee members recognised a responsibility for ensuring such progress and integration of materials, the real work, on a large scale, was done by clinical nurses themselves, with encouragement and facilitation by management and education.

Despite the suspicion and antagonism with which guidelines were received, enough clinical nurses suggested ways in which they could be improved. Members of the committee were grateful for this information – at least in some areas they had not been ignored. Strong statements of dissatisfaction, accompanied by notes of guidance for change, were far more acceptable than apathy.

Revising the format

Armed with suggestions for a changed format, the committee began the formidable task of revision in 1986. This was almost more difficult than beginning with a blank sheet. The original philosophy remained intact, but presentation of the guidelines now evolved into a staged format of assessment, planning, implementation and evaluation. The original objectives, sometimes the results of agonising search for the right expression, remained; so too did the bibliographies, but each has been updated and refined. The result is Objectives for Care, a source book for all nurses, midwives and health visitors, working in any practice setting. This book is the product of an energetic group who were convinced at the outset of the value of the task which confronted them. Some of us had little idea of its enormity, but the team effort involved was its most encouraging aspect.

The second edition of this book has now been published.

Objectives for Care 2nd edn, *is available from Wolfe Publishing, Brook House, 2-16 Torrington Place, London WC1E 7LT. Tel: 071-636 4622.*

References
NERU (1986) Report of the Nursing Process Working Party. King's College, London.
Pretchard, A.P. and Walker, V.A. (1984) The Royal Marsden Hospital Manual of Clinical Nursing Policies and Procedures. Harper and Row, London.
Henderson, V. (1969) Basic Principles of Nursing Care. ICN, Geneva.
Open University (1984) A Systematic Approach to Nursing Care – An Introduction (P553). OU Press, Milton Keynes.

9
Writing the off-duty

Brian Gilchrist, MSc, RGN

Lecturer, Department of Nursing Studies, King's College, University of London

Writing the off-duty is, for many people, one of the most frustrating managerial tasks that the sister or charge nurse has to undertake. The need to satisfy simultaneously the needs of the nursing service, the school of nursing, the ward workload and, not least, the individual requests of the ward staff, mean that many hours (often outside work time) are spent every year in juggling these seemingly incompatible demands into a workable rota.

There is no perfect solution to this dilemma, and it is not the author's intention to suggest one. Rather, this paper highlights many of the conflicting factors which must be taken into account, and in doing so will provide the novice with some useful guidelines.

The constraints have been divided into a number of sections, although they are arbitrary and may overlap.

Legal constraints

These are factors which are set down by statute, or by outside bodies over which the manager has no control, but which must be known and understood. They include conditions of employment agreed by the Whitley Council (contained in the Nurses and Midwives Handbook, and updated periodically by 'letters' issued by the DHSS) such as the maximum hours to be worked, the 37½ hour week and any legal requirements such as the need for trained staff to check controlled drugs.

Also included in this category are individual contracts of employment which have been specially negotiated, and which might include agreements about hours or, for example, specific days of the week that the person has been employed to work.

Local constraints

These are factors which have been agreed locally or which form part of managerial rulings that are intended to ensure satisfactory working practices. In some hospitals many of these will be guidelines only, and may be changed with the agreement of the nurse concerned; in others, they may not be altered without the express permission of senior management. The nurse writing the off-duty will need to keep all of the following factors in mind.

Format of the off-duty

Number of consecutive days to be worked   Many hospitals now state that no more than a certain number of days in a row can be worked unless there is good reason, such as the request for a certain day off. This, of course, is a maximum and individual wards may decide that within this guideline they wish to nominate some lower number.

Split days off   Is this permitted at all? If so, there may be some restriction on how many times a month this can occur.

Weekends   There may be an agreement, formal or informal, about the number of weekends off that the staff should receive each month. This might not be the same for all levels of staff, but might apply, for example, only to trained staff, or to the ward sister. In addition, there could be provision for a Friday or a Monday to be routinely added to make a long weekend possible. The situation is further complicated by staff who rotate through night duty, which may affect their allocation of weekends for that particular month.

Night duty   Where there is a system of internal rotation the frequency of night duty should be closely monitored to ensure that the planned format is maintained, and that there are the correct number of days off before and after each group of nights allocated.
   One further factor that needs to be taken into consideration is the extent to which it is permitted to request holidays during the time of their next night duty, if indeed it is permitted at all.

Daily working hours   Set hours may be worked each day, or there may be a facility to vary them so that the ward is covered adequately at certain busy times. If there is an agreement about the number of early and late duties to be worked by each member of staff each week, then these will need to be adhered to once the off-duty is written. It must be remembered that the off-duty does not always start on a Monday.

Days preceding leave days   Some hospitals try (and many staff request) to roster an early duty before a day off, and a late one after. The manager needs to decide whether this should be a set policy, or simply a desirable practice.

Pattern rosters   In some areas there may already be a 'pattern roster' in use, in which the duties are set down month by month, and the names are simply inserted. Other patterns include a set pattern such as four on, two off, and so on. While such patterns may have some advantages, particularly in terms of predicting days off some time in advance, there does need to be a mechanism which allows staff to change duties, and which allows the manager to alter the pattern if, for example, the lines are not all filled at a particular time.

Holidays There may be set times when certain groups of staff, particularly students, are on holiday. The amount of notice that permanent staff have to give must also be taken into account, as do any limits on the number of staff that can be on holiday at any one time.

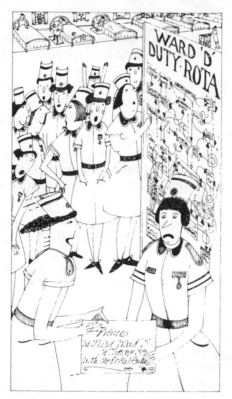

Busy days In surgical wards in particular, it is possible to predict the days on which more staff are going to be required to cope with operations, premedications and admission days. In other wards this may be a little more difficult, but factors such as consultants' acute take days can usually be predicted some time in advance.

Acting up On the days when the ward sister 'acts up' for the nursing officer, there would need to be adjustments made to the off-duty to ensure adequate coverage should she be called away from the ward for long periods of time.

Agency nurses Most units now have a policy regarding extra agency nurses to replace shortfalls in established posts, and it may even be possible to write them in to the off-duty without any further approval. However, financial controls generally mean that approval needs to be sought, and if the nursing officer is unable to supply an agency nurse because of either finance or unavailability, then the ward will still need to be safely covered.

Overtime   Is overtime permitted at all? Does it have to be approved in advance?

Local emergency plan   The ward may be part of the local plans for a major emergency, and the staffing levels would need to reflect this.

ENB rulings   National Board inspectors will look very closely at the level of student nurse supervision, and in some cases will even insist on a particular mix of staff grades and qualifications, eg the number of RSCNs covering a paediatric ward.

Night duty   The restrictions which are placed on the number of nights students are permitted to do, or their frequency, may be different from those which apply to trained staff, and ward managers are informed about this by the allocation office.

Examinations   Many students complain that their off-duty affects their performance during examinations. Some schools of nursing will have rulings about the number of days off before exams, or restrictions on night duty, particularly before finals. It is difficult for the person writing the off-duty, however, if the school does not have a mechanism for informing the wards of such dates.

Time in school   There may well be a local ruling about having the weekend (or at least Sunday) off before a week in school, as well as the weekend following a school block. This can create problems if the student then requests a further weekend for a special occasion, thus disadvantaging those students who have not had their 'quota' of off-duty weekends. Other factors which need to be taken into consideration include any rulings about night duty immediately preceeding school, and odd study days that might be scheduled for particular students.

Staff constraints
This is possibly the most difficult area of all, because it is in this area where the greatest potential for conflict lies, and where there is the greatest risk of upsetting staff. It cannot be emphasised enough that many potential problems can be avoided by the simple act of discussing any problems with the nurse concerned *before* the final off-duty is published. A sympathetic, understanding approach will often result in an acceptable solution being reached quickly, with a minimum of upset.

Staff/skill mix
Unfortunately, this is another factor which is often out of the control of the ward manager because of a number of outside influences. The ward establishment is generally reviewed after a close examination of the

workload of a particular ward. In many cases there may be a shortfall simply due to a lack of nurses in post, or because the levels were set at a time when the workload was very different. If this is the situation then the manager would need to make his or her superior aware of the situation, and be prepared to put the case for having the establishment altered.

Such action is clearly demanded by the UKCC Code of Professional Conduct and it may be argued that failure to do so might constitute an "act or ommission . . . detrimental to the safety of patients/clients," although this has yet to be tested. Nevertheless, the responsibility of the ward managers to "act always in such a way as to promote and safeguard the wellbeing and interests of patients/clients" is a strong argument to advance in favour of appropriate staffing levels.

The allocation of learners to the ward is also outside the control of the ward manager, but will clearly have a considerable impact on the construction of the off-duty.

The actual skill mix on a day-to-day basis forms one of the most important factors that needs to be taken into consideration when the off-duty is being written, both in terms of quality and quantity. The mix must include all the necessary expertise, as well as provision for the adequate supervision of junior nursing staff and auxilliary staff.

Another, often controversial, factor that needs to be taken into account at this point is the policy of the hospital with regard to the amount of responsibility that can be expected, or demanded, of the enrolled nurse. Careful attention needs to be paid to the level of knowledge and expertise that is needed to properly manage a ward.

Individual staff

Part-time or fixed duty staff   Some members of the ward staff may work only set hours or days of the week. Such people are generally not totally inflexible, and may be prepared to change occasionally where a particular need arises. Such requests should be the exception rather than the rule, however, and need to be approached sensitively. More advantage could be taken of part-time staff, and any move towards flexible hours, crêche facilities and job sharing will add to the potential solutions available for ward staffing.

Personality conflicts   Although obviously undesirable, it is sometimes the case that some members of staff are not compatible with each other. Although this should always be the subject of separate management action, part of the solution may be to ensure that contact is kept to a minimum, at least initially; alternatively, the parties may be rostered together at the same time as a senior member of the staff so that the problem can be identified and resolved. Such conflicts can be especially counterproductive on night duty, and should be avoided if possible in that situation.

Staff supervision   Many hospitals now have a staff development programme which may include an element of clinical supervision as part of the requirements of the course. This may mean that the duties of the student and her supervisor may need to be coordinated.

The introduction of various 'mentor' schemes has also increased the pressure to ensure that the student and her mentor are working together for a certain proportion of the time available. It may also be useful for the sister to have worked at least one duty with every student so that when the ward reports are prepared the sister has some knowledge of the student concerned, and is fully responsible for the report, which may be actually written by a staff nurse.

Other situations that need to be taken into account include students who have particular learning needs or those who have been identified as requiring extra supervision and guidance.

In-service education   In addition to the obvious needs of the learners, consideration also needs to be given to the necessity for the trained staff to attend study days, or to have the facility to attend courses for further or higher qualifications. Although such a programme may have been approved by senior management, it may have considerable implications for the off-duty if the leave is needed on a regular basis.

Staff preferences   If a pattern roster is in use, then there will need to be some facility for the staff to change duties.

Where there is no pattern, some sort of request system is generally available. A consistent, written policy is essential for such a system to work properly, and it must take into account such things as who (if anyone) has priority, what length of notice must be given, how many requests are allowed, how much time is given following the publication of a ward change of allocation list, what facilities there are for urgent requests and, most importantly, what the policy of the ward is on changing shifts once the off-duty has been published.

There may have to be variations to cater for particular situations, eg Christmas and New Year, and in these situations the main concern is generally to ensure that everyone is given a reasonable share of both the 'good' and 'bad' duties. Some staff may have a preference for a particular duty for example, to accommodate a regular evening class.

Ensuring cooperation

It can be seen, then, that those writing the off-duty should take into account many different factors, a large number of which are outside their control. Despite this, writing the off-duty is an extremely important part of ward management, and although it does become easier with experience, it still requires the goodwill and cooperation of all staff.

To gain this cooperation, it is perhaps useful to keep a few simple points in mind:
1. Be flexible. The more rigid a structure you attempt to impose, the

more likelihood there is that you will make the whole task more difficult
– within the legal constraints, there is considerable scope for variation.
2. Communicate with the staff as much as possible. Many nurses are

Starts 4/4/88																											
DATE SISTER BROWN	D	D	A	D	/	/	/	A	D	D	/	A	m	on	D	D	A	D	/	/	/	A	D	D	/	A	on	on
SISTER S/N GREEN	/	A	D	A	D	m	m	D	/	A	D	D	/	/	/	A	D	A	D	m	m	D	/	A	D	D	/	/
S/N WHITE	A	D	A	A	D	/	/	/	A	D	A	D	m	on	/	/	N	N	N	N	N	N	/	/	/	/	/	/
S/N BLACK	/	/	N	N	N	N	N	N	/	/	/	/	/	/	/	A	D	A	A	on	on	D	/	A	D	D	/	/
S/N JONES	A	D	D	D	A	m	on	/	/	N	N	N	N	N	N	N	/	/	/	/	/	/	A	D	A	A	on	on
S/N SMITH	D	/	A	D	D	/	/	A	D	A	D	/	/	/	/	A	D	D	A	A	on	on	/	/	N	N	N	N
Student Nurse 1.	/	A	D	A	D	A	D	/	/	A	D	A	D	A	D	/	/	A	A	D	A	M	/	/	N	N	N	N
2.	A	D	/	/	A	D	A	D	A	A	D	/	/	/	/	A	D	A	D	A	D	/	/	A	D	A	D	A
3.	N	N	N	/	/	/	/	/	/	A	D	A	D	A	A	D	/	/	A	D	A	A	D	A	D	/	/	/
4.	M	/	/	N	N	N	N	N	N	N	/	/	/	/	/	A	A	D	D	A	D	D	/	/	A	D	A	
5.	D	/	/	A	D	A	D	M	/	/	N	N	N	N	N	N	N	/	/	/	/	/	/	A	A	D	A	D
6.	/	/	A	D	A	D	A	D	/	/	A	D	A	D	M	/	/	N	N	N	N	N	N	N	/	/	/	/
7.	D	A	A	D	/	/	/	/	A	D	A	D	A	D	/	/	A	D	A	D	A	D	/	/	A	A	D	A
8.	/	A	S/o	M	D	/	A	A	D	S/o	M	/	/	A	A	A	S/o	M	/	/	A	A	D	S/o	M	/	/	A
9.	A	D	S/o	M	/	/	A	A	D	S/o	M	D	/	/	A	D	S/o	M	/	A	D	A	A	S/o	M	/	A	D
10.																												
11.																												
12.																												
13.																												
14.																												

A fixed rota showing staff nurses working one in six and students working one in eight nights.

happy to negotiate around a request if they are reassured that they will
be able to have the time off that is crucial, and are often prepared to
offer a sensible compromise which will suit all staff and the ward's needs.
3. Remember that nurses are people. Some people do seem to complain
more than others, but you cannot expect a nurse to contribute her best
to your ward if you roster her six nights leading up to a major exam –
what is more likely to happen is that she will take a 'sickness break'.
4. Above all, use your common sense. Would you work the off-duty
that you have written? Every line of it? If the answer to either of these
questions is 'No' then why should you ask others to?

Many computer programmes are now being developed which can
assist the ward manager in this task, and these may be very useful tools.
However, the output still needs to be examined closely because, although
they may generate an off-duty which is mathematically sound, there
may be other, more human, factors to take into consideration.

Finally, it is often a very useful exercise to get other members of the
trained staff to take turns at writing the off-duty from time to time. Apart
from introducing them to an important managerial skill, another point
of view may help to improve the overall standard of the off-duty and it
certainly helps acquaint them with the many problems involved.

Writing the off-duty

So how should you proceed? There is no one system that is any better than the rest, but here are some suggested guidelines:

You will need: a sharp pencil; a large eraser; an appropriately ruled sheet of paper; a quiet place where you will not be interrupted; an hour or two; plenty of patience. *In this order:*

1. Write in all the people who have permanent shifts.
2. Write in any other fixed shifts, eg those in school or on holiday.
3. Write in the requests.
4. Add the night duty, and the days off.
5. Now write the off-duty for the trained staff.
6. Add the students last. (This is not because the students are the lowest priority but because trained staff supervision must come first.)
7. Check the numbers for each shift, and adjust according to ward needs.
8. Display the proposed rota for a day or two to allow for a certain amount of negotiation to take place before the final copy is sent to the manager. This will prevent upset and wasted time later on.

There is a certain amount of satisfaction associated with completing a workable roster, but be assured that however good it looks, something or someone is sure to come along and require changes. The only solution in this situation is to keep cool!

Reference

DHSS. The Nursing and Midwifery staff negotiating council conditions of service and rates of pay (The Nurse's and Midwife's Handbook). Standard conditions which are regularly updated.

Bibliography

Matthews, A. (1982) In charge of the ward. Blackwell Scientific Publications London. A useful, practical reference work for all ward managers.
Rowden, R. (1984) Managing Nursing. Ballière Tindall London. Particularly strong on industrial relations aspects of human management.

10

Visiting: should you be more involved?

Judith Ralphs, BSc, RGN
Charge Nurse, St Thomas' Pain Management Centre, London

Visitors are a common sight in most wards. Nurses often have mixed feelings about their presence, commonly using an influx of visits as an excuse for a quick cup of tea, while the patients are momentarily distracted from their illnesses and engrossed in family and friends. As nurses, we assume all visits are welcome, but have little informed knowledge of how patients find these times. Yet we have all visited people in hospital and know the atmosphere can be awkward and artificial.

The 'good' visitor	The 'bad' visitor
1. Visits in ones and twos, stays only for half/one hour, generally in the afternoon when patient is up and washed but not yet too tired.	Visits in large groups, stays too long with little regard as to how the patient is feeling.
2. Really wants to come and see the patient.	Makes his visit appear a duty, or spends the time chatting to others, ignoring the patient.
3. Able to sit and relax looking at ease with the patient, feels free to knit or watch TV.	Appears tense, sits on edge of seat, or paces up and down ward looking at watch.
4. Does not pity the patient, but able to laugh and joke, treating the patient as normal.	Dwells on patient's illness, reluctant to be light-hearted, or appears desperately cheerful. – 'You look marvellous', when it is clear the patient is looking pale and ill.
5. Talks about outside matters, family news, gossip. Many patients prefer to talk about anything but their illness – a most unpopular topic.	Reluctant to talk about old times in case of upsetting the patient.
6. Aware of patient's practical needs, ie taking away dirty washing, mouldy fruit.	Patient feels visitor is coming for his own needs, ie 'to have a good moan'.
7. Gives patient choice about next visit. (Half the sample liked planned visits but often were never asked by their visitors.)	Assumes he may come again and that the patient will always be pleased and well enough to see him.

Table 1. What makes a 'good' or 'bad' visitor?

Changing opinions

Opinions about visiting hospital patients have changed over the years. Somerville Hastings believed half an hour a day was enough (1963), the object being to soothe and encourage the patients, not to interest or amuse the visitors (or, it can be supposed, the patient!). Cartwright (1964) found in her study of ward life, that visiting time was enjoyed greatly and broke the monotony and boredom of the hospital routine.

One hospital visiting report, undertaken by the University of Hull in 1966, goes further: "Visiting hours are not merely an interruption of ward routine, they are a means by which a patient is kept in touch with the outside world, which he understands, making it easier to fit in on his return."

Important part of the day

This author's interest has developed through two studies undertaken on patients' views on hospital life. The first study, undertaken, as an undergraduate nurse, investigated ward routine: it was found that visiting hours, along with meal times, were to patients the most important and looked-forward- to part of the day. This finding prompted the author to look at this subject further, as part of an ENB course, 'Care of the Dying'.

A number of patients (18) at St. Christopher's Hospice were asked their views about having visitors. The hospice has open visiting apart from on Monday, which is a rest day; thus there is little external control on visiting.

It was found that most patients appreciated having visitors, but felt there could be improvements. From the results of this study, it was concluded that some people are naturally good at visiting and enjoyed by the patient, whereas others made their visits rather tiresome to all concerned.

Table 1 summarises the information gathered from the two studies, and illustrates aspects of the 'good' and the 'bad' visitors.

Although these studies involve terminally ill patients, the views expressed are valuable to those involved with general patients as the patients in this sample did not class themselves as 'the dying', but wanted to be treated as normal. In any case, most wards have some terminally ill patients.

Keeping in touch

As Gattis (1974) writes:

"Deep subjects are still in the minority, they are still people with a past and a present history, and therefore will want to talk about these things, to keep in touch with the outside world, which is all part of living."

This is all very interesting, but is there a nursing role? This author believes that there is.

Problem	Aim	Action	Evaluation
1. Patient tired by too many visitors	Visitors come in ones and twos for half hour only.	Ask next of kin to arrange with visitors to ring him/her before visiting. If a large group of visitors arrives, ask them to visit two at a time.	Now only two small groups of visitors daily. Able to enjoy these times as not tired out.
2. Visits appear awkward with visitor ill at ease.	Patient and visitor enjoy time together.	Informally ask patient about visiting time; does he think there is a problem? If he does, discuss causes and what would help: nurse joining in. visitor and patient 'do' something together, eg walk in garden. Be friendly to visitor so does not feel a stranger.	How are they now interacting? Body language looks relaxed.

Table 2. Two possible problems that could be added to a care plan.

Grollman (1974) writes:

"Visiting is like a medicine; useful and pleasant at certain times, but can become toxic at higher levels."

Thus nurses can help prevent visiting times – and visitors themselves – from becoming toxic, and make it a pleasant and useful occasion.

Nursing intervention

Perhaps nurses should see it as part of their symptom control.

Four nursing interventions are suggested:

1. Enquire how each patient is finding visiting times – this can be done informally, eg at bath times. Be alert to any hints given, as patients may feel guilty if they have mixed feelings about their visitors. Observe how patient and visitor interact together: do they look relaxed and as if they are enjoying their time together?

2. Assess if there is a problem, eg too many visitors, awkward silences. If a problem is identified, add it to the patient's care plan, along with the aim.

3. Give practical help. Some of the things nurses have done on the author's ward are:

i. Discuss ideas at report time;

ii. Have a gentle word with visitors as they enter;

iii. Place a polite notice at patient's door;

iv. Join in awkward conversation – lighten the tone if necessary;

v. Give patients a rest, with periods of time free from visitors. Obviously, all of these things should be done with sensitivity and in consultation with the patient.

4. Evaluate. Informally ask patient how he is now finding visiting times. Observe if visitors have made the desired changes in behaviour.

Table 2 is an example of two possible problems that could be added to a care plan.

Although many visitors are a pleasure, the author believes nurses do have a role to play in their handling. Involvement with managing visiting time will help patients enjoy visitors' time on the ward and to get the most possible out of such important times.

References

Cartwright, A. (1964) Human Relations and Hospital Care. Routledge and Kegan Paul, London.

Gattis, J.W. (1974) in Barton, D. (ed) Death and Dying. Chapter 10. Wavery Press, Baltimore.

Grollman, E.A. (1974) Practical Guide for Living. Beaver Press, Boston.

Somerville Hastings, A. (1962) Visiting in hospital. *British Medical Journal*, No. 5338.

University of Hull (1966) Department of Social Administration. Hospital project visiting report. Unpublished.

11

A crucial journey which needs a standard: transportation of critically ill patients

Jenni Frost, BN, RGN, RM, DipN, PGCE, RNT
Nurse Lecturer (Continuing Education), University of Wales College of Nursing and Midwifery, Bodelwydden, Clywd

Lynne Moran, RGN, FETC
Sister, Accident and Emergency, Ysbyty Gwynedd, Bangor

Movement of critically ill patients to a hospital following sudden illness or injury is usually referred to as 'primary transport', a role generally undertaken by the ambulance service and paramedics, supported occasionally by hospital-based and medical teams or locally-sited general practitioners (Ledingham and Banks, 1980). Transportation from one hospital to another, for whatever reason, or within the same hospital, is referred to as 'secondary transport' (Waddell, 1975).

Risks of secondary transportation

There appears to be no form of standardised system for either equipment or nursing practice in the United Kingdom for secondary transportation of critically ill adults (Bion *et al*, 1988), with the result that specialised care could be denied to patients who might have benefited from it during that transfer. This research also shows that most journeys are inadequately prepared for, hurriedly undertaken, noisy and traumatic, often leading to a discontinuation of vital monitoring or therapy. Further research by Ledingham and Banks (1980) shows that deleterious changes do occur in the cardiovascular and respiratory systems in patients being transported to intensive care units (ICU), and Gentlemen and Teasdale (1981) draw attention to the fact that cerebral anoxia is a likelihood when transporting critically ill people to neurosurgical units. Parks (1985) stated that the transfer of a patient between hospitals or even within the hospital itself is a critical event in an already critical illness, a view backed up by Bion, Wilson and Taylor (1988) who show that life-threatening complications do occur when critically ill patients are transferred in conventional ambulances. This reiterates Waddell *et al* (1975) who had previously looked into the effects of ambulance transportation on critically ill patients.

Bion, Wilson and Taylor (1988) used a modification of the acute physiology and chronic health evaluation or APACHE 11 scoring system, the sickness score being calculated from data collected immediately before and after transfer. Mean sickness scores were then tabulated and showed highly significant (p<0.0001) differences between survivors and non-survivors. Waddell (1975) also looked into the effects of movement of critically ill patients within the hospital environment itself. The incidence of serious side-effects due to intrahospital movement showed a high incidence of negative conditional changes directly accountable to patients being moved. It was found that even simple monitoring, traction and suction therapy was extremely difficult in narrow corridors and lifts.

Prior to transfer

1. Stabilisation of the patients:

Airway and oxygen requirements	Constant vital sign monitoring
Checking of blood gases	Correction of acidosis
X-ray requirements	Maintenence of temperature
Need for assisted ventilation?	Continuation of drug administration
Arterial cannulisation/central line	Need for a nasogastric tube?
Intravenous fluids (peripheral lines?)	Catheterisation
Minimal handling or transfers between bed and trolleys	

2. Notify relatives of transfer:
Give full explanation and reasons for transfer
Give reassurances
Give them details of receiving hospital/unit

3. Obtain consents from next-of-kin:
(Especially if the patient is under-age or unconscious) for operations/investigations/procedures

4. Collect copies of all documents
Case notes/X-rays/investigation reports/charts/nursing process documents/care plans/models/medication charts etc.

5. Do not arrange for transfer ambulance or police escort until almost ready to leave:
This prevents two costly facilities being held-up with forseeable delays

6. Notify the receiving hospital of time of departure and approximate time of arrival

During transfer

1. Continue to closely monitor the patient

2. Do not discontinue any therapy or treatments

3. Keep bed or trolley transfers and handling of the patient to a minimum

4. Reassure and talk to the patient, even if unconscious

5. Take the journey *safely,* smoothly and unhurried. Stop the ambulance if the patient deteriorates suddenly or treatment changes are called for.

The equipment checklist below has been adapted from Dawson and Babington's research of 1987 and Halliday *et al* (1985):

1. Adapted York ambulance trolley	7. Blood pressure monitor (Tycos)
2. Syringe pumps - IVAC 700	8. Two emergency boxes
3. ECG and defibrillator (Lifepack 5)	(See Tables 2 and 3)
4 Respirometer (Spirox H)	9. Oxygen supply
5. Thermometer (Libra Medical ET 100)	10. Ventilator (Draegar Oxylog)
6. Suction (AMBU Uni-suction)	

Table 1. Aims of mobile intensive care.

Parks (1985) perhaps holds a possible solution to the transportation dilemma. He states that the risks of transportation can be greatly diminished if suitably experienced professionals undertake the task with the help of equipment that is reliable and designed to work in difficult environments. Not all peripheral hospitals and rural communities, however, possess ICU trained medical and nursing staff, and such is the upsurge of the operating department assistant's role that this will continue to be an eroding role of the nurse.

This equipment and expertise already exist within the field of neonatal intensive care. All regional and subregional units have mobile, portable incubators and life support systems, staffed by neonatal flying squads, which go out to peripheral midwifery units, when summoned, to stabilise and transfer critically ill premature infants (MacNab and Smart, 1990). A solution for adult patients might, therefore, be to establish a similar mobile unit, staffed by ICU flying squads or paramedic teams, with an equipment and general requirement checklist which could be individualised for each patient.

Trolley design

A great deal has been published since the 1960s on setting up adult mobile coronary care units (CCU), but with the advancement of paramedics in the ambulance service the original concept of mobile CCUs has been superseded. However, two articles were published in the 1980s on the design of a mobile ICU, based upon a modified hospital trolley (Aitkenhead *et al*, 1980) or a modified York ambulance trolley (Dawson and Babington, 1987). Aitkenhead *et al*'s design unfortunately required a modified ambulance in which to carry the mobile unit. This not only added to the cost, but also severely reduced the flexibility of the system. Dawson and Babington's design, however, fitted into an unmodified ambulance, ensuring the trolley could be carried by any ambulance, thus reducing the costs and ensuring rapid deployment of the service. Their design encorporates all the equipment required for life support, and allows for the continuation of vital signs and therapies. Although designed primarily for the transportation of patients between hospitals, it proved invaluable in intrahospital movements in an unhurried, more stable and controlled manner with the least harm to the patient. This unit was set up in 1984, performs well, requiring no major modifications, and could form the blueprint for the manufacture of more mobile ICUs.

A further innovation has recently occurred with the setting up of 'Bart's Careflight' in 1989. This is a fully supported and medically supervised helicopter transfer system, set up between St Bartholomew's Hospital and the City of London, and will assist with the movement of critically ill patients who require medically supervised, secondary transfer between hospitals anywhere in the UK. They are designed to carry one adult or child and are fully equipped and staffed for critical patients' care. Similar assistance can also be obtained from the RAF or army medical teams.

Laryngoscope
Magill forceps
Portex endotracheal tubes, varying sizes
Syringes and needles
Artery forceps
Catheter mounts
Oropharyngeal airways
Anaesthetic facemasks
Laerdal self-inflating resuscitation bag or
  water circuit
Yankaeur sucker and catheters
Suction tubing
Lubricating jelly
Elastoplast strapping and tracheostomy
  tape and Sleek
OpSite dressings
Mini tracheostomy set

Table 2. Emergency box 1.

Ventflon intravenous cannulae x 2 each
  size
Chest drain trochars and cannulae x 2
Intravenous giving sets x 2

Haemacel 500mls x 2
8.4% sodium bicarbonate 250mls
0.9% normal saline 1000mls
ECG electrodes and gel
Defibrillation shock pad

Drugs

Atropine	Adrenaline
Isoprenaline	Calcium gluconate
Lignocaine 1.0%	Verapamil
Practolol	Aminophylline
Frusemide	Hydrocortisone
Methohexitone	Suxamethonium
Water for injection	

Other drugs for the individual patient

Table 3. Emergency box 2.

Aims of mobile ICU

A list of aims of mobile intensive care (Table 1) is found in Halliday *et al*
(1985). Although this book specialises in neonatal intensive care, the
authors believe the aims are just as relevant to adult critically ill patients
as to premature sick infants, and could form the basis of a general
aims/requirements checklist.

The trolleys outlined above become an integral part or mobile
extentions of the ICU, requiring minimal technical expertise when not in
use, but vital when the need arises. Routine daily checks per shift
change is all that is required of the ICU staff, and this leads to
familiarisation with the workings of the emergency equipment, valuable

Patient transfer - checklist

Transferring nurse	Status...........................	Date..................................	Time....................................
Observations on transfer:	Temp.................................	Pulse.................................	Resp....................................
	Blood pressure....................	Time.................................	CVP....................................

Patient	Reason for transfer	Next of kin
Name: DoB:		
Address......................................	Consultant:...	Tel:...............…...
....		Family contacted: Y/N Status...........
....	Ward:	Police notified: Y/N
....		Relatives interviewed: Y/N
Tel:................ Religion...........	Hospital tel:......................................	Status of relative...

Documentation

	(Tick)
Nursing orders	☐
Nursing charts	☐
Case notes	☐
X-rays/scans	☐
Consent form - (adult)	☐
Consent form - (minor)	☐
Investigation results	☐
Drug charts	☐
Fluid regime	☐
Dialysis programme	☐
Transfer letter	☐

Fluids/drugs/treatments prior to transfer

Comments on patient status

Investigations prior to transfer	U/E	K
Blood gases prior to transfer	PaO_2	Pco^2
	B.Ex.	HCO_3
Blood grouping	Cross match	Y/N
Dextrostix	Serum glucose	

Respiration/ventilation

Oxygen:%................. Sat:%...................

Spontaneous resps ☐	Assisted ventilation ☐
Rate of resps ☐ per min	IMV ☐ IPPV ☐ CPAP ☐
Intubated ☐	Tube size ☐
Date/time intubated..	
Tracheostomy ☐	Tube size...
	Cuffed Y/N
Date/time tracheostomy changed...	

Fluid balance

Arterial/central line -   Y/N
Peripheral lines (number/fluid)
Arterial line (infusing)
Central line (type and fluid)

Urinary catheter	Y/N	Type...............
Peritoneal dialysis	Y/N	(infusing)
Nasogastric tube	Y/N	drainage (mls)

Chest drains (N° mls).

Circulation

(circle)

Cardiac monitoring	Y/N	Rhythm..............
Cardiac catheterisation	Y/N	Type...................
		Size...................
Pacing wire	Y/N	Frequency..........

Arterial pressure:
Normal medication of patient:

Nutrition

Total parentral nutrition	☐
Nasogastric feeding	☐
Orogastric feeding	☐
Nil-by-mouth	☐ Diet ☐

Girth measurement:..
Frequency:..

Locomotor

Glasgow coma score	
Adelaide coma score...	
Norton's scale	Frequency performed....................
Splints - *in situ*	
Traction	Weights
Skeletal survey performed	Y/N
Intracranial monitoring	Y/N

Senior sister (Name)

Ambulance arranged	Y/N
Helicopter transfer	Y/N
Police escort	Y/N
Notified receiving hospital	Y/N
(i) Time of departure	
(ii) Expected time of arrival	

Signature.......................................

experience during an emergency and thus would assist in the lowering of the risk factors when transporting patients.

A far greater way to diminish the risk factors involved, however, would be to staff these trolleys with an ICU flying squad or paramedic team, as is the case in neonatal ICU, with the receiving specialised unit extending their skills to the outlying, peripheral hospitals and collecting their patients for transfer, in a similar way to 'Careflight'. This would totally dispense with unskilled and inexperienced practitioners transferring patients and hopefully the conclusion of detrimental factors and side-effects to the patient.

References
Aitkenhead, A.R., Willis, M.I., Barnes, W.H. (1980) An economical mobile intensive unit. *British Medical Journal*, **280**, 1219-21.

Bion, J.F., Wilson, I.H., Taylor, P.A. (1988) Transporting critically ill patients by ambulance: audit by sickness scoring. *British Medical Journal*, **296**, 170.

Dawson, A.D.G. and Babington, P.C. (1987) An intensive care trolley - an economical and versatile alternative to the mobile intensive care unit. *Anaesthesia and Intensive Care*, **15**, 2, 229-33.

Gentleman, D.W. and Teasdale, G. (1981) Adoption of Glasgow. *British Medical Journal*, **283**, 408.

Halliday, H.L., McCure, G., Reid, M. (1985) Handbook of Neonatal Intensive Care. Balliere Tindall, London.

Ledingham, I., McA. and Banks, J.G. (1980) Movement of the critically ill patient. Special Report. *Hospital Update*, 43-49.

MacNab, A. and Smart, P. (1990) Lightweight monitoring equipment for paediatric transport. *Intensive Therapy and Clinical Monitoring*, **11**, 3, 92-96.

Parks, G. (1985) Transporting critically ill patients. *Care of the Critically Ill*, **1**, 6, 18-22.

Waddell, G. *et al* (1975) Movement of the critically ill patient within hospital. *British Medical Journal*, **2**, 417-19.

12

Making the most of the ambulance service

Fred Robinson

Assistant Divisional Ambulance Officer, Cumbria Ambulance Service

Every day the ambulance service carries thousands of patients to, from and between all parts of the health service. Although everyone knows the service exists it often seems that many healthcare professionals are unclear about its organisation, needs, problems and demands.

This chapter explains the general working and organisation of the service, so other professionals will be better equipped to make efficient use of it. This will not only help the ambulance service, but, more importantly, help provide patients with the best possible service. It will also help other parts of the health service improve their performance by ensuring patients are where they need to be at the right time.

Organisation

All ambulance services are organised on health service regional or district boundaries, and are accountable to and managed and funded by that region or district, although in some areas one district manages the service on behalf of a number of others.

The service exists to provide transport to, from and between NHS treatment centres for patients who cannot, for health reasons, travel by their own or public transport. Transport must be authorised by a doctor, midwife or dentist, and it must be made on health grounds rather than economic or social reasons such as lack of public transport, or the patient not having access to a car. The Departments of Health and Social Security have special provisions for patients with financial or social needs.

Patients are grouped by two main categories – urgency and need, and these are further divided into sub-groups as follows:

Urgency

Emergency   Any request which, if not attended without delay, would result in loss of life or serious deterioration of a patient's condition. The term should never be used to 'hurry up' the service when the request is outside its definition of emergency.

Urgent   A request which, while not an emergency, has a time limit, which usually means a pick-up of within one or two hours.

Non-urgent or routine A request with no emergency or urgent needs. This is usually used for outpatients, discharges and transfers, which can be planned 24 hours or more in advance.

Need

Stretcher (Str) A patient who must lie down during the journey and/or requires ambulance nursing care.

Sitting case two (S/2) A patient who needs to be lifted into the ambulance by two people, or who needs the assistance of two people to get in. Also a patient who needs care and attention during the journey.

Sitting case one (S/1) A patient who can get into the vehicle with the help of one person and will not require care and attention during the journey. Help here means ascending and descending steps into the vehicle, and general movement.

Wheelchair case (Chr or T/lft) Patients who need to travel in their own wheelchair. A specialised vehicle is provided for these patients, and since these vehicles are not common, they should not be requested unless they are really needed. They should not be requested to supplement a shortage of wheelchairs in the hospital, for example.

Ambulance staff

There are three grades of ambulance staff, who have different levels of skill and responsibility.

Basic grade Qualified to carry patients who do not fall into the urgent or emergency categories or stretcher cases.

Qualified These staff are qualified to carry out all ambulance service functions. They have been trained to cope with any type of case, and diagnose and treat on their own initiative.

Extended trained Qualified ambulance men or women who have skills above those of qualified status. They can intubate, infuse and defibrillate as needed, and can also administer a limited range of drugs. They receive no additional pay for these skills at present.

Coordinating requests

All ambulance services operate a central control, which coordinates and allocates all requests for transport. Urgent and emergency requests are dealt with by operational control, while non-urgent ones are passed to a planning department for coordination.

Resources are always limited, so the use of the ambulance service should be as efficient as possible. Requests for transport should be made with reasonable advance warning wherever possible, as resources allocated for short notice requests can result in overtime payments or a reduction in emergency response capacity. It can also mean patients missing hospital appointments or not being discharged, and tying up a bed unnecessarily. Most services operate a time limit on requests for non-urgent transport, such as midday the previous day, or 24 or 48 hours before it is needed. Requests made later than the deadline may be refused.

Many district hospitals have an ambulance liaison officer, whose job is to coordinate requests for transport, and as far as possible, ensure the best possible service for all its users. Requests from that hospital or group should be made through the liaison officer, who is also a useful source of information and advice on the service. If you are ever in any doubt about an aspect of the ambulance service, ask the liaison officer.

Diverse duties

The ambulance service has many diverse duties, including social services work, attending major accidents, and planning. It also carries out duties at public events, and carries private patients, for whom a charge is made.

Other duties can include house-to-house removals, upstairs-to-downstairs, putting people back to bed, and many more. Some of the work has legal implications, such as transporting people to psychiatric hospitals, when they are committed under the Mental Health Act.

Long distance journeys also come under the ambulance service's remit, whether by ambulance, train or air, and are paid for by the service. The cost of a helicopter is enormous, running into thousands of pounds, so requests for these should only be made if they are absolutely essential for the patient.

If patients are accompanied by an escort, provided either by themselves or the hospital, the ambulance service will carry him or her with the patient as long as they are prebooked. The service is not, however, responsible for returning escorts, although it will try to do so.

In rural areas, car transport is often used, usually known as the hospital car service (HCS) or similar. This service is provided by members of the public, who use their own cars to transport non-urgent patients. Although these people are volunteers, their mileage rate usually more than covers their petrol costs. Volunteers are not usually given much training, so they can only be used to transport patients who do not require care and attention during the journey.

Requesting an ambulance

It is far easier for everyone concerned if all the information is to hand when a request for transport is made. Apart from being time consuming, it is frustrating for ambulance personnel to constantly have to ask the same questions over and over again.

The service must be informed of contagious and infectious cases when the request for transport is made, for the safety of both the crew and other patients. Confidential information can be passed on to the ambulance service with confidence, as it has strict rules governing the maintenance of confidentiality.

Special needs should also be mentioned and discussed with the ambulance service or the liaison officer when a transport request is made, so that they can be taken into account when the transport is being arranged, and any problems are quickly ironed out.

As with all areas in the NHS, the ambulance service has limited resources, and these should be used carefully. It has a diverse and complex role, which often falls between being a hospital service and an emergency service like the police or fire brigade. Ambulances are not at the beck and call of any one department – the service has many calls upon its limited resources, so it helps to stay calm when requesting transport, even when the pressure is on. Requests are dealt with as quickly and efficiently as resources allow, and by clearly stating the nature of their request and any special needs, and not getting annoyed if there will be a delay in providing transport, other healthcare professionals can help us provide the optimum service for patients.

13

An opportunity we must not miss: computers and nursing practice

Melanie Hodkinson, BSc (Hons), D.N. RGN
Greater Care Nursing Home, Northern Ireland

As technology has advanced in recent decades, the nursing profession has incorporated many new devices and ideas to enhance patient care. Computers are one area which is becoming (and in some cases already is) a considerable asset to nursing, both for ward- and community-based care. While it is easy to imagine using computers for nurse education or administration, some nurses find it hard to accept that they can be used on the wards. Nurses must learn to view computers in a positive light, and take advantage of the valuable support they offer in providing effective ward-based care.

Computer benefits

So what is a computer and what are its functions? Computers are "any machine which can accept data in a prescribed form, process the data and supply the results in a specified format as information, or as signals to control some other machine or process." (Oxford Dictionary, 1979). Computers have four functions, explained in greater detail by Burnard (1990). Briefly these are:

- Calculate data - like a simple calculator it can add, multiply, subtract and divide.

- Communicate data - the computer can communicate with the user via a visual display unit (VDU) or print-out, or with other machines, via telephone cables.

- Enable user control by giving access to the programming facilities, so the user can regulate the outcome.

- Store data -this can be done by loading information onto a magnetic disk, which either is 'hard' or a 'floppy'.

Although nursing already uses computerised technology in a small way to enhance competency of care, the profession must become computer literate and identify areas where personal computers can aid nursing care. Personal computers used efficiently at ward level can reduce the amount of nursing time often - as much as 40 per cent - spent on non-nursing clerical duties (Staggers, 1988).

If, for example, all hospital departments were linked through a mini computer system, electronic 'memos' could be dispatched from and to wards enabling tests to be booked or cancelled, and results requested without having to spend time telephoning (Jydstrup, 1966).

Ward sisters are in an excellent position to make full use of personal computers, especially with regard to their clinical, educational and administrative roles. By pre-programming the computer, they could automatically reorder commonly used ward items such as syringes, lotions or drugs, thus cutting out the weekly re-ordering routines.

A pre-programmed disk containing information such as ward policy or types of nursing care peculiar to specialty, could help orientate new or temporary members of staff to the ward. If ward sisters were able to link up to a nursing research unit via computer, they would keep up-to-date on relevant research, particularly with regard to new products or nursing procedures.

The ward sister's educative role may be eased using computer assisted learning packages (CALPs) which help students learn with the computer at their own speed and ability. Computers, being available on a 24-hour basis, allow students greater access to theoretical knowledge, reducing the time ward sisters need to devote to individual learners. CALPs are not limited only to use by students, but also help trained staff keep up-to-date with, or consolidate, various aspects of nursing.

Hospital computers' role

Computers must and will come into the profession: their speed and storage abilities alone far outweigh those of any human being. It must be realised, however, that a program's accuracy is only as good as the skills of the programmer. Adequate resources and facilities must be made available to ensure nurses learn the linguistics and skills of computer useage.

Personal computers used in nursing administration may enable managers to efficiently and effectively forsee staff shortages, store and retrieve clinical progress reports on students, and ensure objective rotation of trained staff for study days. As managers in both public and private medicine become increasingly aware of the costs and resources required by their departments, they may use computers to estimate the projected needs and costs of nursing in a particular department or district.

Nursing has been defined as 'a science of caring' (Dunlop, 1986). Computers, although invaluable in assisting care planning, administration and educational areas, will never be able to replace the humanistic approach to caring and communicating with patients.

Nurses, therefore, have nothing to fear about the prospect of losing their jobs to a computer. If used correctly, computers can only enhance the profession releasing nurses from clerical and administrative roles to provide direct nursing care to patients or clients.

The nurse's role will continue to change and adapt, as it has done in the past, encompassing new technology to assist patient recovery or peaceful death. Most of these new skills have been gained initially to assist other professions. If nurses do not grasp the potential computers have to enable them to nurse with greater skill and dexterity, then history will undoubtedly repeat itself - nurses will learn little about computers or their application to nursing, but just enough to enable them to assist other medical and paramedical groups. The choice is still ours.

References
Burnard, P. (1990) So you think you need a computer? *Professional Nurse*, 6, 2, 119-20.
Dunlop, M.J. (1986) Is a science of nursing possible? *Journal of Advanced Nursing*, **II**, 6, 66I.
Jydstrup, R.A., Gross, M.J. (1966) Cost effectiveness of information handling in hospitals. *Health Service Research*, **I**, 3, 235-71.
Oxford Paperback Dictionary (1979) (2nd Ed.). Oxford University Press, Oxford.
Staggers, N. (1988) Using computers in nursing. *Computers in Nursing*, 6, 4, 165.

Bibliography
Baly, M. (1986) Nursing and Social Change. Heinneman, London.
    Gives a history of nursing and its latest developments.
Davison, R.B. (1968) A Guide to the Computer. Longman, London.
    An introduction into the field of computers.
The bimonthly journal *Computers in Nursing* gives up-to-date information on the subject.

Resource
Management

14

What is resource management?

Shirley Williams, RGN, RHV
Director of Nursing Services (Community Services), Oxford H.A. Formerly Director of Nursing Services, Radcliffe Infirmary, Oxford

A major complaint voiced by nurses is that they have an ever increasing workload without any commensurate increase in staffing. As a result they are unable to provide what they consider to be an acceptable standard of care. There is considerable evidence to support the claim that workload has risen both in volume and intensity.

- Shorter length of stay has resulted in a rise in the dependency of those patients who are in hospital.
- Quicker throughput may mean the patient due for admission arrives before the patient occupying his or her prospective bed has been discharged. This means the nurses have more patients than beds (and staffing establishments are traditionally set on bed numbers).
- Increasingly sophisticated medical procedures often require added nursing support.

Not surprisingly, the increase in the number of patients treated has resulted in a marked rise in expenditure, particularly in non-staff items such as drugs, X-rays and prosthesis. This has generated considerable alarm in government circles.

Cash limits

In an attempt to control what appeared to be runaway expenditure, 'cash limits' were introduced whereby district health authorities were instructed to ensure they contained their spending within the funds they were allocated. Many health authorities simply passed this directive down the line, and in some cases budget holders found themselves being reprimanded for 'overspending' when they had no idea what money they had been allocated, nor what they were expected to achieve with it.

As a result of cash limits, hospitals found themselves between a pincer movement. On the one hand they were under pressure from the Department to maximise use of their resources, with particular reference to such things as theatre time, while on the other hand they were being reprimanded for expenditure above that which had been allocated by the department, but which had been incurred as a result of the very increase in efficiency which the hospital had been instructed to undertake. The NHS enquiry tried to address this dilemma, and Griffiths said it was necessary for "each unit to develop management budgets which involve clinicians and relate workload and service objectives to financial and manpower allocations".

There was, however, a major obstacle preventing the achievement of Griffiths' aim. The NHS had no idea of the cost of individual components of treatment and care. Previously it had not been deemed necessary to have a pricing policy, since there had been no requirement to 'bill' a patient. However, if Griffiths' ideas were to be realised it would be essential to identify how money was being spent; and work has been going on in this area in a number of pilot sites, on a system of management information known as resource management.

The resource management initiative involves the following:

- Agreeing clear objectives with doctors, nurses and other hospital managers.
- Agreeing with them budgets related to their workload and objectives.
- Giving them greater control over the day-to-day use of resources.
- Providing better information on the actual cost of clinical activity and services used by clinicians and patients.
- Holding budget-holders accountable for their performance.
- Reviewing outcome.

The resource management system will, where these basic principles are applied to a specialty or clinical service, base the information on an individual patient episode, linking the costs to discharge diagnosis, and perhaps ultimately a diagnostic group. Doctors and nurses can then not only understand the potential of their overall budgets to manage their service, but the effects their case-mix has on this.

Thus, with resource management we move from attempting to cope with an unplanned, demand-led workload within a cash limited financial allocation to a position where there is agreement about the amount of work which can be accomplished within available resources. It is imperative that nurses play an assertive proactive role in agreeing workload related budgets, since it is us and only us who can make the necessary statements about what constitutes nursing workload. The way in which we nurses approach this will be determined by our own understanding of the nature of nursing work.

What is nursing?

If we believe nursing consists of the execution of a series of largely predetermined tasks, we are likely to think it appropriate to deploy any nurse to carry out any task in any area. With such a philosophy it is possible to separate the responsibility for the proficient completion of the task from authority over the resources to carry them out. This position is clearly reflected in traditional nurse management arrangements, where ward sisters are held responsible for standards of care on their wards, but have minimal control over the composition of their establishment or deployment of their staff. Their day duty plans can be overridden by the nursing officer or duty nurse who has authority to redeploy their staff; and their responsibility for and authority over night duty is often either tenuous or a subject of outright hostility between themselves and the night sister. In a traditional system the duty nurse, both on day duty and at night, has resources of her own in the shape of a pool or team, which she deploys on a shift by shift basis at her own discretion.

In a task orientated hospital, the approach to resource management would be to devise a system where all tasks were identified and timed and all nursing resources were controlled centrally so that they could be deployed on a shift by shift basis in response to the predicted task-constituted workload and then be 'costed' at patient level. Many hospitals are taking this approach and indeed the production of computerised nurse deployment systems to support them is a new growth industry.

So where should a ward sister start when implementing a resource management system? A report from the Department of Health's Nursing Division (1988) reviewed the issues. It is first helpful to draw up three component functions that could make up a ward based management information system – the functions are:

- workload assessment;
- ward nurse tracking (recording past, present and planned future shift and work patterns of individual staff);
- care planning support.

Workload assessment
Systematic methods of assessing the demand for nurse manpower date back to the late 1950s. A vast amount has been written in the UK and America dealing with the various issues arising in this area of nursing demand, with conflicting claims as to the which is the best approach. It is vital to have some understanding of these issues before designing a resource management system.

Clearly, to decide how many nurses should be on a particular ward at a particular time is not simply a question of measurement – some judgement is also necessary, but existing approaches can vary a great deal in the level of detail they require. Some simply focus on 'nursing tasks', while others go into more detail, classifying patients into dependency groups. Greater complexity and detail does not necessarily bring greater accuracy, however. Schroeder at al (1984), in a trial between two systems found an easy to establish and simple to operate one gave essentially the same results as a more cumbersome task orientated system. They recommended that nurses avoid adopting expensive, detailed task orientated staffing tools, and depend on systems developed in-house by their own nursing staff, which the staff are happy using. This view has also been endorsed by the NHS Management Board (Peach, 1987).

The question of whether the resource management systems should be used to formulate nursing process care plans is a contentious one. It is unlikely that nurses would willingly accept the idea that workload derived task specifications could or should play a role in care planning. Part of the philosophy of individualised care planning is to move away from the mechanical, task-based approach to patient care. It is probably wise, therefore, to keep the care planning process separate from the resource management system, otherwise the system may end up fulfilling neither of the functions for which it is intended. However, since nursing workload is generated by a patient's need for care, the level of nursing resource required will be reflected in his care plan. The amount of care he actually receives will be determined by a combination of the level of total nursing resources available and the priority of his needs against those of other patients who have a call on the same resources. Whilst not strictly part of resource management, it is important to identify any discrepancy between care needed and care received if we are to include the added dimension of quality.

Use of computers

Computers can be useful tools in resource management, and their use can have a number of advantages. Information retrieval is quick and easy, and all the information is easily stored without taking up precious space. However, individual ward sisters need to ask whether using a computer will be better for them than a preprinted form to be completed by hand. When nurses are busy and documentation is not seen as a priority, it is just as easy to produce misleading and incomplete computer records as it is hand written ones, so computers should not be seen as a way of imposing a discipline which guards against this. If they are to be used, it should be because the ward sister (and the rest of the staff) feel computerisation will genuinely allow them to operate their resource management system more efficiently and effectively.

Government commitment

The recent White Paper (DoH, 1989) makes it clear the Government is committed to the expansion of the resource management initiative. It is imperative that nurses ensure the opportunities it affords are used for the benefit of patient care, and that the exercise does not merely become a costing mechanism to help the accountants ensure that 'the money follows the patient'.

It is important that hospitals understand the implications of introducing resource management. Merely introducing modern information systems to record clinical and operational activities will achieve nothing except perhaps lots of pretty pie charts. At whatever level a hospital decides it is best to run its clinical services – involving doctors, nurses and other professionals – it must be based on the principle that the people responsible for care need to be given clear areas of responsibility. This must be supported by an agreed budget which is related to a level and quality of service that can be reasonably be provided within the funds available.

An appropriate management philosophy – and a proper structure within the unit to support it – is an essential prerequisite for the successful introduction of resource management.

References
DoH (1988) *The Resource Management Initiative and Ward Nursing Management Information Systems*. DoH Nursing Division and Operational Research Services, London.
DoH (1989) *Working for Patients*. HMSO, London.
Peach, L. (1987) Nurse manpower planning. Letter to regional and district general managers. Ref DA (87)**12**.
Schroeder, R.E., Rhodes, A., Shields, R.E. (1984) Nurse acuity services: CASH vs GRASP (a determination of nurse staff requirements). *Journal of Nursing Administration*, **21**, 2, 72-77.

15

Making resource management work

Jan Chalmers, RGN, RCNT
Critical Care Manager, Radcliffe Infirmary, Oxford

Resource management was implemented at the Radcliffe Infirmary based on our belief in the value of professional judgment and the importance of building teams to facilitate a high standard of individualised patient care. We believe decisions regarding patient care and the authority over resources to provide that care should be made as near to the bedside as possible.

The changes in our nursing structure described in this chapter were made in line with this philosophy. We moved from a task orientated approach to what we believe to be the much firmer ground of professional practice.

Professional practice is based on the nurse's responsibility to identify individual patient needs. The example used to illustrate this in a recent Nurses and Midwives Advisory Council's circular suggests the question ceases to be "How quickly can I take the temperature of all my patients?" and becomes, "Which patient's temperature do I need to monitor and how frequently?" Acceptance of professional practice has a profound effect on the way nursing is managed, particularly in the choice of level at which responsibility and authority for decision making is placed.

Key role of ward sisters

Ward sisters   At the Radcliffe Infirmary, each ward has one sister or charge nurse who works primarily on day duty with a 24-hour, 365-day-a-year responsibility for the quality of nursing on the ward. This also involves occasional night duty when required.

Ward sisters have 'ownership' of non-staff expenditure and the staffing resources for the ward and the authority to decide how nursing staff on the ward will be deployed and what the skill mix will be (see Table 1). In addition, they negotiate an agreed workload for the ward with medical staff, so controlling non-emergency admissions to the ward.

Senior ward sisters   Wards are grouped together in specialty units, for example elderly care, neurosurgery etc. The sister (or charge nurse) in charge of one of the wards within a particular specialty unit is responsible

```
REPORT NUMBER  ORG/0042SCS                    OXFORD REGIONS BUSINESS INFORMATION SYSTEMS (ORBIS)                    PAGE:      84
MR:   CV RI - OPTHALMOLOGY                          BUDGET MANAGER'S SUBJECTIVE REPORT :                             DATE:  10/01/91
69 MONTHS ENDING 31/12/90                           COST CENTRE 20970 THEATRES - OEH                                TIME:  08:49:35

COMMENTS:

          STAFFING                                                                    FINANCE
  CURRENT  CURRENT  AVERAGE
  MONTH    MONTH    Y.T.D.
  BUDGET   ACTUAL   ACTUAL          SUBJECTIVE         ANNUAL  ------ CURRENT MONTH -------   ----------- YEAR TO DATE -----------
  WORKED   WORKED   WORKED                             BUDGET   BUDGET   ACTUAL   VARIANCE      BUDGET   ACTUAL   VARIANCE  CF
  WTE      WTE      WTE     CODE   DESCRIPTION          £        £        £        £            £        £        £        %

  1.00     1.00     0.45    122505 GRADE G NURSE       19472    1623     1410     213-         14607    15354     747     5.1
  1.00     1.00     0.81    123005 GRADE F NURSE       16804    1400     1159     241-         12600    12097     503-    4.0-
  2.50     2.28     2.20    123505 GRADE E NURSE       33514    2792     2503     289-         25128    23131    1997-    7.9-
  2.53     1.52     2.50    124005 GRADE D NURSE       18983    2646     1454     1192-        11040    21610   10570-   95.7
  2.39     0.44     0.20    124505 GRADE C NURSE       21852    1821      322     1499-        16389     1291   15098-   92.1-
  0.00     0.00     0.00    156410 OPERAT DEPT AS BG       0       0        0        0             0        0        0     0.0
  0.00     0.00     0.00    156415 OPER DEP ASS TRAI       0       0      113      113             0      391      391     0.0

  9.42     6.24     6.16    PAY TOTAL                  110625   10282    6961     3321-        79764    73875    5889-    7.4-

                           301506 DRUGS-STORES ISSU        0       0        5        5             0       18       18     0.0
                           310505 MEDICAL GASES            0       0        0        0             0      105      105     0.0
                           311005 DRESSINGS-PURCHAS        0       0        0        0             0       20       20     0.0
                           311006 DRESSING-STORE IS        0       0      766      766             0     1010     1010     0.0
                           311503 MSSE-PURCHASES-DI        0       0       23       23             0    10375    10375     0.0
                           311504 MSSE-PUR-NON DISP        0       0        0        0             0      503      503     0.0
                           311510 MSSE-STORES ISSUE        0       0      197      197             0     1668     1668     0.0
                           311565 OPTICAL EQUIPMENT        0       0       33       33             0      378      378     0.0
                           311580 SURGICAL INST DIS        0       0        0        0             0     9650     9650     0.0
                           311581 SURGICAL INST-GEN        0       0        0        0             0     1613     1613     0.0
                           311582 SURG INST NON DIS    38300    3192        0     3192-         75536        0    25536- 100.0-
                           311587 SURG INST-OPHTHAL        0       0        0        0             0     2833     2833     0.0
                           311589 SURG INST-ORTHOPA        0       0        0        0             0       93       93     0.0
                           311590 SUTURES                  0       0     1310     1310            0    10949    10949     0.0
                           311592 SYRINGES                 0       0       22       22             0       22       22     0.0
                           311740 LENS IMPLANTS        114860    9571     3137     6434-        76568    41750    34818-  45.5-
                           311750 OTHER PROSTHESIS         0       0       23       23             0      246      246     0.0
                           312045 PLIERS/INSTR.ORTH        0       0      443      443             0      443      443     0.0
                           313045 MED EQUIP MAINTEN        0       0       69       69             0       69       69     0.0
                           315100 PAT APPLI OPTICAL        0       0       78       78             0       78       78     0.0
                           316005 LABORATORY EQUIPM        0       0        0        0             0      452      452     0.0
                           316006 LAB EQ-STORES ISS        0       0        0        0             0       25       25     0.0
                           322011 STAFF UNIFORMS SI        0       0        0        0             0       36       36     0.0
                           322020 GLOVES-DISPOSABLE        0       0      383      383             0      383      383     0.0
                           324506 BED&LINEN-DISP-SI        0       0        0        0             0        9        9     0.0
                           330506 PRINT&STATION-SI         0       0        0        0             0       10       10     0.0
                           332505 STAFF ADVERTISING      100       8        0        8-           64        0       64- 100.0-
                           333005 TRAVELLING EXPENS        0       0        1        1             0        1        1     0.0
                           333020 TRAVEL EXP-STANDA        0       0       98       98             0      164      164     0.0
                           333030 TRAV EX-PASS MILE        0       0        1        1             0        1        1     0.0
                           343072 TRANS.OF TRANSFPA        0       0      160      160            0     1075     1075     0.0
                           385500 ALL OTHER EXPENDI        0       0        0        0             0      113      113     0.0
                           391005 SER REC OTHER HA         0       0      160-     160-           0        0        0     0.0

                           NON PAY TOTAL             153260   12771     6496     6275-        102168    84093    18075-  17.7-

  9.42     6.24     6.16    COST CENTRE TOTAL        263885   23053    13457     9596-        181932   157967    23965-  11.2-
```

Table 1.

for coordinating the activities of the other sisters in the unit. Designated 'senior ward sister', they are assisted by a junior sister in their own ward.

Each senior sister is a member of the specialty team responsible for monitoring and planning work in the specialty unit. Other members of the team are the consultant, an administrator and an accountant. The specialty teams meet quarterly to review workload and expenditure

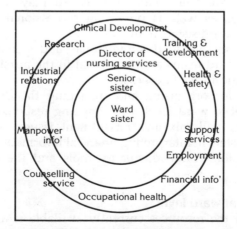

Figure 1. The ward sister is the centre of the devolution of authority to ward level.

under the chairmanship of the unit general manager. The senior sister also acts as the specialty unit's spokesperson, representing its interests either to the director of nursing services (DNS) or to other professional groups in the hospital. Senior sisters have direct assess to the DNS, to whom they are professionally and managerially accountable.

This access to the DNS means the conventional (and often non-clinical) role of nursing officer has been discontinued at the Radcliffe Infirmary. The responsibility and authority awarded to ward sisters has removed a tier of management which previously dealt with the central deployment of staff in the hospital. (See Figure 1). Traditional nursing officer posts (whose holders expected to directly influence clinical practice) were redesigned as support roles to facilitate the introduction of resource management.

Preparation and support of staff

The key to the successful implementation of resource management at ward level is the adequate preparation and ongoing support of ward sisters, who are responsible for the smooth working of the system.

By abolishing the nursing officer role and subsequently reorganising and redeploying nursing personnel within individual wards, we released resources for four new posts. Two clinical practice development nurses were appointed, and these are clinically involved with all wards in the hospital, helping them develop their clinical practice at whatever pace is appropriate for the nursing team involved. Clinical practice development nurses also organise workshops, undertake research and act as personal 'mentors' for individual nurses and ward teams.

The two other new posts were designed specifically to support organisational development and the introduction of resource management and it is to these posts that I and my colleague, Kate Woods were appointed. We were both expected to play a leading role in managing change, as well as providing professional and managerial support to all the ward sisters in the hospital.

These two posts provided professional and personal support to individuals and ward teams and were vital to the nursing system. Each has its own specific areas of expertise:

• Responsibility for organising and managing the devolution of the nursing budget to ward level, with ongoing responsibility for yearly budget setting, skill mix and recruitment issues and support and guidance for sisters in interpreting financial information.

• Responsibility for workload, quality tools and the development of trained staff.

Budget control at ward level

A knowledge of the resources currently available is a prerequisite for effective budgetary control at ward level. A first step was to help each ward sister identify the total size of her nursing establishment - a matter about which many ward sisters were unclear. After a nursing establishment for each ward was agreed upon, it was important to reassure the sisters that there could be no change to this without their approval.

After gaining the confidence of a particular ward sister in this way, we discussed whether or not the skill mix in the ward was fully suited to its patients' needs. It was evident that on some wards the mix was not ideal, either because of changes in medical practice or because of a failure to recruit appropriately trained nurses. On one ward, a senior ward sister was assisted by a total of only three whole time equivalent (WTE) trained nurses, and had seven nursing auxiliaries. After discussion, she changed the skill mix within her overall budget by appointing three additional trained nurses and redeploying five of the seven auxiliaries. This resulted in a new skill mix which was better suited to changed medical practices and her current nursing requirements.

A simple device which helped nurses assess the scope for modifying the skill mix within a fixed budget was a table showing how many hours of a particular grade equated (in salary cost terms) to how many hours of another grade (Table 2). Reference to the table showed, for example, that on average the salary of one Whole Time Equivalent (WTE) Grade

Payscales	A(<18) 1.00	A(>18) 1.00	B(18) 1.00	B(18+) 1.00	C 1.00	D 1.00	E 1.00	F 1.00	G 1.00	H 1.00	I 1.00
A(<18)	1.00	1.26	1.31	1.45	1.70	1.94	2.22	2.55	2.91	3.23	3.56
A(>18)	.79	1.00	1.04	1.16	1.35	1.54	1.76	2.02	2.32	2.57	2.83
B(18)	.77	.96	1.00	1.11	1.30	1.48	1.70	1.95	2.23	2.47	2.72
B(18+)	.69	.87	.90	1.00	1.17	1.33	1.53	1.75	2.00	2.22	2.45
C	.59	.74	.77	.86	1.00	1.14	1.31	1.50	1.72	1.90	2.10
D	.52	.65	.67	.75	.88	1.00	1.15	1.32	1.50	1.67	1.84
E	.45	.57	.59	.65	.76	.87	1.00	1.15	1.31	1.45	1.60
F	.39	.49	.51	.57	.67	.76	.87	1.00	1.14	1.27	1.40
G	.34	.43	.45	.50	.58	.66	.76	.87	1.00	1.11	1.22
H	.31	.39	.40	.45	.53	.60	.69	.79	.90	1.00	1.10
I	.28	.35	.37	.41	.48	.54	.62	.72	.82	.91	1.00

Table 2. Whole time equivalent trade-off matrix for the clinical Grading Structure, calculated as cost based mean of all points of scale. The horizontal payscale reference shows the post to be traded at 1.00 W.T.E. The vertical payscale reference shows the different values that can be "bought".

A nursing auxiliary over 18 years of age is equivalent to 0.65 WTE of a Grade D staff nurse/enrolled nurse or 0.57 WTE of a Grade E staff nurse.

Using a fixed annual budget

Sisters are not held to account every month since the agreement is based on an estimated annual workload. This is important. Previously, if sisters had an establishment of 10 nurses, they would have been required to ensure this number was not exceeded, but they now have the authority to 'spend' the equivalent of 10 salaries over a full year .and are encouraged to use their discretion over the way this is used. For example, one month a sister may have a vacancy but because none of her staff are on maternity or sick leave, the ward can function safely and satisfactorily. The following month she may theoretically have 10 nurses in post, but with one on maternity leave and several off sick she needs to 'buy' more nursing hours for her patients, either through overtime payments or by employing bank nurses. By doing this, the sister can provide nursing care for the same overall workload in each month by using only nine salaries during the first month and 11 salaries during the second.

There are many similar ways in which ward sisters can make flexible use of resources within a fixed annual budget. If, for example, over a period of several months they have been unable to recruit up to the full level of their establishment, they could use the money saved to buy a hoist to assist the depleted nursing team when lifting patients.

The ward sisters receive financial information every month to help them manage the resources for which they alone are responsible. This information gives details of budgeting and expenditure from the beginning of the year to date.

Consolidating the new role
If ward sisters are to fulfil their new role, it is essential that they are given adequate preparation to enable them to relate with other disciplines. The preparatory programme consisted of a negotiation skills workshop, a resource management module set up by the local polytechnic and a series of assertiveness sessions to develop their role in multidisciplinary teamwork and to gain increased personal confidence. With the help of these aids, staff were fully able to undertake their new roles brought about through the implementation of resource management.

16

Managing a budget at ward level

Wanda K. Shafer, RGN, Cert. Man. Studs.
Outpatient Manager, Hillingdon Hospital, Uxbridge

Managing a budget at ward level requires a systematic approach in order to do it well. The essential elements are:
● Good information which is readily available.
● Resource people to provide the much needed support.
● Authority to implement changes.
● A forum which provides evaluation in an ongoing fashion.

Good information
The manager must have a comprehensive knowledge of the current expenditures for the ward.

Computer print-outs of central supplies, stock levels, pharmacy stock levels, inventory of furniture and equipment (asset registry), staff levels and the costs often associated with other departments, i.e., advertising, radiology, theatre, TSSU, etc. These latter costs are often forgotten when budgets are devolved to ward level. Having this information is crucial to the understanding of how the speciality unit/ward relates to the hospital.

Current information regarding staffing levels, skill mix, patient dependency, patterns of workload (i.e., 5-day beds, day cases, ward attenders etc.) is necessary to determine if you are utilising your human resources effectively.

It is extremely important to be aware of any anticipated changes in medical practice which would have an effect on the unit i.e., a purchase of new equipment in theatre or a new minor operation/diagnostic procedure which can be carried out in the outpatient department. These changes can have an affect on the dependency level of the patients on the ward. A change of consultant could have a major knock-on effect which is sometimes not considered in advance.

Nothing can be more important than good communication. Sharing your information, thoughts and asking questions keeps everyone aware of what is happening. It also encourages staff to participate in the problem solving process which strengthens the team and improves the quality of the services you are offering.

Resource people

Central supply   The Radcliffe Infirmary uses a topping up service for those items most frequently used on the ward, i.e., tapes, syringes, needles etc. The level is or can be controlled by the ward.

When I first observed my stores expenditure as a new Senior Sister, I was quite shocked. I wanted it decreased, but I did not want to decrease quality. Initially, I spent what seemed an eternity in "the cupboard", so much time that staff began referring to it as "Sisters office". Once I knew what was on the shelf Mike, the person responsible for topping up, provided a complete list indicating what quantities, when and where they were ordered with a total expenditure for the year.

I spent several hours sorting through this and with Mike's help we set new stock levels. As treatments or needs change, the levels are adjusted. We have also begun to do some "comparison shopping".

Pharmacy   Anyone who has even looked at a ward budget knows that the one area always high in expenditure is Pharmacy. There seems little that can be done. However, you must investigate to ensure there is not high wastage.

We first looked at our ward stock levels, which again, are maintained on a topping-up system by the Pharmacy. It has been my experience that nurses are "be prepared" people. We had stock items which were never touched but were there "just in case". Many times these items would expire and be replaced having never been used. This sort of "shelf wastage", as I refer to it, is very costly.

With the assistance of the pharmacist, and the perseverance of the team leaders, we now have our stock levels in a reasonable state.

Clinical Practice Development Nurses   The highest expenditure in any ward budget is staffing. It is, therefore, always being challenged. The manager must understand and be able to defend her staffing levels. The only way to be able to firmly say your levels are correct is to start at the beginning by developing a ward philosophy, determining how you will organise your nursing (i.e., team nursing, primary nursing, task, patient allocation) and choosing/developing a model of nursing.

Patient   dependency: Resource   Management   Project   Nurse Continuing on from the above, you must now determine what dependency level of patient you have. The Oxford Nurse Management System is based on the work carried out by Dr Sue Pembrey in 1979. It establishes patient need, planned nursing hours, available nursing hours and the cost of nursing care for each patient. The ward staff develop this information utilising their ward philosophy and nursing care plans along with the immense support from the Resource Management Project Nurse. Once this information is available on the computer, it is then possible to look at skill mix to ensure that you have it correct.

Personnel officer   Some of the hidden costs, that can become quite high, have to do with an area of personnel, ie, advertising, annual leave, sick pay, training. It is very important to consult the personnel officer whenever you have a question in these areas.

Medical staff   It cannot be stressed enough that managing a budget at ward level requires team work. Working with the medical staff is imperative and therefore it is up to the ward manager/senior sister to keep communication channels open. This is sometimes a difficult area.

Accountant   A very useful resource person is the accountant, but do keep in mind that they are not always familiar with hospitals, nurses or the fact that there is a human life at issue not a product.

Director of Nursing Services   The Director of Nursing Services is always there and is always needed for consultation, challenge and the ability to offer the personal support to keep you going.

Clinical service manager/Administrative assistant   Whatever your institution may refer to them as, they are indispensable. A non-nursing input that allows you to delegate non-nursing tasks to them. The type of support you need when you are not quite certain who you need to consult – they just seem to always know the answer!

Implementing change
Having all this information and reams of computer print-outs will be of no use if you do not have the authority to implement change. You must be aware at the start what you will have the authority to change and what procedures you must follow. Understanding change and its effect is important for all concerned. Introducing too much too quickly can often produce unwanted results.

Again, keeping all staff informed and involved is essential. Many ideas for change or improvement are initiated by the ward staff. If they are allowed to implement change they will also be willing to accept the responsibility for evaluating the effectiveness of the change.

It is apparent to me, after nearly two years in post, that being ward-based with some clinical involvement is beneficial as it provides the opportunity to see first hand how things are working on the ward and the sorts of issues that arise in the course of the day. Communication channels are also easier to maintain when you are visible.

Evaluating progress
Each specialty unit has a quarterly Management Budgeting meeting. The agenda for this meeting is derived from the accountants financial information pertaining to the specialty. The meeting is chaired by the Unit General Manager and attended by the senior sister, senior

consultant, the accountant, the clinical services manager and, if it is a surgical specialty, the theatre manager. This forum allows for reviewing the current situation and highlighting areas that may need extra attention.

In the ENT specialty unit we have determined that extra meetings are needed to address some of our problem areas. We have therefore set up a meeting between the Management Budgeting meetings. We use this forum as an investigative/problem solving meeting and involve members from the multidisciplinary health care team. These have proven useful as we can then report back to the quarterly meeting with our results.

I have only been able to touch on some of the aspects involved in managing a budget at ward level. With each gain that is made, some new areas become apparent which require attention and the whole process begins again.

References
Bagust, A. (1990) Dispel that old myth. *The Health Service Journal,* **6,** 1000–1001.
Brechbiel, K. (1990) Getting a grip on your unit's budget. *American Journal of Nursing,* **90**(1) 42I–42L.
Brechbiel, K. (1990) How to justify your staffing. *American Journal of Nursing,* **9**(5,)28.
Cardin, S. (1990) What's in a (manager's) name? *American Journal of Nursing,* **90**(5)28.
Chalmers, J. (1990) Making resource management work. *Professional Nurse,* **5**(4,)178–80.
Haynes, M. (1987) Make every minute count: How to manage your time effectively. *Crisp Publications,* Los Altos, California.
Williams, S. (1989) The Radcliffe revolution. *Nursing Times,* **85,**18.
Wood, K. (1990) Resource management in action on the ward. *Professional Nurse,* **5**(5,)492–94.

17

Showing where the money goes: cost-effective care in ICU

Karen Ballard, RGN
Sister, ICU, St Peter's Hospital, Chertsey

The nurse practitioner role is centred around delivering the best possible care to patients and their families. The recent proposals outlined in the government's White Paper (DoH, 1989) have raised awareness among nurses that resource management will soon become their responsibility - indeed many ward-based nurses have already taken on the system.

In setting up effective systems of resource management, Griffiths (1983) said each unit must "develop management budgets which involve clinicians and relate workload and service objectives to financial and manpower allocations". A major problem in meeting Griffiths's aim has been that the NHS has no real idea of the individual costs of care. The clinical nurse's role has not been shown to realistically extend to full accountability for the cost of care, and it is vital that whatever changes do occur in the NHS, the quality of care remains paramount. There is little doubt that nurses will become more involved in budgeting care, but valuable nurse manpower must not be misused. Views about nurses' primary role are changing, and a conflict exists between the traditional role of carer at the bedside and the developing role in such areas as resource management. These issues must eventually be solved, and it is up to us as nurses to ensure the solution does not put efficiency and cost-effectiveness above quality of care.

Increasing awareness
In order to prepare for the change to resource management, staff in the intensive care unit (ICU) at St Peter's Hospital, Chertsey decided to find ways of delivering the most cost-effective care without compromising the quality of that care. Many methods can be used to carry out nursing procedures, and these involve diverse pieces of equipment, take variable amounts of time and may result in different levels of effectiveness for the patient. When considering cost-effectiveness, the priority must remain to ensure the patient receives the highest standard of nursing care possible, and our prime consideration had to be that patient safety was in no way compromised. Apart from the potentially devastating effect sub-standard

care could have on our highly dependent patients, savings made at the expense of safety are usually a false economy. Patients may well develop complications as a result of cheaper but poorer quality care, and may cost the NHS more to treat. For example, if pressure relieving aids are not used, particularly with the highly dependent patients in ICU, they may well develop pressure sores, which were estimated to cost the NHS £15,000,000 per year to treat five years ago (Johnson, 1985). Appropriate use of short-acting sedation can be more expensive than longer acting drugs, but can mean the patient requires less time on the ventilator and is highly dependent for less time, making the care cheaper to provide.

Equipment costs

When assessing costs, it is important to consider the amount of nursing time that can be saved when using more expensive items. It is essential that nursing manpower is put to the most appropriate use and this may mean that a more expensive item is indicated. For example, the cost of intravenous infusions with pre added drugs such as potassium or heparin can cost around 40% more than buying the infusion fluid and drugs separately. When you consider the savings in nursing time, the cost of the two methods can be calculated to be roughly the same.

We decided that a good starting point in gaining an awareness of the costs of care would be in concentrating on our use of equipment - of course there are other facets to resource management, such as staffing and skill mix, but we felt equipment costs were an area in which we could all help make savings simply by becoming more aware of the costs of items we used. We began by researching the prices of all items, from the 2.5 pence plastic apron to the £60 pressure monitoring catheter.

Our original assumption that this would be a relatively easy task was far from true - it turned out to be a lengthy process involving staff from stores, pharmacy and the suppliers themselves. Issues to consider included the fact that some companies charge a 25 per cent cancellation fee for standing orders, some prices included VAT or needed a carriage charge to be added, and some companies give discounts for large orders. Eventually, however, we managed to work out reasonably accurate prices for the items we used, and set about displaying them for all to see. Every box, container or cupboard now gives the price of all items it contains, so all the staff - including doctors - can see the cost of the items they use. This alone has generated some interesting conversations about the best choice of equipment for various procedures, and has made staff stop to think before opening items that are not really required.

In finding the prices of equipment, we realised we used many items that could be obtained more cheaply: intravenous (IV) giving sets ranged from 85 pence to £3.70. We could now select the item which gave us the quality we required at the most cost-effective price. The criteria we established for giving sets were: accuracy (20 drops/ml), luer lock connections, whether they needed burettes, and whether they were the appropriate standard. For example, blood giving sets are expensive because they incorporate a filter, which is not necessary when only administering crystalloids.

The quality of urine bags is vital if urinary tract infections are to be minimised by using systems that prevent the reflux of urine. When we looked at the range, we found that cheaper bags were available, but these would have to be changed more frequently, and could be detrimental to patients if they did not give the protection they needed.

Staff awareness

Displaying the prices also made staff more aware of the possible unnecessary wastage caused by poor planning of patient care. For example, some patients will inevitably require multiple infusions, such as inotropes, parenteral feeding and sedation, within 24 hours of the first line being inserted. These patients could have a multiple lumen central line inserted, rather than a single line which would have to be changed for a multiple one within 24 hours, wasting £10.00. Constant reminders of the cost of waste makes all staff more aware of the necessity to plan the care they deliver more effectively.

Care delivery

Having individually priced all the items we use, we began to explore different methods used to deliver care, such as the administration of drug infusions, eye care, bronchial saline lavage and the use of water humidification. Arriving at accurate costings for nursing procedures was extremely difficult, as so many variables require consideration. We took account of factors such as nursing time, the need for more equipment, possible effects on the patient, patient comfort and increased wear and tear on existing equipment, and calculated the most cost-effective methods of carrying out procedures without compromising patient care. It has already been demonstrated (Cousins, 1988) that savings of up to 35 per cent can be made by using the Pall 0.2 micron IV filter, which allows IV disposables to be changed every 96 hours, as opposed to every 24. There are added advantages in that the patient is better protected from microbial and other particulate contamination, endotoxins and air emboli, while nursing time is also saved, and our calculations confirm the figure of 35 per cent savings.

Recent studies (Chalon *et al*, 1984) have shown the Pall heat and moisture exchanging filter in the ventilator circuit acts as an efficient humidifier, and avoids the hazards presented by water humidifiers (Gallagher *et al*, 1987). When we compared the cost of humidification in a ventilated patient using a heat and moisture exchanging filter with installation of saline into the endotracheal tube prior to suction, we calculated that savings of £4,164.65 per bed per year were possible.

Questioning procedures

Although we initially set out to explore the financial aspects of patient care, this involved looking closely at the quality of care being delivered. By questioning our procedures in an effort to be more cost-effective, we were able to improve the quality of patient care. Making the best use of resources in the NHS must be considered by all those working in the services, so patients can receive the best possible care. It has been shown by the studies within our unit that savings can be made without compromising the care we give, but it is essential that where savings are made, budget-holders can use the money saved within their unit, to buy new equipment, fund staff study leave or improve the staff skill mix. This will provide the incentive so desperately needed for staff to make themselves cost-conscious and cost-effective.

References

Chalon, P. et al (1984) The Pall ultipor breathing circuit filter: an efficient heat and moisture exchanger. International Anaesthesia Research Society, New York.

Cousins, D. (1988) Cost savings in IV therapy. *Care of the Critically Ill*, **4**, 1, 30-35.

DoH (1989) Working for Patients. Department of Health, London.

Gallagher, J. et al (1987) Contamination control in long-term ventilation. *Anaesthesia*, **42**, 476–81.

Griffiths, R. (Chair) (1983) NHS Management Enquiry. DHSS, London.

Johnson, A. (1985) Blueprint for the prevention and management of pressure sores. *Care; The British Journal of Rehabilitation and Tissue Viability*, **1**, 2, 8–13.

Quality Assurance

18
Defining quality assurance

Lynn M. Dunne, MA, RGN, RCNT
Quality Assurance Adviser, Richmond, Twickenham and Roehampton Health Authority

The New Collins Concise English Dictionary (1985) defines as follows:

Quality: a distinguishing characteristic or attribute; the basic character or nature of something; a degree or standard of excellence; having or showing excellence or superiority.

Assurance: a statement or assertion intended to inspire confidence; freedom from doubt; certainty.

Standard: an accepted or approved example of something against which others are judged or measured; a principle of propriety, honesty and integrity; a level of excellence or quality; of recognised authority, competence or excellence.

Monitor: to check (the technical quality of); a person or piece of equipment that warns, checks or keeps a continuous record of something.

Quality of nursing care embodies a certain degree of abstraction. It expresses reality and yet is also synonymous with aspects of desirability. Making the necessary distinction is often difficult especially in relation to individuals, as judgements may be clouded by subjectivity due to individual beliefs, values, expectations and cultural background. To overcome this problem it is suggested that effectiveness of care is measured using specific criteria, statements of performance, behaviour or circumstances (standards), derived from broad goals (values), which represent the views of the department and are acceptable to all concerned.

First nursing standards

The current wave of interest in nursing, quality assurance began in the early '80s. However the idea itself of measuring the quality and effectiveness of nursing care is not at all new. From 1854 to 1870 Florence Nightingale led the impetus for systematic evaluation of both the process of nursing care and its outcome in terms of patient wellbeing. When she and her team of nurses arrived at the Barrack Hospital, Scutari in 1854 the mortality rate was 32 per cent, within six months the mortality rate had fallen to aproximately two per cent, arguably the best performance indicator for the effectiveness of her nursing care.

Florence Nightingale also established what might be described as the first nursing standards in *Notes on Nursing* (Nightingale, 1860), in which she stated that the first rule of the hospital was that it should do the patient no harm. The book went on to describe the importance and benefits of cleanliness and fresh air for patients and underlined the need to prevent overcrowding in hospitals to control infection amongst patients. This point is still relevant today, as many hospitals continue the practice of 'hot-bedding' for daycases. Nightingale also highlighted the importance of nurses being able to observe patients keenly, so that they might detect and report changes in a patient's condition. (Quite apart from the educational ramifications, how often is this point taken into consideration when designing new hospitals?)

Establishing quality assurance programmes

Efforts to establish quality assurance programmes began in 1918 in the USA. Rapid growth and development of nursing quality assurance activity took place there throughout the seventies and interest reached Britain towards the end of the decade. This was reflected by the publication of two discussion documents, 'Standards of Nursing Care' (RCN, 1980) and 'Towards Standards' (RCN, 1981), by the Royal College of Nursing.

Characteristics of quality

The two documents attempted to identify the characteristics of high quality nursing care. 'Standards of Nursing Care' (RCN, 1980), addressed the question "what constitutes good nursing care?", and the committee agreed that both the process and the outcome of nursing care should be taken into consideration and that by using collective professional judgement it would be possible to determine whether or not good nursing care had taken place. Good nursing care was defined as being planned, systematic and focused on the individual. The nursing process must obviously be used to evaluate the quality of nursing care.

Evaluating quality

There are now numerous tools available to evaluate the quality of nursing care in various clinical settings. It is still helpful to take one step further back and consider the model or framework from which a quality assurance programme can be developed. Figures 1 and 2 illustrate the models of quality assurance used by the American Nurses' Association and the Registered Nurses' Association of British Columbia, Canada. Both take a similar approach.

The first step in any quality assurance programme is to identify values and a philosophy/ideology for the department and individuals concerned. These will act as the cornerstone for the programme. In America and Canada this means a printed statement (often referred to as a mission statement) that can be found in every nursing office and ward. The mission statement clearly outlines what nursing (in that particular hospital/clinical setting) will and will not do. The next stage is the identification and formulation (writing) of valid, acceptable nursing

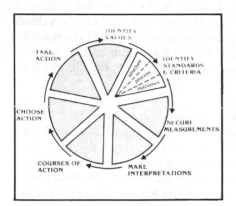

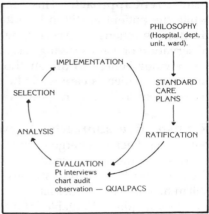

Figure 1. Adapted from the American Nurses' Association model for quality assurance programmes.

Figure 2. The Registered Nurses' Association of British Columbia model for quality assurance.

standards (in Canada these were expressed in standard care plan format as opposed to a list of formal statements which is more popular in the USA). These standards cover such areas as nursing manpower levels, equipment, clinical practice, nurse education (ie ward learning climate) and patient responses to the nursing care delivered.

Evaluating present practice

Having agreed upon their standards the nursing department's next step is to measure present practice against the desired, pre-set standard to determine whether or not the service provided is acceptable or whether some form of remedial action and in-service education needs to be taken. The appropriate course of action is then selected and implemented and the problem/remedial action reassessed to see whether or not the problem has been resolved. Should further action be required, intervention takes place at the appropriate stage of the quality assurance model. Thus the cycle of quality monitoring is continuous, aiming to consistently improve or maintain a high standard of nursing care.

There are three common approaches that can be taken when developing a system to monitor the quality of nursing practice:

Prospective approach To a certain extent this type of assessment is something of a paradox. You may well be wondering how care can be evaluated before it is given. In reality prospective quality monitoring tends to be the prior identification of types or groups of patients — ie the next 20 patients admitted who are deemed to be at risk from developing pressure sores using the Norton Score (Norton, 1975). Once the patients have been identified evaluation of their care will take place either concurrently or retrospectively.

Concurrent approach   This is an evaluation procedure that takes place while the patient is still in hospital. It tends to focus on the quality of the nursing actions themselves (the process of nursing) and involves direct observation of nurses giving care, questioning patients and chart audit. An obvious benefit to this method is that information can be used to improve a patient's care while he or she is still in hospital should it be found wanting in any respect.

Retrospective approach   A review of care that takes place after a patient has been discharged from hospital. Audits of patient records and charts is the most usual method. Obviously this approach does not have the benefits of concurrent studies (influencing care whilst the patient is still in hospital) but it does allow a comprehensive evaluation of the whole case to take place. Valuable information can be gained about successful nursing care that staff would wish to repeat and likewise unsuccessful nursing intervention that staff should avoid in future.

Whatever method is chosen, the emphasis should be on solving known or suspected problems revealed by the monitoring process which affect patient care or the nursing service detrimentally and cannot be justified.

The quality assurance programme may be designed by an individual or an elected committee but it is important that it is owned and accepted by the staff implementing nursing care to patients. Including some or all of the staff involved in patient care areas (depending on the size of the hospital) in developing the programme would certainly provide a broader perspective and hopefully increase commitment and participation.

Thorough planning

Thorough planning is essential to strengthen and secure the programme and allow participants to be directed and supported.

Many nurses harbour negative feelings towards quality assurance programmes. They are often suspicious of management's motives for such an exercise, fearing cost cutting measures. There is a certain reluctance among the profession to review the care given to patients (as can be seen in its failure to get to grips with evaluation of planned patient care since the adoption of the nursing process by the General Nursing Council in 1977), and personal performance. This is hardly surprising in a system where few hospitals even today practise employee appraisal. It may help to point out to staff that they are already carrying out some quality monitoring activities, nearly all clinical areas have some form of quality control (infection control, review of domestic services), thus proving that quality assurance is not such an alien and theoretical topic.

It is important to distinguish between quality assurance and quality monitoring/control (Figure 3). Quality monitoring is a crucial part of any quality assurance programme and is the process whereby current practice is compared with pre-determined standards. It is however not quality assurance (freedom from doubt concerning the degree of excellence).

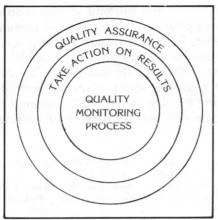

Figure 3. The relationship (and difference)
between the quality monitoring process and
quality assurance adapted with kind
permission from Lang (1974).

Quality assurance is only present when current nursing practice has been compared with the standard and appropriate action has been taken successfully to remedy the problems identified.

Running quality assurance programmes

Staff frequently need help to realise that unless action is taken on the results of quality control and monitoring, then quality assurance cannot be achieved (Figure 3). Involving ward staff in developing the programme and utilising their experience and skills by asking them to act as assessors/ observers is important in overcoming negative feelings and running a meaningful programme. Management must be committed to replacing any staff taken away from clinical areas to participate in the programme, or to pay the necessary overtime.

Quality assurance programmes should only deal with problems that will have a positive effect on patient care or nursing practice when resolved and which can be remedied within existing, available resources (realistic problem solving). Likewise, the prioritising of problems will depend on their effects on patient care and resources. The causes of selected problems must be identified and options outlined for action. Finally the programme must include documentation of problem resolution and indicate to what extent the desired change has been achieved.

The completed quality assurance manual should be available in all nursing departments, with the relevant evaluation reports and action plans. Improvements and problem resolution should be noted and praised and management should be quick to highlight staff who have made particular efforts in this direction. Feedback and knowledge of results regarding a department's quality assessment should be as fast as possible to maintain staff motivation and commitment.

The aim of every nurse and nursing service is surely to provide the highest quality nursing care possible given the presenting situation and resources. It therefore follows that each nursing service must strive to develop a quality assurance programme that accurately measures the level of goal attainment within its clinical areas. To design a successful programme, time must be spent planning well defined goals and objectives, reviewing existing activities that attempt to measure quality and building on them with the cooperation of nursing staff at all levels.

References
Lang, N. (1974) A model for quality assurance in nursing. In: *A Plan for Implementation of Standards of Nursing Practice*. Kansas City Mo: ANA 1975.
Nightingale, F. (1860) *Notes on Nursing*. Dover Publications Inc., 1969, New York, USA.
Norton, D. (1975) *An Investigation of Geriatric Nursing Problems in Hospital*. Churchill Livingstone, Edinburgh.
Royal College of Nursing (1980) *'Standards of Nursing Care' a discussion document*. RCN, London.
Royal College of Nursing (1981) *'Towards Standards' – a discussion document*. RCN, London.

Bibliography
Meisenheimer, C.G. (1985). *Quality Assurance: a complete guide to effective programmes*. (1st edition). Aspen Systems Corporation, USA.
  Bought in USA, may be difficult to obtain in the UK.

19

How do we set nursing standards?

Lynn M. Dunne, MA, RGN, RCNT

Quality Assurance Adviser, Richmond, Twickenham and Roehampton Health Authority

Nursing standards are valid, acceptable definitions of the quality of nursing care, and cannot be valid unless they contain a means of measuring (criteria) to enable nursing care to be evaluated in terms of effectiveness and quality. When standards are written without criteria (eg 'the patient will not suffer postoperative pain'), the effect is similar to using a ruler without measurements marked on when making a scale drawing. The measurements would have to be guessed, would undoubtedly be wildly inaccurate and they would certainly vary enormously from one individual to another (Mason, 1978).

Implicit in Florence Nightingale's famous statement that the first requirement of a hospital is that it should do the patient no harm (Strauss, 1967) is the idea that nursing care should be of a high standard and through her continued scrutiny of nursing practice she strove to attain this goal. More recently in the UK the Royal College of Nursing, concerned with the promotion of nursing and the ability of its members to provide and maintain an adequate standard of care to their patients, published two authoritative documents on setting, monitoring and evaluating standards of care within the nursing profession (RCN, 1980; RCN, 1981).

What is nursing care?

It is important that before trying to evaluate their individual or collective performances, nurses should have a clear understanding of what 'nursing' and 'nursing care' actually mean. Nursing departments can accept a well known definition of nursing such as 'The unique function of the nurse is to assist the individual, sick or well, in the performance of those activities contributing to health and its recovery (or to a peaceful death), that he would perform unaided if he had the necessary strength, will or knowledge; and to do this in such a way as to help him gain independence as rapidly as possible' (Henderson, 1979). Alternatively they can opt for an in-house definition (mission statement) (Dunne, 1986) that has been ratified by the nursing staff. Which they accept is purely a matter of choice, but it must reflect the values of the nursing service concerned.

The concept of nursing care standards is immediately complicated as the phrase becomes synonymous with both the quality and effectiveness of care. The word 'standards' has both qualitative and quantitative connotations, it may be something that serves as a basis for comparison (a yardstick) or a measure of the level of performance (output) required of an individual. Previous studies of the effectiveness of nursing care have concentrated on the quantitative aspects; however current emphasis is on a more holistic approach, attempting to evaluate the more discrete qualitative issues in nursing care eg interpersonal and communication skills.

'Standards of Nursing Care' (RCN, 1980) suggests that the most suitable method of deciding what constitutes good nursing care is by identifying desired nursing behaviours. Observation of current nursing practice and comparison with predetermined standards would enable nurses to judge whether or not good nursing care had taken place. The report defines desired nursing behaviour as being planned, purposeful, systematic and goal directed, ie the use of the nursing process. 'Towards Standards' (RCN, 1981), in considering how to formulate nursing standards, felt that the writing of checklists, norms and ratios was inappropriate and instead identified eight key factors for professional nursing standards (Table 1).

1.   A philosophy of nursing.
2.   The relevant knowledge and skills.
3.   The nurse's authority to act.
4.   Accountability.
5.   The control of resources.
6.   The organisational structure and management style.
7.   The doctor/nurse relationship.
8.   The management of change.

Table 1. Prerequisites for the professional control of standards of nursing care.

Accountability

Of these eight factors, accountability is the most central to the formation of professional standards. Nurses must also be clear about the extent of their authority, and responsibility and accountability must be matched with the necessary authority to carry out the job effectively. Senior nurses must be prepared to provide the nurse with the tools to do the job — ie manpower, equipment. Devolving accountability to individual nurses may well be the long term answer to improving standards of nursing care but the profession should ask itself if this move is really appropriate now, in a system that still entrusts the majority of its 'basic care' to untrained/unqualified individuals?

Having looked at what nursing standards are and the key areas related to them, how do we set these standards? In his review of the evaluation of the quality of medical care, Avedis Donabedian outlined three approaches (studying the structural variables, studying the process of care and reviewing the outcome of care in patients); these approaches are still widely used by nurses in the field of quality assurance, as most areas of nursing fall into one or more of the three categories (Donabedian, 1966). The three categories when applied to evaluating the quality of nursing care may be defined as follows:

Structure standards   These regulate nursing practice and include the organisation of nursing services, recruitment, selection, manpower establishments, provision of necessary equipment, buildings and include all the processes of licensing, eg National Board educational visits to approve facilities for learner/post basic education. They generally tend to indicate minimum expectations or levels of service, eg there will always be at least one RGN on duty on the ward at all times.

Process standards   These look specifically at the actions performed by nurses and define the quality of the implementation of nursing care. Nursing departments should develop process standards for all nursing interventions (nursing procedures). Nursing procedures and process standards, although similar, are not the same thing.

Outcome standards   The patient's response to planned care, ie the expected change in a patient's condition following nursing intervention, is an outcome standard. Nursing action may result in positive or negative outcomes for a patient (positive outcomes being beneficial and appropriate nursing intervention, and negative outcomes inappropriate nursing care). Outcome standards frequently include some measure of the patient's satisfaction with the care. Many authors define a further category:

Content standards   These describe the nature of nursing that is communicated to other groups or disciplines and the basis of nursing decisions, ie information that must be recorded in nursing notes and reported to the multidisciplinary team, communication and teaching of patients and their families or friends (Mason, 1978).

Writing standards
Many standards set for a nursing service will concern clinical work (direct nursing care given to patients), and tend to be written in the form of principles of nursing practice (the foundation of but not quite as detailed as a nursing procedure). The seven steps outlined below can be used when writing any nursing standard (structure, process, outcome or content); here they are illustrated using the example of the process standards set for performing endotracheal suction of a ventilated patient.
1. Select the area of nursing for which the standard is to be written and identify the type (structure, process, outcome, content) eg **process standard:** endotracheal suction of a ventilated patient.
2. Identify the objectives for the standard stating explicitly what you intend to achieve. The objectives may be nurse centred or patient centred:

Nurse-centred objectives
a. To apply suction to the patient without introducing infection into the respiratory tract.
b. To prevent trauma to the respiratory tract.
Patient-centred objectives
c. The patient will not experience hypoxia during the suction procedure, ie PO_2 of no less than 11kPa.
d. The patient will not experience anxiety or distress during the suction procedure.
3. Specify the nursing action essential to achieve the objectives, eg:
a. Wash your hands; use sterile equipment and an aseptic technique.
b. Apply suction only when withdrawing catheter.
c. Hyperoxygenate patient prior to the procedure (if prescribed) with ventilator or re-breathing bag for one minute prior to suction procedure.
d. Do not apply suction for more than 15 seconds; suction only until secretions are removed.
4. Where possible specify a time frame for each action, eg apply suction for no more than 15 seconds.
5. Write up the standard in a logical order, eg i. Define subject. ii. Identify objectives. iii. List standards.
6. Review the work done to eliminate ambiguous or irrelevant information that cannot be evaluated, eg suggestions for procedure technique.
7. Test the new standard for acceptability and validity.

Who should write the standards?
In order to decide who should write these standards, it is useful to identify the size of the task, the types of standards to be written and the resources available, eg nurse managers, educationalists and clinical specialists, and to use them as effectively as possible. It is essential that the meaning of any nursing standard is shared, accepted and understood by those who have written it and those expected to implement it.

Examples of nursing standards that should be found currently in any hospital would include a nursing practice and policy manual that is based on current nursing research findings, the use of specific ward learning outcomes for learner nurses in ward areas, the practice of individualised patient care through the use of the nursing process, adherence to National Board training requirements, staff ratios of trained staff: learners and compliance with the UKCC code of professional conduct.

Location of standards
Once written, all nursing standards should be easily accessed and referred to by the nursing staff either before, during or after nursing intervention. Formulating and measuring nursing standards is not akin to setting a closed book exam or an attempt to catch individuals out, so it is only right and proper that staff should know what is expected of them before their

action and its effects on patients are critically evaluated on either a collective or individual basis.

High quality nursing care does not happen by accident, it must be planned for and evaluated against pre-set standards so that nurses can recognise and repeat good nursing care and avoid mistakes in the future (McFarlane, 1979).

Nurses have a responsibility to society, themselves and their colleagues in the health care services to ensure they provide the highest quality care possible in the presenting situation and resources. Nursing standards are the key to any successful quality assurance programme as they define valid, acceptable, measurable levels of performance and outcome against which current nursing practice must and will be judged and evaluated.

References
Donabedian, A. (1966) Evaluating the quality of medical care. *Millbank Memorial Fund Quarterly*, **4**, 166–203.
Dunne, L. (1986) Developing quality assurance. *The Professional Nurse*, **2**, 2, 47–9.
Henderson, V. (2979) *Basic Principles of Nursing Care*. (11th edition). International Council of Nurses. Geneva, Switzerland.
McFarlane, J.K. (1979) Take aim and shoot for goal. *Nursing Mirror*. (supplement). 19.4.79. xx–xxviii.
Mason, E.J. (1978) *How to Write Meaningful Nursing Standards*. (2nd edition) John Wiley and Sons Inc, USA.
  NB Bought in USA. J. Wiley outlets in UK.
Royal College of Nursing, (1980) *'Standards of Nursing Care'* – a discussion document. RCN, London.
Royal College of Nursing, (1981) *'Towards Standards'* – a discussion document. RCN, London.
Strauss, M.B. (1967) *Familiar Medical Quotations*. (1st edition) J.A. Churchill Ltd, London.

20

Quality assurance: methods of measurement

Lynn M. Dunne, MA, RGN, RCNT

Quality Assurance Adviser, Richmond, Twickenham and Roehampton Health Authority

Attempts to define quality assurance (Dunne, 1986) and how a nursing service might set acceptable standards of nursing care (Dunne, 1987), have already been made. In the next phase a method of measuring current nursing practice against pre-determined standards must be developed. The four methods reviewed here: Qualpacs, Nursing Audit (Phaneuf), the Rush-Medicus System and Monitor, are among several currently available.

Qualpacs

The Quality Patient Care Scale (Qualpacs) was developed by Mabel Wandelt and Joel Ager at the College of Nursing, Wayne State University, Michigan, USA in the early 1970s, a time that saw a rapid increase in knowledge and literature about quality assurance in North America.

It is a tool based on evaluation of the *process* of nursing (ie how nursing care is delivered to patients), by direct observation. The scale itself lists 68 items of nursing care, arranged under six subsections as follows:

Psychosocial: Individual Actions directed towards meeting the psychosocial needs of individual patients.

Psychosocial: Group Actions directed towards meeting the psychosocial needs of patients as members of a group.

Physical: Actions directed towards meeting physical needs.

General: Actions that may be directed toward meeting either psychosocial or physical needs of the patient or both at the same time.

Communication: Communication on behalf of the patient.

Professional implications: Care given to patients reflects initiative and responsibility indicative of professional expectations.

Two or more trained observers evaluate all interaction between nurses and patients in a clinical area for two hours. Any one of the 68 items is scored on a scale of one to five (Table 1).

Wandelt and Ager advocate that Qualpacs observers complete an orientation programme which allows sufficient time for them to become familiar with the background to the Qualpacs; the cue sheets for each section, individual items and spend some time (two days is suggested) discussing what standards are acceptable and becoming familiar with the

```
1 = Poorest care
2 = Between
3 = Average care (that expected of
    a newly qualified RGN)
4 = Between
5 = Best care
```

Table 1. Qualpacs scoring method.

actual use of the rating scale.

The use of Qualpacs evokes a mixed response from nurses. Those who are against it express doubts about the tool as a reliable, objective method, saying it is both subjective (as it is the opinion of the observer as to whether poor, average or best care has taken place and that is highly dependent on previous experience and personal values). The counter argument to this is simple: if you reject Qualpacs on the basis that it is subjective and therefore unreliable it is tantamount to saying you reject the professional judgement of nurses in matters related to nursing practice (for previous experience and personal values are the basis of professional judgement also), which in turn opens Pandora's Box on such issues as the necessity to have a nurse(s) in charge of nursing.

Many groups and individuals (particularly trade unions) fear that as Qualpacs looks at individual nurses and the care they give to patients, the opportunity exists to use the findings in a disciplinary manner if poor or unsafe practice is observed. Certain steps can be taken to overcome these potential problems. First, only nurses with a clinical involvement should order a Qualpacs assessment or act as observers and second, feedback should be direct between the observers and the ward nurses. Management should not have access to a Qualpacs assessment as part of an investigation or disciplinary procedure. This approach has been used successfully at Burford Nursing Development Unit and is now used throughout Oxfordshire Health Authority.

In its favour it must be said that as a direct observation tool, Qualpacs provides an opportunity to improve care and benefit patients while they are still in hospital. Many people involved in quality assurance feel that direct observation of nursing care is the most effective way of evaluating its quality and is critical to the success of any quality assurance programme.

The Phaneuf Nursing Audit

This audit was developed by Maria Phaneuf in the mid 1970s and, as the name suggests, is an audit of nursing care taken from the patients' notes. Phaneuf herself described nursing audit as a process orientated approach to appraise the nursing process as reflected in the patients' records.

The Nursing Audit reviews 50 separate criteria which are grouped under seven headings as follows:

1. The application and execution of the doctor's legal orders.

2. The observation of symptoms and reactions.
3. Supervision of the patient.
4. Supervision of those participating in care (except the doctor).
5. Reporting and recording.
6. Application and execution of nursing procedures and techniques.
7. Promotion of physical and emotional health by direction and teaching.

The first part of the nursing audit consists of a patient details form (similar to many hospital admissions slips) which Phaneuf suggests can be completed by a member of clerical staff, eg ward clerk, as professional nursing knowledge is not required. The second part of the nursing audit is the evaluation of the patients care using his/her inpatient notes. The criteria are evaluated using yes/no/uncertain categories and scored accordingly. To arrive at the final score the total of the individual component scores is multiplied by the value of the 'does not apply' scores. The quality of nursing care is described in Table 2.

Score			Quality of Care
0	— 40	=	Unsafe
41	— 80	=	Poor
81	— 120	=	Incomplete
121	— 160	=	Good
161	— 200	=	Excellent

Table 2. The Phaneuf Nursing Audit Scoring Method.

Nursing Audit has been widely criticised by many nurses who argue that nurses frequently give care that is not documented and conversely often document care that is never given to the patient. I suggest this somewhat cynical view of nursing practice is neither a typical nor fair representation, despite the profession's many faults, and that Nursing Audit has a useful role to play in evaluating quality as it is quick, simple and comprehensive. Familiarisation and training for assessors is easy too. The biggest barrier to using Nursing Audit in the UK is documentation as audit is only feasible in clinical areas using a systematic approach.

Many feel that Nursing Audit can be a useful part of a quality assurance programme. Burford Nursing Development Unit have successfully combined Qualpacs and Nursing Audit in their quality assurance programme (to overcome the criticisms of using each method independently) thus enabling nursing care to be evaluated as it is given to patients and retrospectively via the nursing records.

Rush Medicus System

The Rush-Medicus System was also a product of the early 70s (1972) and was the result of a collaborative project between the Medicus Systems Corporation and Rush Presbyterian St Luke's Medical Centre in Chicago and the Baptist Medical Centre in Birmingham, Alabama.

The conceptual framework chosen for the system was the Nursing Process which had been implemented at Rush Presbyterian St Luke's Medical Centre and the concept of patient needs. The nursing process was defined as the comprehensive set of nursing activities performed in the delivery of a patient's care; assessment of the problems or needs of the patient, planning for care, implementing the plan of care and evaluating/updating the plan of care.

It was hoped to develop a system that would evaluate all these areas. The concept was further enhanced by evaluating whether patient needs were actually being met in accordance with the care plan.

Once the conceptual framework was decided it had to be broken into logical components. Six objectives and 32 sub-objectives were outlined, which the project team believed defined the nursing care process succinctly and with a degree of detail not achieved in previous programmes. The next step was to develop criteria that would evaluate each of the sub-objectives. A total of 357 criteria were developed (Master Criteria List).

The Master Criteria List is held on a computer programme which will produce up to 76 different questionnaires that can be used for patients in accident and emergency departments, labour and delivery wards, psychiatry, nursery, recovery and general medicine and surgery, according to their dependency group. In addition there are nine questionnaires which can be used for the parents of babies in the nursery and 18 ward based questionnaires that can be used in all clinical areas.

Ward areas tend to be evaluated three-to-four times per year in hospitals using the Rush-Medicus System in the USA. Quality monitoring takes place over a calendar month during which 10 per cent of the patient throughput is sampled.

Patients forming part of the quality assessment are selected using a random number table and their permission is then obtained verbally before proceeding. Nurse observers tend to be either staff nurses working at ward level who have completed the necessary observer's training course and belong to the hospital nursing quality assurance observers 'bank', or a small permanent team of observers who carry out all the nursing quality monitoring for the whole hospital.

The Rush-Medicus System has the advantage of having been extensively tested during its development (19 hospitals across the USA). It is now widely used by many hundreds of hospitals throughout the USA and Canada which form a users group that feeds in results to provide comparative scores and allows the tool to be updated. The disadvantages of the system are that it is large and time consuming to administer (most hospitals using Rush-Medicus have a full/part time coordinator) and a computer is a prerequisite to run the programme effectively.

Monitor
Of all the quality assurance systems mentioned in this chapter Monitor is probably the most familiar. It was developed by Goldstone, Ball and

Collier, (1984) as part of the North West Region Staffing Levels Project and is the adaptation for the UK of the Rush-Medicus System.

Monitor consists of four patient questionnaires each related to one of the four patient dependency categories and a general ward based questionnaire. As with the Rush-Medicus System patients are allocated a questionnaire according to their dependency group. The authors recommend that either a random sample of three patients per dependency category are selected or the whole ward be included. Each questionnaire is divided into four sections:

- Assessment of nursing care.
- Meeting the patient's physical needs.
- The patient's non-physical needs are met.
- Evaluation of nursing care objectives.

Sources of information for the question answers include direct patient questioning/observation, patient's records/charts, observation of the clinical environment and questioning of nursing staff.

Answers to questions are scored (Table 3) and a final score is obtained by deducting the non-applicable responses and then dividing the total score by the number of applicable questions and expressing this as a percentage. The authors suggest a score of 70 per cent is desirable. It is recommended that Monitor be carried out in wards once a year.

Answer	
Yes, Yes always, Yes complete	= 1
Yes sometimes, Yes incomplete	= ½
No	= 0

Table 3. Scoring Method For Monitor.

Monitor has been criticised for suggesting a desirable score. Many feel it is better to allow individual ward sisters and nurse managers to decide what is appropriate for their units. For many, a score of less than 100 per cent on knowledge of cardiac arrest procedure or fire drill is unacceptable, while a temporary lapse in other areas, eg evaluating nursing care objectives may be acceptable in a given set of circumstances, such as high vacancy factor/high proportion of new appointees. It has also been criticised for its method of selecting a patient sample, which differs considerably from the Rush-Medicus System of randomly selecting 10 per cent of the patient monthly turnover, irrespective of their dependency groups. Administration is time consuming, particularly in the scoring of the questionnaires, which if done manually can take one person about two working days to complete.

In its favour it must be said that Monitor is a quality monitoring tool developed by a British team who understand the NHS and nursing in the UK and while it is easy to criticise with hindsight, at least North West Region did more than just talk about quality assurance. Monitor has now been adopted by several health authorities in Britain which enjoy a support and update service from Suppliers, Newcastle Polytechnic.

Which programme
Quality Assurance is here to stay, of that there can be little doubt. Hospitals considering implementing a quality assurance programme have two distinct choices; they can either create their own in-house programme or adopt a programme that is commercially available. There are advantages to both. In-house programmes can produce a high level of commitment, creativity and cohesion; bought-in programmes avoid the exercise of reinventing the wheel and have an easily identified price tag and running costs with no hidden extras. Whatever method is chosen by nursing managements it must accurately reflect and measure the quality of care delivered to the patients within the relevant clinical areas.

References
Goldstone, L.A. Ball, J.A. Collier M.M. (1984). MONITOR – An Index of the Quality of Nursing Care for Acute Medical and Surgical Wards. (2nd Impression). Newcastle Upon Tyne Polytechnic Products UK.

Pearson, A. (1983). The Clinical Nursing Unit. (1st Edition). Heinemann Medical Books Ltd, London.

Phaneuf, M. (1976). The Nursing Audit. Appleton-Century-Crofts. New York. USA.

Wandelt, M. and Ager, J. (1974). Quality Patient CAre Scale (QUALPACS). Appleton-Century-Crofts. New York. USA.

Bibliography
Burford Nursing Development Unit. A Compendium of Articles Published in British Nursing Journals by Staff at BNDU (1983–84). (Available on application to BNDU Burford, Oxfordshire).

21

The Stirling model of nursing audit: its relationship to standard setting and quality assurance

Moya J. Morison, BSc, MSc, BA, RGN
Clinical Audit Co-ordinator, Stirling Royal Infirmary

Every organisation has a responsibility to monitor the quality of its activities, to identify areas where quality is below an agreed standard and take appropriate remedial action to guarantee the customer a specified degree of excellence of a product or service. This is quality assurance. Quality control is the means by which quality is assured (Table 1). Nurses have long been concerned with assuring their patients a high quality of care, and have employed many methods of quality control including informal peer review, standard setting, monitoring and evaluating practice, and systematic audit using generic tools such as Monitor (Goldstone *et al*, 1983) and Qualpacs (Wandelt and Ager, 1974).

Quality control is the means by which quality is assured
• Informal peer review
• Standard setting, monitoring and evaluation
• Audit

Table 1. Quality control.

Pressures on healthcare professionals to introduce audit are coming from the government, royal colleges and hospital management as well as from within the professions themselves. 'Working for Patients' (DoH, 1989) recognises the most effective studies are likely to be internally generated with local peer group review of the data under analysis. It advocates a 'bottom-up' rather than 'top-down' approach, but with the proviso that management can initiate an independent professional audit, for example where there is cause to question the quality or cost-effectiveness of the service.

Redfern and Norman (1990) argue that a preoccupation with cost-effectiveness threatens to swamp nurses' traditional concern with quality of care and underline the importance of clinical nurses becoming familiar with the concepts and complexities of measuring quality. This chapter aims to explore the nature of nursing audit and its relationship to standard setting and quality assurance, and to describe how one Scottish Unit is developing a philosophy of, and a method for, nursing audit which builds upon the standard setting and quality assurance initiatives already underway.

Chart audit

What is audit? In its oldest sense auditing means: "an examination of accounts by an authorised person or persons" (Chambers 20th Century Dictionary). Churchill's Illustrated Medical Dictionary (1989) defines medical audit as: "Detailed retrospective review and evaluation of medical records by skilled staff to assess the care that was provided". Unless the notes are highly structured, this is a time consuming exercise because of the difficulties in retrieving information, yet review of practice by reference to records is now an established system for medical audit in the USA (Hopkins, 1990), and is the basis of several generic nursing audit tools such as Phaneuf's Nursing Audit (1976).

The assumption with all audits of records is that the quality of care and the quality of documentation are related. This is not always so (Mayers *et al*, 1977). A nurse may give competent technical care in a compassionate manner and have excellent interpersonal skills, but may be poor at documenting the care given. Conversely, several studies have shown that the care actually given may fall far short of that painstakingly prescribed in individualised care plans. Furthermore, nurses soon learn how to document care in a way which favourably influences the audit results (Jelinek *et al*, 1974), and Hegyvary and Haussman (1976) argue that chart audit only serves to improve documentation, not care. Despite all these arguments, auditing nursing records can be useful as part of a quality assurance programme if other measures of care are also recorded.

A broader perspective

A broader definition of medical audit given in 'Working for Patients' is: "The systematic, critical analysis of the quality of medical care, including the procedures for diagnosis and treatment, the use of resources and the resulting outcome and quality of life for the patient".

Within this very broad definition, many operational methods can be developed. An audit can be carried out retrospectively or prospectively. It can include record or chart review, patient and staff interviews, the use of questionnaires, direct observation of activity or any combination of these. Generic (preformulated) measuring instruments can be used. The uses, advantages and disadvantages of some of the most widely available generic nursing audit tools are reviewed by Pearson (1987), Dunne (1987) and Sale (1990). Alternatively, an audit tool can be developed locally to gain insights into a perceived problem. The tool can include items to measure the criteria and level of performance previously agreed in a locally generated standard relating to the problem.

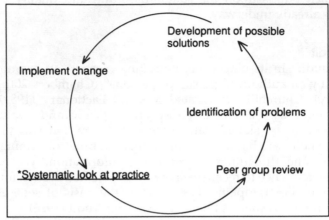

Figure 1. The audit cycle.

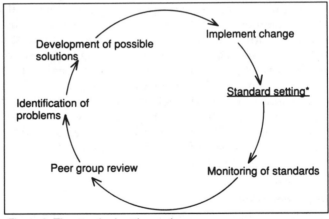

Figure 2. The standard setting cycle.

The principle stages in the audit cycle are summarised in Figure 1; similarities with the standard setting cycle (Figure 2) are immediately apparent. Both have quality assurance as their primary aim and involve:

• peer group review of data;

• problem identification;

• the development of solutions to the problems identified;

• implementing change aimed at overcoming these problems.

There are, however, certain differences. Standard setting involves agreeing ahead the criteria for the process, including an acceptable level of performance and monitoring this, while in a purely audit study there need be no predefined expectations of the process. Audit involves a systematic look at what is actually happening - different practices may be compared but there need be no advanced decision about what constitutes best practice. In reality many standard setting projects have an audit component and in most, if not all, audit studies there are implicit normative standards.

Introducing nursing audit locally

The Strategy for Nursing, Midwifery and Health Visiting in Scotland (SHHD, 1990) highlighted as a key objective the establishment of a system of nursing audit, in tandem with continued development and monitoring of standards of care. We at Stirling saw this as an opportunity to review our priorities in nursing quality assurance initiatives, and out of our deliberations came our model of nursing audit (as depicted on the wallchart) in which we defined audit and explored the audit process and its relationship to standard setting initiatives already well under way.

When developing our strategy we:

- agreed a management statement,

- identified key objectives,

- prepared an action plan and timetable for our short-term goals.

Appropriateness
Meeting the actual needs of individuals, families and communities

Effectiveness
Achieving the intended benefit

Acceptability
Satisfying patients' reasonable expectations

Continuity
Of care and care provider(s)

Accessibility
Availability not unduly restricted by time, distance or finance

Efficiency
Maximising outcomes with the available resources

Table 2. Dimensions of quality of healthcare (based on Shaw, 1986).

We had to agree what we felt nursing audit was, what we were aiming to achieve by it, the nature of the audit process and how to build on the standard setting and quality assurance initiatives already underway. We decided on a definition of nursing audit which would be compatible with that of our medical colleagues, with its emphasis on a critical look at the quality of care and outcomes and quality of life for the patient. We discussed the dimensions of quality as described by Shaw (1986) (Table 2), and using Donabedian's (1969) framework of structure, process and outcome, summarised the key factors to consider when measuring quality of care (Table 3). These aims are what we hope to achieve through nursing audit:

- to improve the quality of patient care;

- to make the most efficient use of resources;

- to foster in nurses a critical questioning approach to their activities and the needs of their patients.

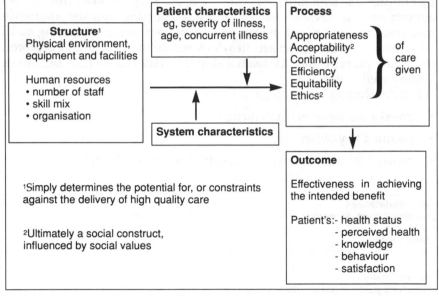

Table 3. *Some factors to consider when attempting to measure quality of care (based on Donabedian , 1969; Shaw,1986; Hopkins, 1990).*

Creating a climate for audit

A major objective is to create a positive climate for audit, involving the maximum number of practice based nurses in a small way without impinging on their time spent with patients.

It is natural and understandable that people should initially resist being involved in audit. One definition of audit is "a calling to account", which has many negative connotations, and people may feel threatened. Resistance to audit, or to any change, manifests in many ways: rarely as outright aggression, more often as lethargy while paying lip service to the change. Things only get done by the enthusiasts.

It is therefore vital to create a positive climate for enquiry from the outset and to address issues of confidentiality fully and frankly with staff, discussing ways of maintaining patient and staff anonymity. More positively, audit should be regarded as an important component of nurses' continuing professional development, helping them individually to identify their strengths as well as their continuing education and training needs.

Creating a climate for enquiry involves organising an education programme to ensure the nursing staff understand what they are trying to do and how to set about it. Nursing staff themselves should identify and decide the priorities for local audit projects.

Priorities for audit

When deciding our priorities for audit, we felt it was important to ensure we chose topics where the nurse's intervention had most influence on outcome for the patient. We are for instance looking at pressure sore prevention, wound care in the community, nursing care of dying patients and pain control, beyond merely the giving of analgesia. Some topics selected and seen as priorities for audit are summarised in Table 4.

- Pressure sore prevention

- Care of the dying patient

- Bereavement counselling for relatives

- Information giving

- Pain control

- Wound assessment

- Maintaining a safe environment for the confused or aggressive patient

- Source isolation: barrier nursing

- Chemotherapy

Table 4. Some topics seen by staff as priorities for audit.

Integrating nursing audit with standard setting initiatives already underway was identified as a high priority. The essence of the Stirling model is the integration of the two approaches (Figure 3). Quality assurance can start with standard setting or a prospective look at current practice or both concurrently. An example will make this more clear.

We are interested in pressure sore prevention in non-ambulant patients brought to the A&E department, as research has identified these patients to be at high risk. A standard has been written on pressure sore prevention in A&E and a monitoring tool to compare observed practice with the agreed standard is being developed. We have decided to carry out an audit at the same time to help us identify:

- how many high risk patients arrive in A&E over a month and whether there is any pattern to the time of the day the injuries are sustained;

- patients' primary diagnosis;

- how long patients wait in A&E before transfer to the ward;

- the pressure relieving equipment currently available and whether it is in use.

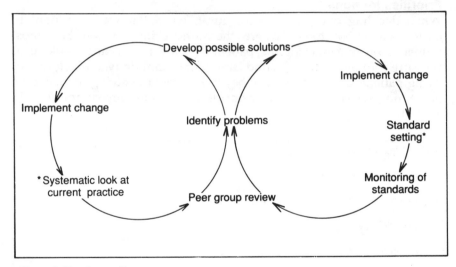

Figure 3. Nursing audit.

It may be helpful to think of our model of nursing audit (Figure 3) as a pair of spectacles which allow nurses to look systematically at their practice and its effectiveness. The audit 'lens' has its ancestry in healthcare research. The standard setting 'lens' represents the existing work on nursing standard setting and quality assurance. Each has a great deal to offer on its own, but together they provide a useful conceptual framework of nursing audit within which a variety of operational methods can be developed. Two lenses give a more three dimensional view of nursing practice than looking at practice through one.

The Stirling model is helping us to understand what we are trying to do, the stages in the audit process, and the relationship between nursing audit and standard setting. It is evolving, as the concept of audit in the NHS is itself evolving, in the light of our experience, but no doubt we have still got a great deal to learn.

References

Department of Health (1989) Working for Patients: Medical Audit (Working Paper No. 6), HMSO, London.

Donabedian, A. (1969) Some issues in evaluating the quality of nursing care. *American Journal of Public Health*, **39**, 10, 1833-36.

Dunne, L.M. (1987) Quality assurance: methods of measurement. *The Professional Nurse* , **2**, 6, 187-90.

Goldstone, L.A., Ball, J.A., Collier, M. (1983) Monitor: an Index of the Quality of Nursing Care for Acute Medical and Surgical Wards. Newcastle-upon-Tyne Polytechnic, Newcastle-upon-Tyne.

Hegyvary, S. and Haussman, R. (1976) Monitoring nursing care quality. *Journal of Nursing Administration*. **6**, 9, 6-9.

Hopkins, A. (1990) Measuring Quality of Medical Care. Royal College of Physicians of London.

Jelinek, D., Haussman, R., Hegyvary, S. (1974) A Methodology for Monitoring Quality of Nursing Care. US Department of Health, Education and Welfare, Bethesda, Maryland.

Mayers, M., Norby, R.B., Watson, A.B. (1977) Quality Assurance for Patient Care - Nursing Perspectives. Appleton-Century-Crofts, New York.

Pearson, A. (Ed.) (1987) Nursing Quality Measurement: Quality Assurance Methods for Peer Review. John Wiley, Chichester.

Phaneuf, M. (1976) the Nursing Audit. Appleton - Century - Crofts, New York.

Redfern, S.J. and Norman I.J. (1990) Measuring the Quality of Nursing Care: A Consideration of Different Approaches. *Journal of Advanced Nursing*, **15**, 1260-71.

Sale, D. (1990) Quality Assurance. Essentials of Nursing Management Series. MacMillan, London.

Scottish Home and Health Department (1990) A Strategy for Nursing, Midwifery and Health Visiting in Scotland. HMSO, Edinburgh.

Shaw, C.D. (1986) Introducing Quality Assurance. Paper No. 64, Kings Fund, London.

Wandelt, M. and Ager, J. (1974) Quality Patient Care Scale. Appleton-Century-Crofts, New York.

Bibliography

Scottish Home and Health Department (1988) Quality Assurance in Nursing: Report of a Working Group of National Nursing and Midwifery Consultative Committee. HMSO, Edinburgh.

Royal College of Nursing (1989) A Framework for Quality. Royal College of Nursing Standards of Care Project. Royal College of Nursing, London.

22
Choosing the right tools for the job: standard setting in pressure sore prevention

Cathy Ingram, BSc, RGN
Clinical Practice Development Nurse, Elderly Care, St Thomas's Hospital, London

Maggie Woodward, RGN
Clinical Nurse Manager, St Thomas's Hospital, London

Elderly people nursed in hospital are at varying risk of developing pressure sores, most of which can be prevented if appropriate nursing care and pressure-relieving equipment are provided. The elderly care unit at St Thomas's Hospital attempted to ensure adequate provision of pressure-relieving mattresses for its elderly patients. A standard setting exercise was implemented to establish whether appropriate mattresses were being used, and the Waterlow scoring system was chosen to assess people's risk of developing pressure sores. This chapter gives an insight into the problems nurses face at grassroots level in establishing research-based practice, focusing on the experiences and results – negative and positive – of implementing a standard setting exercise.

The unit consists of four acute admission and rehabilitation wards caring for elderly residents of inner London. It is developing rapidly with a high turnover of patients, a high percentage of whom are old and very old. In 1989/90 the clinical nurse manager and clinical practice development nurse noted that a number of the standard hospital mattresses needed replacing, which inspired them to look further at the use and need for different forms of mattresses and cushions, and also at the general approach to the management of pressure area care. Table 1 lists the areas of concern that were uncovered following discussion with staff and informal review of practice.

Standard setting
Addressing many of these issues would have required considerable expenditure of time and money. However, it was felt that the problem of the time lapse between admission and a pressure-relieving mattress being available could be resolved by forward planning, without the need for substantial expenditure. The first-line pressure-relieving mattress used in the unit is the large cell Ripple mattress, as this is the one most readily available in the hospital. These are obtained from the central sterile supply department CSSD, where they are cleaned,

1. 11% of standard hospital mattresses were in a poor condition and replaced immediately from excess stocks.
2. Generally perceived but unquantified lack of pressure-relieving equipment, particularly for patients at high risk. Plenty of large cell Ripple mattresses that are costly to maintain.
3. No funds to buy new equipment or quantifiable evidence to argue for funds.
4. Time lapse of often 12-36 hours or more between admission and a pressure-relieving mattress becoming available. This would also disrupt the patient's transfer onto a new mattress.
5. More patients were being admitted with severe tissue damage, particularly extensive/deep sores.
6. Uncertainty among nurses as to most appropriate prevention/treatment, and subsequent inconsistency in care. No written guidelines to assist staff.
7. Routine calculation of the Norton score, this was not actively used in planning and implementing care.
8. Nursing staff provided a good standard of pressure area care, but efforts were limited by the high vacancy rate (18 vacancies at E grade).

Table 1. Recognition and identification of the problem.

maintained and stored. Many people admitted to the unit fall at home and may, therefore, have already spent considerable time lying on hard surfaces at home and/or in A&E. Minimising the delay in providing pressure relief is, therefore, essential to prevent further tissue damage (Hibbs, 1988).

It wa decided to adopt a more proactive strategy for prevention, with the aim of admitting all patients onto large cell Ripple mattresses. They would then be assessed in the usual way, and if at low or no risk and not requiring the Ripple, the mattress could then be removed. Prolonged use of the mattress could be arranged for people at high risk or a suitable alternative obtained for those requiring a higher degree of pressure relief. This would also reduce the disruption to frail patients, who could remain on the Ripple mattress and would not need to be transferred after admission. It was decided to pilot this scheme on one ward initially, as there was some uncertainty as to how it would affect the hospital supply of Ripple mattresses.

The process of setting standards was introduced in 1989 and, in light of this, it was decided to document this latest change in practice as one

Standard of care no.:

Topic: pressure area care   Sub topic: prevention   Achieve standard by: Review standard by: Contact person:

All empty beds shall be made up with a clean and functioning Ripple mattress in preparation for each new admission

Structure	Process	Outcome
• Adequate supply of clean, working mattresses and motors (Supply to be unit/ward based)	**Ward receptionist to:** • check that 5 clean Ripples are available for use each day • phone CSSD for further supplies if necessary	All patients receive a degree of pressure relief until their true needs can be fully assessed
• Clear plastic bags (to return broken mattresses in)	• phone CSSD if any broken Ripples need picking up from ward • record how many are delivered to ward each day/week on form provided	Improved knowledge of cost of care
• Teepol and wipes (to clean mattresses)	• order wipes from RDC	
• Identifiable system for returning and replacing broken mattresses	**Nurse /auxiliary/housekeeper to:** • clean mattress with Teepol after patient discharged	
• Form to document number of mattresses used	• ensure mattress functioning • place clean/working mattress on bed before 'making up'	
• Storage area for clean mattresses and motors	• remove broken mattress and place in red box in sluice in plastic bag, ready for return to CSSD	
• Ward receptionist 5 days a week	• order Teepol from pharmacy	
• Nurse/auxiliary/housekeeper available at all times	**Primary nurse to:** • fully assess patient within 24-48 hours of admission and remove mattress if not required	
• Storage area for broken mattresses and motors awaiting collection – ie, red box in sluice area		

Table 2. Documentation of the standard.

of the unit's first standards (Table 2). The standard was discussed with the staff of the ward concerned and implemented shortly afterwards.

As this was one of the first experiences at standard setting by the clinical practice development nurse and clinical nurse manager, some mistakes were made from which lessons were learned. It was thought that, in terms of its practicality and day-to-day relevance, it would be useful for staff to see and use the written standard, and it was hoped this would improve their knowledge and understanding of the process of standard setting and how standards can be useful to practising nurses at ward level (Dunn, 1990).

Since they were not involved in writing the standard (i.e, 'bottom-up' approach; Kitson,1990), staff initially felt they were being criticised for their pressure area care. This was quickly overcome by explaining that the ward was chosen to pilot the standard because the staff did have a good grasp of the issues involved in pressure area prevention. The second problem was monitoring and evaluating the standard; informal monitoring revealed that the standard *was* being implemented – empty beds were made up with a Ripple mattress but there were difficulties in obtaining the mattresses as the stocks in CSSD were variable and, on occasions, they were not available when required. The data compiled, however, revealed useful information on the cost of providing Ripple mattresses; for example, the cost for one month was approximately £97, while an individual mattress cost £13.50 to be cleaned, repaired or checked. A clear method of evaluating the standard had not been identified, but continuing studies of pressure area care on the unit meant the standard's effectiveness was apparent a number of months later.

Further work
To address the other issues outlined above, a full multidisciplinary working party was set up. This included a consultant physician, clinical nurse manager, clinical practice development nurse, physiotherapist, occupational therapist, dietitian, pharmacist and a nurse representative from each ward within the unit. The working party members each had their own areas of expertise; a review of literature was also undertaken. Discussion of specific risk factors within the group brought about suggestions for simple changes of practice.

Choosing an assessment tool   One of the group's first activities was to look at tools used on admission to identify the degree of risk of developing pressure sores. Following a search of the relevant literature (Spenceley, 1988; Pritchard, 1986), the Waterlow Pressure Prevention/ Treatment Policy (Waterlow, 1985) was chosen for the following reasons:
• The scoring system is simple and quick to use, but is also comprehensive, encompassing risk factors such as nutrition, neurological deficit and tissue malnutrition, which were significant to the client group and are often not included in other scoring systems.

- The total score increases with increasing risk, and this seemed more logical than some other scoring systems.
- The total score is categorised into at-risk, high risk and very high risk, providing some guidance as to the equipment required and degree of nursing intervention.
- Nursing interventions can also be guided by analysis of risk factors which significantly contribute to the total score. These can then be incorporated into the patient's care plan; for example, if appetite and continence are significant risk factors (potentially contributing six to the total score), these can be highlighted as separate problems on the care plan, rather than being referred to in the more 'routine' care plan phraseology, such as 'at risk of pressure sores'.
- The score also provides guidance on the related care of patients and of any existing pressure sore. It was hoped the use of the Waterlow score would help to address issues 6, 7 and 8 outlined in Table 1 ie, provide more detailed guidance to staff for planning and implementing care and therefore helping to overcome the problems associated with the high vacancy rate.

Quantifying the problem   The group's next activity was to identify the number of people at risk and subsequently estimate the need for pressure-relieving equipment of various types (issues 2 and 3 in Table 1). The method chosen included:

- calculate the Waterlow score for each patient;
- document the pressure relieving equipment in use, and
- document the incidence and grades of pressure sores.

Unfortunately in October 1990, data could only be obtained on two wards due to time constraints, but the survey has recently been repeated on all patients in the unit (August 1991).

Results and discussion

Table 3 shows the result of the survey on two wards, ward A being the site for the standard setting exercise. The results showed that all the people on this ward who were at high risk had a pressure-relieving mattress, unlike many of those in ward B who did not, including one person at very high risk. This demonstrated clearly the value of the standard

Total no. of patients		Waterlow score 15+	20+	With pressure-relieving mattress 15+	20+
Ward A	24	13 (54%)	7 (29%)	13 (100%)	7 (100%)
Ward B	24	11 (45%)	5 (20%)	5 (45%)	4 (80%)
Total	48	24 (50%)	12 (25%)	18 (75%)	11 (92%)

Table 3. Results of survey 1 (August 1990).

setting exercise. Table 4 shows the results of the August 1991 survey, indicating high numbers of at-risk patients in all categories.

The Waterlow policy recommends that people with a Waterlow score of 10+ should be nursed on a pressure-relieving mattress such as Vaperm or Spenco, those with a score of 15+ on a (*fully functional*) large cell Ripple and people with a score of 20+ on a mattress such as a Pegasus, low air loss bed or a Clinitron unit.

The Waterlow policy does not give guidance on chair cushions, and this issue is being addressed separately as many patients are more at-risk when sat in a chair for long periods. The Working Party is now finalising written guidelines for staff on:
• use of equipment;
• pressure sore prevention;
• ward management.

Mattresses currently available to the unit consist of numerous large cell Ripples, occasional Spencos, and low air loss beds and four Pegasus mattresses. Additional Pegasus mattresses and Clinitron beds were available by rental. The large cell Ripple has traditionally been used for people in all categories as the availability of alternative mattresses is extremely limited. The findings of the survey of all four wards revealed:

• approximately 18 patients at any one time required a high degree of relief such as Pegasus low air loss or Clinitron mattresses;
• approximately 20 patients required moderate relief such as a large cell Ripple;
• approximately 30 patients required a pressure-relieving mattress such as Spenco or Vaperm.

The results of the 1990 survey (Table 3) enabled the ward managers to confidently argue a case for the purchase of new equipment for patients at very high risk of developing pressure sores. This was accepted in the last round of budget setting as a legitimate claim for expenditure, but this funding has never materialised. As a result, the unit relies on renting equipment for patients at high risk, which is inevitably more expensive in the long term, and is unable to provide a pressure-relieving mattress for all patients at risk. The clinical practice development nurse and

Total no. of patients		Waterlow score			With pressure-relieving mattress
		10+	15+	20+	
Ward A	24	19 (75%)	12 (46%)	9 (37%)	13
Ward B	24	18 (72%)	7 (21%)	3 (12%)	7
Ward C	24	14 (70%)	6 (30%)	3 (15%)	7
Ward D	20	22 (90%)	13 (54%)	3 (12%)	11
Total	92	73 (79%)	37 (40%)	18 (19.5%)	38 (41.3%)

Table 4. Results of survey 2 (August 1991).

clinical nurse manager will use the 1991 (Table 4) survey to present further evidence for the cost-effectiveness of the strategy.

The use of the large cell Ripple as a first line pressure-relieving mattress is now being reviewed. It has proved expensive to maintain, and stock is not available to cater for both at-risk and high risk patients. For the large number of patients in the at-risk category, the use of alternatives such as low pressure sponge mattresses, toppers or other alternating pressure relieving mattresses may be more appropriate and cost-effective in the long term, so the initial standard and alternatives available are in the process of being reviewed. Current reliable research into the comparative relief offered by different mattresses is, however, extremely limited (Clark, 1991).

The difference in the percentage of patients at risk in the two surveys may be explained by the seasonal difference in the nature of patients – nurses often intuitively feel people are more dependent in the autumn and winter months. More research is required in this area, however.

Reduced incidence

Incidence of pressure sores was significantly reduced on the second survey (October 1990, 29 per cent; August 1991, 18 per cent), and it is hoped that both the use of the Waterlow score and the subsequent heightened awareness of nursing staff has contributed to this. It is recognised that people still remain at risk following discharge home, so all people with a Waterlow score of 15+ are now referred to the district nursing service so a care plan can be implemented in the community.

The introduction of the Waterlow score across the unit has been welcomed by some, but others remain sceptical. It has provided detailed information about each patient's individual risk and their significant risk factors, and has enabled staff to identify accurately and confidently the range of pressure-relieving equipment required on the 92 bedded unit, while demonstrating its potential use as a tool for auditing the standard of pressure area care. The results have also enabled the unit to assist community staff in estimating pressure-relieving equipment required in the community. The setting of the standard allowed staff to easily focus on one aspect of patient care by identifying the systems required, and resulted in improved care and use of equipment.

References
Clark, M. (1991) A comparison of the pressure redistributing attributes of a selection of bed mattresses used to prevent pressure sores. *Journal of Tissue Viability*, **1**, 3, 65-67.
Dunn, C. (1990) Who cares? *Nursing Standard*, (Quan Newsletter) **5**, 9, 6.
Hibbs, P. (1988) Pressure Area Care for the City and Hackney Authority. C&HHA, London.
Kitson, A. (1990) Quality matter and standard setting. *Nursing Standard*, **4**, 44, 32-35.
Pritchard, V. (1986) Calculating the risk. *Nursing Times*, **82**, 60, 82.
Spenceley, P. (1988) Norton v Waterlow. *Nursing Times*, **84**, 32, 52-53.
Waterlow, J.A. (1985) A risk assessment card. *Nursing Times*, **89**, 27, 49-51.
Waterlow, J.A. (1987) Calculating the risk. *Nursing Times*, **83**, 39, 58.

Bibliography
King's Fund (1989) The Prevention and Management of Pressure Sores Within Health Districts. King's Fund Centre, London.
   A general guide to pressure sore prevention strategies.
Morison, M.J. (1989) Early assessment of pressure sore risk. *Professional Nurse*, **4**, 9, 428-31.
   Discusses nursing assessment for pressure sore risk.

The Waterlow Card
Copies of the Waterlow Card are available direct from Judy Waterlow at: Newton, Curlands, Taunton, Somerset TA3 5SG.
Cost: 20p per card, plus postage and packing (50p for up to 24 cards; 24-49 £1; 50-99 £1.40; 100-149 £2; 150-249 £2.50; 250-349 £3).
Cheques payable to: Tissue Viability Society.

23

Qualpacs: a practical guide

Paul Wainwright, SRN, MSc, DANS, DipN, RNT

Professional Adviser, Welsh National Board for Nursing, Midwifery and Health Visiting

There are several quality monitoring tools available to nurses, including Quality Patient Care Scale, also known as Qualpacs (Wandelt and Ager, 1974). We shall discuss here some of the practical problems involved in putting Qualpacs to work in the ward.

Commitment

The first point to be clear about if you want to measure the quality of care in your area of practice, with Qualpacs or any other tool, is that you and your colleagues really want to do it. To ask nurses to expose their practice to observation and criticism by others is asking a lot, and if there is no commitment to look constructively at the result, the whole exercise will be pointless. The decision to use any quality measuring tool should only be taken after thorough discussion with all the staff involved, including the area manager. An involved and supportive manager is an invaluable ally, who may be able to provide material help with things like photocopying, typing, or extra cover for a meeting of all the ward staff. He or she may offer moral support, share some of the risks and offer a different perspective if things get difficult. The manager may also be able to put you in touch with other helpers, perhaps someone in the school or at district headquarters, who you may not know about. You may even have a standards officer or quality assurance manager to whom you can go for help.

Is Qualpacs the tool for you?

Having thrashed out such questions as: ''do we really want to measure quality and why?'' and: ''what are we going to do with the results of our measurements?'', you can think about which tool to use. Perhaps the most important task at this stage is to decide what quality nursing means to you and your colleagues. Unless you are sure of your values you cannot begin to set standards or measure quality.

If your ward or team has not got a written statement of your nursing philosophy, with some statements about beliefs and values, this is the first step. Measuring quality is a subjective business, involving choices. If no-one agrees beforehand what their preferences are, the result would be like organising a night out at the local Indian restaurant and expecting everyone to enjoy the food, even though nobody else but you likes spices.

Preparing the ground

Assuming you have a philosophy which everyone supports, the next job is to read everything you can find about tools in general. The bibliography at the end of this chapter will help.

Qualpacs involves watching the care being given, as well as some consideration of charts and records and other aspects of communication. It attaches great importance to individual patient care and involvement and expects the nurse to have good interpersonal skills. If you and your colleagues share these values, Qualpacs may well be the tool for you. However, be wary of measuring only the things you think you are good at. You may get a shock if you find out you are not as good as you thought (which is a good thing to know), but you may also be tempted not to look at things where you know you are weak.

If all the nurse-patient interaction in your area is excellent, but the standard of record keeping is poor you might be well advised to use a chart audit of some sort, either instead of, or as well as, Qualpacs.

Validity and reliability

The concepts of validity and reliability are discussed briefly in Figure 1. You will also find a more detailed discussion in the text of Qualpacs and in Barnett and Wainwright (1987).

Subjectivity: If I stand at the end of the bed and look at a patient I may form all sorts of impressions and opinions about him, but these will be subjective judgements based on my experience, knowledge, beliefs and values. Indeed, to say: subjective judgements, is tautology, since judgements are by definition subjective. Much of the work of any profession is based on subjectivity, because no matter how many hard facts you may possess about something, you will always have to exercise judgement when deciding what to do about it. This is not something to be ashamed or frightened of. It is simply a matter of recognising the importance of professional judgement and making sure that it is based on as much good evidence as possible.

Objectivity: The opposite of subjectivity. An accurate thermometer correctly used will give an objective measure of body temperature. No opinion or judgement comes into it.

Validity: To say that a measure is valid is to say that it actually measures what it claims (or is being used) to measure. Thus a clock can give a valid measurement of time and a thermometer can give a valid measurement of temperature.

Reliability: A reliable instrument is one which gives the same result consistently if it is used repeatedly to measure the same thing, by the same or by different people. If a thermometer records a patient's temperature as being sometimes a degree more than it really is, and sometimes a degree less, then it is not reliable. Neither is the clock which sometimes gains and sometimes loses. Of course, some tools may give different results depending who is using them. It is important that all users agree to use the same methods, otherwise the results will be unreliable through no fault of the tool. A tool may be reliable, but not valid, as for example a clock which is always ten minutes fast.

Figure 1. Definitions of subjectivity, objectivity, validity and reliability.

Having decided you want to use Qualpacs, the next thing to do is to read the items in the questionnaire and the cues once again. This time you and your colleagues need to ask yourselves: "do we really understand what this item means? How will we recognise this behaviour when we see it, and what represents good and bad performance?" I would advise you not to alter the wording of any of the items in the questionnaire, but you are at liberty to make minor alterations or additions to the cues that go with it. This will enable you to give examples that relate to your area of practice. It will also ensure that everyone in the team has the same understanding of the items.

At this stage, if you have not already done so, you will have to decide who are to be the observers who will carry out the exercise. There is no rule about this, other than that they must be practising nurses who know something about your area of work and, above all, are acceptable to the staff to be monitored. An adverse report is easily rationalised away if it can be suggested that the observers did not know what they were looking at. The observers could be members of staff in the area concerned who will monitor their colleagues at work, from another similar area, from a neighbouring unit, hospital or district, managers, teaching staff, or anybody else who is acceptable, available and willing. Preparing for and carrying out the exercise will require some commitment and time from the observers, so you may need to negotiate with the relevant managers, to release them from duties or provide cover for them.

Training the observers
The observers will then have to be trained to use the tool. This does not take long, perhaps three days in total, but will require some organisation. A friendly tutor or helpful in-service department could be invaluable. Training should include:
- introducing the concept of quality measurement;
- introducing Qualpacs;
- giving everyone time to read through the items and cues;
- discussion of the concepts of validity, reliability and objectivity;
- discussion of the items and cues so that everyone understands and agrees them;
- discussion of the five point, best-nurse-poorest-nurse scale;
- discussion of practical problems — where to sit when observing, how to cope with rapid activities, ensuring privacy and so on;
- practice sessions in clinical areas other than the one to be monitored;
- debriefing sessions to compare scores and establish reliability.

The objective of the practice sessions is that if two or more observers watch the same patients getting the same care without comparing notes at the time, when their scores are checked afterwards they should be very close to each other. The Qualpacs text discusses this and suggests the degree of correlation that should be obtained. If you are not sure about things like correlation coefficients you can probably find a statistician in your district headquarters, or the school of nursing, or at a local college, who will help.

Many modern scientific calculators have a correlation function built in, which makes life simpler. If, having done all this you find your observers produce very different scores, they need to sit down together and go over their notes from the session, comparing their responses to the various situations and finding out where they differed. They should then repeat the exercise and check that their scores are now close enough to be acceptable.

Rating the procedures

The trickiest thing for newcomers to using tools like Qualpacs is the concentration needed to watch a nurse do something, split it up into four or five different components, find those items in the questionnaire, and rate how well they were done. For example, while bathing a patient, a nurse may pay attention to him, treat him in a kind and friendly manner, choose appropriate topics for conversation, utilise the nursing procedure as an opportunity for patient interaction, give the patient information, respond appropriately to him, observe changes in his condition and react accordingly, adapt the procedure to meet his needs, involve him in decision making, record information about him or communicate it to others, as well as maintaining his privacy and dignity and observing acceptable standards of hygiene and cleanliness and making him feel safe!

All of these (and more) are noted separately in Qualpacs, and the same nurse may do them well one minute and poorly the next, with the same patient. She may also change from patient to patient. However, with practice it is possible to record a surprising amount of detail with great accuracy.

Using the tool

It is essential to plan ahead and make sure everyone involved in the project knows what is happening. You will probably have discussed the project with your manager at intervals, but have a final session to go through all the arrangements. Pick an ordinary day: you are not trying to prove how hard you work or how short staffed you are, so don't choose the morning when there are three lists and two ward rounds all at the same time. Pick the patients to be monitored, randomly if possible, though the final choice will be partly governed by their condition, the layout of the ward, and their willingness to take part. Explain to the patients what is going to happen and ask their permission. Explain what is happening to other staff — domestics, porters and doctors — so that they are not worried by the sight of people with clip-boards busily writing down everything that happens. Don't be afraid to cancel at the last minute if unforseen problems crop up. Introduce the observers to the patients and make sure that everyone knows they are observers, and that they cannot help with care or do anything for patients except in dire emergency.

The report

There is no point in spending a lot of time and effort — and therefore money — on an exercise like Qualpacs if you don't intend to use the findings. There must be a commitment from the start to respond constructively to criticism and use the report as the basis for change and improvement. Nevertheless, the staff will have found the experience of being observed quite uncomfortable and will be apprehensive about the outcome. A useful tactic to prepare for the feedback session is to ask the staff to jot down the points they think are going to come out in the report.

Most people have a reasonable degree of insight into their strengths and weaknesses, and will probably err on the critical side if asked to appraise themselves. It should then prove possible to start the feedback with the positive aspects, and you may be able to say of the bad points: "it was better than you expected, though there is room for improvement". People are much more likely to accept that they have faults and to look for remedies if they have identified the faults themselves, and have the opportunity to find their own solutions.

A serious undertaking

Measuring the quality of care in your area is not a task to undertake lightly. This chapter has touched on many of the problems, but has deliberately skimmed the surface in many areas, assuming that you will get hold of Qualpacs and some of the many other articles about it, and read this article in conjunction with them. I do strongly recommend that you seek help from people you trust and spend a lot of time preparing and planning before you do anything. That said, if you wish to recognise your professional responsibility to evaluate the quality of what you do, I wish you well!

References

Barnett, D. Wainwright, P.J. (1987) A measure of quality. *Senior Nurse*, **6**, 3, 8–9.
Dunne, L.M. (1987) Quality Assurance: methods of measurement. *The Professional Nurse*, **26**, 187–190.
Wandelt, M. and Ager, J. (1974) Quality Patient Care Scale (QUALPACS). Appleton Century Crofts, New York.

Bibliography

Barnett, D. and Wainwright P.J. (1987) Between two tools. *Senior Nurse*, **6**, 4, 40–2.
Barnett, D. and Wainwright P.J. (1987) The right reflection. *Senior Nurse*, **6**, 5, 33–34.
Burford Nursing Development Unit. (1983-84) A compendium of articles published in British nursing journals by staff at BNDU. Available on application to SNDU, Burford, Oxfordshire.
Burnip, S. and Wainwright, P.J. (1983) Qualpacs at Burford. *Nursing Times*, 36–38.
Dunne, L.M. (1987) How do we set nursing standards? *The Professional Nurse*, **2**, 4, 107–9.
Kemp, N. (1986) What is quality assurance? *The Professional Nurse*, **1**, 5, 124–126.
Kitson, A.L. (1986) Indicators of quality in nursing care: an alternative approach. *Journal of Advanced Nursing*, **11**, 133–144.
Kitson, A.L. and Kendall, H. (1986) Rest assured. *Nursing Times*, 29–31.

Kitson, A.L. (1986) Taking action. *Nursing Times,* 52–54.
Wainwright, P.J. (1987) Peer review: in Pearson, A. (Ed), Nursing Quality Measurement, 15–24. John Wiley and Sons.
Wilson-Barnett, J. (1986) A measure of care. *Nursing Times,* 57–58.

Recruiting and Managing Staff

24
Get the best from staff recruitment

Hilary Shenton, RGN, Managing Director, Raine
Christine Hamm, RGN, Director, Raine

However attractive the conditions of employment and working environment, and however good the morale, teamwork and opportunities for professional development at your place of work, people will inevitably leave and vacancies will need to be filled. With the current shortage of nurses, employers have to work hard to make their posts attractive. It is also important to make sure appointments are appropriate to the needs of existing staff. Here we will consider the issues arising from staff vacancies and how to fill them most efficiently.

Staff vacancy

Do you actually have a vacancy?   If someone resigns, it is often the immediate reaction of their colleagues that the post must be refilled. But you do not necessarily have a vacancy when someone leaves: this can be an opportunity to restructure the department so that other staff have increased responsibilities which they are pleased to accept, or the post could be filled by promoting another member of staff, creating a vacancy, or an opportunity for restructuring, elsewhere. It is a good idea to spend at least a couple of days to consider the situation and to look at the needs and skills of others in the department and of the client group. It may be a good opportunity to offer another member of staff training so that they can develop the skills to fulfil the new post in a few months.

Seek out views   The next step is critically important to the success of both the recruitment process and the future employment. The views and needs of *all* relevant colleagues, most importantly those who will be immediately responsible for the newcomer, *must* be sought. Their thoughts on the exact nature of the job, and the ideal skills, personal qualities and level of experience required are essential.

Increasingly, ward sisters and charge nurses are becoming actively involved in the recruitment process for their immediate ward staff. This involvement may make new demands, but will provide the ward managers themselves with the opportunity to build and maintain the team *they* feel is most appropriate for their clients and colleagues.

The staff to be involved in interviewing must also be identified and included in these discussions; there is no point in one group of interviewers shortlisting a candidate who is rejected by someone more senior with different views of the qualities required. Everyone's views must be known before the post is defined and advertised.

Internal or external appointment?

Again, the decision to consider all applicants, including existing staff, or to only look outside *must* be made before the post is advertised – and *everyone* in the relevant departments must be informed. If you decide to use this opportunity to bring in new skills from outside, it is demoralising for existing staff to apply and be rebuffed.

Similarly, if the post is open to internal applicants, they need to know, and should be given a deadline beyond which the post will be advertised externally, unless suitable candidates have applied.

Job descriptions should contain:
- Objectives of the job.
- Manager to whom the staff member will report.
- The individual duties of the job (list and detail no more than 12).
- Outline, for each of these duties, where responsibilities begins and ends.

Table 1. The job description

The ideal candidate:
- Level of experience required.
- Any special experience required.
- Personal qualities needed such as:
  flexibility of attitudes;
  leadership;
  problem-solving ability;
  ability to communicate well.
- Other requirements, such as flexibility to travel.

Table 2. The personnel specification

Job description and personnel specifications

Draw up a *brief* description of the job, based on the information and ideas pooled from relevant colleagues (Table 1) and also a list of qualities sought in the 'ideal' candidate (Table 2). These should be circulated to those involved with interviewing; the job description should also be sent to candidates called for interview. The interviewing team should also agree about the parts of both specifications on which they are willing to compromise: the absolutely ideal candidate rarely exists!

Advertising the vacancy

Advertising is not the only way of making a vacancy known, but it is the most effective way of reaching a wide selection of potential candidates.

Content   Put the minimum amount of information that will attract appropriate candidates to respond (Table 3). It is essential to describe the job clearly but briefly and to highlight particularly attractive opportunities or facilities (such as a professional development course which is available, or well-equipped ward). Include brief details of the *easiest possible* means of applying for the post. This is usually a (correct!) telephone number, and the name of someone friendly and helpful who will be at the extension given (check that they are not on holiday or on a course during the week after the advertisement is placed) and can get an application in the post first class to enquirers the same day.

Put the minimum information to attract response:
- Job title.
- A sentence to stimulate interest and make potential candidates want the job.
- Details of the easiest means of applying.
- Salary grade.
- Closing date.

Table 3. The advertisement

Design In magazines where there are many advertisements, a large advertisement will attract more attention, and the inclusion of a border or logo may also help to catch the eyes of potential applicants. Advertising is expensive, but so is bridging the gap between staff. Disruption and increased workload on existing staff should also be considered.

Timing How urgent is the re-appointment? If the time scale is not at panic proportions, it is probably advisable to avoid advertising just before bank holiday weekend. If another post is coming up you may decide to delay advertising for a week or two so the two can be advertised together in a bigger space. On the other hand, you may feel it would boost the morale of existing staff to advertise early.

Choose the right medium The only valid measure to assess the effectiveness of magazines or newspapers is the response rate to the advertisements you place. It is also important that the applicants who respond are appropriate for the post, but your wording for the advertisement should ensure this. If you want and need good responses *do not* place your advertisement in a publication where you know you get a very low response rate. You may decide, however, that you want to be seen to be supporting a particular group, and place the advertisement in its journal. Local papers can also be useful.

Handling the applications
If possible, let every applicant know that their application has arrived and is being considered. Inform anyone whose application is obviously inappropriate *straight away*, so that they can get on with more appropriate applications. Once the closing date has passed, let your interviewing team draw up a shortlist for interview. Invite interviewees as early as possible for interview and an informal visit; if candidates

have a long distance to travel, these could both be on the same day.

Informal visits These *must* be informal, and not used as an extra interview. They should give the candidate the opportunity to assess the working environment and the job in a relaxed atmosphere. Their questions should be answered by someone who is enthusiastic about the work; preferably *not* by the person who is leaving.

Interviews Decide who will be interviewing and how long the interviews will be and inform the candidates of this at the start. The interviewing panel should be kept as small as possible – preferably no more than three people – and interviewers must have the views and requirements and the trust of their relevant colleagues.

It is not easy to assess all the professional skills and personal qualities of a candidate in an interview, but it is possible to get a clear idea of the individual's appropriateness for the job, assessed against the qualities you have identified for the 'ideal' candidate. You need to assess their professional skills and level of motivation, which can be done by asking them to talk about their last (or present) job. Ask what they enjoyed most and least, and what they could handle, given more training. Ask them to identify their training needs, as this will help to build a picture of what they would like most to be doing.

Assessing personal qualities such as leadership and problem-solving ability is difficult, but asking how they have handled problems in previous posts will help. Referees' reports are also important here.

Do not be afraid of 'digging too deep' in an interview: as long as you do not ask unfair personal questions, it is reasonable to find out about the candidate in some depth. After all, it is important for them that they find themselves in the 'right' job, too.

References

At least two references should be sought, one from the current or last employer, and one from a previous employer (or, if newly qualified, from the candidate's school of nursing). An *employer's* reference (even from a non-nursing employer if the candidate was not previously in nursing) is more valuable than that from a colleague (Table 4).

Ask referees for:
- Statement of the candidate's duties.
- Length of employment.
- Sickness and absenteeism record.
- Reliability.
- Ability as a team member.
- Professional conduct.
- Other qualities and skills.

Table 4. The reference

It is often possible to gain more frank analysis and information and depth from a referee by telephoning them. Most people are now willing to give references in this way; give them the option to think about it and telephone you back. You could ask for a written reference, and then telephone the referee for a more detailed discussion. Always check that the candidate is happy for you to contact their referees before doing so, and work fast.

Offering the job

Once the interviewers have agreed upon the candidate for the post, act fast and offer the post, subject to satisfactory references. This could be done on the same day as the interview, and, if they have already had an informal visit, you should expect an immediate (or reasonably quick) response. Do not wait until the references are in – you may lose the candidate to another employer.

Making the appointment

Once the candidate accepts the job, keep up the momentum and get the starting date agreed, uniform measured and holidays booked. Write immediately to confirm the appointment, terms, conditions and starting date; people are reluctant to hand in their notice until they have the job offer in writing. Also, inform the other applicants as quickly as possible.

It is hoped that if these suggestions for recruitment are followed and some of the ideas for retaining staff acted upon, it should be possible to build and maintain reasonable staffing levels – even in the specialties where nurses are few and far between, and in work places located in the heart of cities.

25
Job sharing can take the strain out of recruitment

Ann Shuttleworth, BA
Editor, Professional Nurse

Shortage of labour costs huge sums of money in industry – in health care it costs lives. The projected shortage of nurses is already biting in some specialties and areas, and it is essential for health authorities to retain the staff they have, and attract more recruits – and as the number of 18-year-olds drops, different kinds of recruits. However, unlike industry, they cannot simply pay higher salaries to attract people, so they have to find new ways to persuade people to nurse – ways that compete with the money industry has to offer.

Health authorities have begun to move towards greater flexibility in working hours, to try to attract those people – mainly women – whose other commitments make them unable to undertake full-time work. Part-time work is often characterised by low pay, job insecurity, poor promotion prospects and the lack of fringe benefits. Far more appealing to many is job sharing, an idea which began in the early 1970s as more women decided they wanted families without giving up their careers. They often found the part-time work available was low paid and low skilled, and at a lower level than they had been used to.

A voluntary arrangement
Job sharing is an arrangement whereby two (or more) people voluntarily share one full-time post, sharing salary and benefits between them according to the hours they work. As long as each one works 16 or more hours a week, they are eligible for employment protection. Within this definition, job sharing is completely flexible in how the job is shared, and is at the convenience of the employees and employers concerned. Most people suggest a job share with a partner already in mind, although some have been put in touch with each other after applying for jobs advertised as suitable for a job share. Normal contracts are usually suitable with appropriate amendments, but sharers may wish to add clauses to cover such eventualities as one wishing to leave.

Advantages
There are many advantages in job sharing, both for employees and employers. The most obvious advantage for the employee is the

opportunity to work part-time while retaining the advantages and security of a full-time post. This alone makes job sharing attractive both to nurses wishing to work part-time without moving to a lower grade and those who have taken a career break and want part-time work at the grade they had previously attained.

Job sharing also gives more opportunities for jobs to reflect individuals' interests and skills than part-time work. The increased free time is not only a chance to care for children – it can also be used for the pursuit of research or study interests. In a profession as potentially stressful and demanding as nursing, the opportunity to work in a responsible position only part-time alleviates these problems, while job sharers can offer mutual support and different expertise.

There are also numerous advantages for employers (Buchan, 1987). Trained staff can be retained and are less likely to suffer from job related stress, a major cause of absenteeism. Voluntary job-sharers are also likely to have a high level of commitment since they have shown a positive desire for their job by arranging the job-share, rather than opting for a more easily attained post. They are also likely to be more flexible and able to provide additional cover in peak periods. Working shorter hours, they have often been found to be more productive and able to sustain higher levels of activity.

Disadvantages

While the advantages to both employees and employers make job-sharing attractive, it does have potential disadvantages. Employees' earnings will obviously be limited and promotion prospects may be decreased. A tendency has also been found in job sharers to work more than their half-time, and they may experience some loss of job satisfaction. They will certainly have to ensure their managers do not try to give them too much work and the post is subject to the usual appraisal systems. Sharing the control and responsibilities of the job may cause problems, and must usually be resolved by compromise.

Employers have cited potential disadvantages from their point of view, but in practice these are not always significant (Buchan, 1987). The cost of employing two people – providing uniforms and training, and paying for time spent together in handover is higher, but National Insurance may actually be lower if the post attracts a gross pay of less than £350 a week. The handover time is likely to be minimal, and it has been argued that it leads to increased planning and efficiency.

Job sharers' managers may have to spend more time in supervision and work allocation, although no recorded schemes have reported this as a problem. Staff supervised by the job sharers may find difficulty being accountable to two people, especially if they have different ideas on organisation. Problems may also occur if one sharer wishes to leave.

These disadvantages can be overcome given commitment from those involved, as Judith Lathlean (1987) found in evaluating a job shared ward sister post at the Charing Cross Hospital in London. The sisters found initial resistance from their staff, who knew one of the sisters well and the other not at all. Hackney Job Share, an external organisation, came in to explain to the staff about job sharing and diffuse some of their negative feelings. The first few months involved the sisters in high levels of communication in setting up systems, and they found they had to compromise to reach workable agreements on issues in which they differed. Once systems were operating, the ward settled down and the staff gradually became more supportive and understanding.

While the job share described by Lathlean was not without difficulties, on the whole it was successful and illustrates that job sharing is possible for jobs with managerial responsibilities. Lathlean recommends that health authorities consider job sharers in more posts, and take the initiative in creating opportunities for employees to job share.

New ways to Work (NWTW) is an organisation committed to advising people on job sharing and other flexible working ideas, such as annual hours and taking career breaks. Started in 1979 as a voluntary organisation, NWTW are now funded by the London Boroughs Grant Scheme to advise both employees and employers. They are currently involved with the Royal Institute of Public Administration in designing a course on job sharing aimed specifically at health authorities.

Health authority interest

They say health authorities are starting to take a little more interest in job sharing, but they are still lagging behind local authorities in actively promoting job sharing schemes. NWTW feel that health authorities are finding it something of a hurdle to start encouraging job sharers, and most of those employed by health authorities say they have had difficulty in negotiating their posts. There are exceptions, however, including one manager who advertised a post specifically as a job share, and another who has several health visitor job share partnerships.

Obviously, some posts will adapt more easily to a job share than others, and will be more easily broken down. NWTW say, however, that most jobs can be successfully shared, given commitment and flexibility from all concerned. Difficult managerial posts have been shared successfully, allowing people with years of experience to continue to work at the level they are qualified for, rather than leaving employment altogether or working in lower grade jobs. They say it is essential for professional organisations to get involved in encouraging job sharing, as people are most likely to contact them for advice.

Job sharing may not answer all the problems of nurse recruitment, but it could certainly tap an unused and probably frustrated pool of experienced ex-nurses unwilling to return to part-time work at a lower level than they left, and retain many who wish to devote some time to other commitments. If it is to live up to its full potential, health authorities and the nursing unions will have to become more active in publicising the idea and helping potential sharers negotiate their posts.

References
Buchan (1987) A shared future. *Nursing Times*, **83**, 4.
Lathlean, J. (1987) *Job sharing a ward sisters post*. Riverside Health Authority, London.

Useful addresses
New Ways to Work
309 Upper Street
London N1 2TY
Tel: 071-226 4026.

Hackney Job Share Project
380 Old Street
London
Tel: 071-739 0741.

26

Part-time staff: a blessing in disguise?

Jean Fisher, SRN, ONC
Clinical Teacher, St Michael's Hospice, Bartestree, Hereford

As a ward sister with a full-time staff of four, including myself, out of a full complement of 12, to cover the 'day-time' hours from 07.30 to 21.30 hours, all the pleasures and pains of managing part-time staff can certainly be said to be mine. In this particular setting of a small, purpose-built hospice, which is totally charity-run, the stresses and strains – as well as the job satisfaction – encompass both the high and low of nursing morale.

The particular stress encountered here is in coping with pain, and fear, anger and desperation in patients, and also in dealing almost daily with bereaved families. To counteract that the staff has the satisfaction of usually being able to help relieve suffering with good symptom control and that most precious gift – time. More often than not, the nurse may only need an extra five minutes with patients to really make them comfortable or to find out what they are really frightened of.

Those few extra minutes are often just not available to nurses, but to the patient may mean the difference between good nursing and the extra special 'caring' that hospices are all about. All nurses – whether they work in a hospital or hospice – want to give those minutes and they become frustrated when they see less and less time available to spend with patients due to constant pressure and staff shortages. Using part-time staff may provide part of the solution for several problems, including this one.

Increased flexibility

For the employer, one of the greatest advantages of using part-time staff must be increased flexibility. At the hospice all nursing staff (except those employed on the nursing bank) work full shifts in an effort to increase continuity and teamwork. However, there is no doubt that even more flexibility can be obtained (and some considerable financial saving made) by staff working part shifts at peak hours, ie, mornings and 'twilight' shifts. My view is that staff commitment and participation is higher when they are at work for a whole shift and can take part in ward reports, case conferences and decision making.

Almost all continuing education in the form of lectures, video viewing and so on take place in the afternoon during the overlap period. Very few staff off duty at 13.00 hours would be able, or willing, to return at 14.30 hours for a lecture or ward staff meeting. The other important factor in the use of full shift patterns is that staff can be given back 'time owing' during the overlap period. It is known that nurses often work extra time. It is also well known that, more often than not, they do so willingly, to maintain the level of nursing care given to their patients. It is not usually possible for them to be paid for this time. However, this commitment should not be taken for granted – commitment is a two-way process, and therefore 'time off in lieu' should be given at mutual convenience to the unit and the member of staff. The pressure in many areas today usually prevents this, and the extra frustration upon so many others could well become the straw that breaks the camel's back. But 'time off in lieu' might even encourage staff to come in on a day off sometimes for a lecture if that time could be given back during a quiet period.

The other flexibility of part-time staff is that, if necessary, one can *occasionally* ask a part-time nurse to cover an extra part-time shift when unforeseen staffing problems occur. This would obviate the need for agency staff, who are expensive and provide less continuity of care. It is important that staff who are willing to do extra time do not feel that they *have* to do so and that they are not taken advantage of by being asked on a regular basis.

Stress
Stress levels in part-time staff are undeniably lower, which in the hospice situation is vital. The extra time for 'real life' means nurses are more refreshed and have more to offer when they are at work. But what about the effect the number of part-time staff has on the stress levels of their full-time colleagues? In fact, it may *increase* their stress levels a little, in that the onus to provide continuity lies more heavily upon them. However, in many ways this can only be another recommendation for good documentation and the implementation of the nursing process with full-time staff coordinating the nursing teams.

The added stress of working part-time is that it can become more difficult to make useful relationships with patients and their families. However, this may be an advantage if it makes staff less complacent about making contact with patients and relatives. Clinical observations may be much more acute from part-time staff as they have more time away from work and therefore see changes in situations more clearly than staff who are there five days a week.

The small details of the smooth running of the ward are those that break down at times. When the part-time staff nurse hardly ever works the third Tuesday in the month and is therefore not usually required to order stores . . . except when sister is on a day off and the full-time staff nurse is sick . . . then problems can arise. Like most problems there is usually a solution.

Another advantage for employers in taking on part-time staff is ease of recruitment. Present staff shortages and recruitment problems highlight the outdated historical ideal of nurses being single women, working full-time on a vocational basis, with no life away from work. It is now becoming apparent that few nurses fit into this category today. There are many nurses leaving the profession, or not returning after a break, because of management failure to make it either feasible or acceptable to do so. Hopefully, the increase in crêche facilities, 'back to nursing' courses and the moves towards improved continuing education in nursing (UKCC, 1990), together with flexibility of employer and employee will put this situation to rights. If the idea of job sharing (Cole, 1987) does spread, many high calibre senior nurses may be able to stay in or return to their profession.

Common sense

Most of the staff at St Michael's Hospice are married, and some have children. As their sister, I am always grateful for their common sense approach and skills of empathy as, being younger and single, I still have much to learn in certain situations. If nurses seriously want to take the abnormality and mystique out of ward situations (in hospital, nursing home or wherever the wards may be) they should aim to make them as much like the outside world as possible. This means a good staff mix (single and married as well as more men). The single staff also have their own skills. They may often have new ideas and practices to share, which may be varied as single nurses tend to be less settled. Often, married staff – unless their partners are in the Services – stay in one area for a much longer span of time. Herein lies the answers to a manager's prayer – married staff can provide ongoing continuity and single staff bring new ideas. They can bring the best (or perhaps prevent the worst) from Oxford, East Grinstead or Outer Mongolia!

Skill mix is not just a question of the ratio of trained to untrained staff but also of age group, background and professional expectations. A unit where the turnover of staff is as high as that of the patients is as difficult to manage as one where no one has moved for years. All ward sisters know at some time the frustration of training a bright young staff nurse only to find that once you make progress and she becomes able to be your right hand, the obligatory six months or one year is up and she is off to the next rung of the ladder. We have all done it ourselves and accept its inevitability, but there is no doubt that a nucleus of staff who have been in the team for a while makes for smooth running. The management skills required then are to maintain commitment and prevent staleness and the old adage, 'We always do it this way'. Also, it prevents exclusivity and a clique formation that precludes newcomers from being accepted as part of the team. A clear and agreed ward philosophy should help to prevent these occurring, but the situation needs constant and careful monitoring (Teasdale, 1987; DHSS, 1986; Mallin, 1987; Moores, 1986).

Commitment

Diminished level of commitment among part-time staff is an often quoted problem but is, I suspect, a fallacious one. Certainly among my own staff, the level of caring and commitment is as high in part-time as in full-time staff. The personal areas of responsibility and accountability have never been more clearly stated within the nursing profession and this can only decrease the degree of complacency which exists in some members of various professions. The days of the ward sister 'carrying the can' for every occurrence is being replaced at last. This alone must increase the level of motivation in most trained staff. It may be more difficult for part-time staff, particularly those working on night duty, to participate in continuing education, as often the reason for doing night duty is to dovetail family commitments and work. My own staff seem to have most amenable partners, mothers, neighbours, cousins and aunts who can take care of children for a day to allow them to attend a study day or conference.

Motivation in giving care to an agreed standard is not, or should not be, a problem. Most nurses have high personal standards for bedside care. Why are so many leaving the NHS at the moment? Not because their own standards are inadequate, (or at least only in a very small number of cases) but because they feel they cannot practise at what they consider an acceptable standard. It is the frustration, stress and constant pressure which is driving so many out into the private sector, or abroad, or, most sadly of all, out of nursing altogether. Most nurses want to do their best for patients whether they are on duty for two days a week or five. Certainly the bank staff employed by the hospice, who may come in for a half shift to cover sickness perhaps only once a month, give excellent care to patients and their families (West Dorset H.A., 1987).

I am sure that the level of commitment among staff is high when they are in a position to give good care, as part of a caring team, supported by all tiers of whichever structure they are working within. Staff whose input of care is being respected and appreciated will have higher morale. They will give of their best, perhaps not in every shift – which none of us can – but in a more than acceptable majority.

A valuable part to play

Part-time staff have a valuable part to play in any nursing team. They can provide continuity, stability, maturity and empathy, and enhance the 'normality' of ward environment sought by many team leaders.

The situation in which I work may be said by some to be ideal. It is a small unit, with a small team which works very closely together. It is not attached to a hospital and is not bound by the conservative and short-term views found in some health authorities. The system of part-time staff working full-shift days has been most successful. Working in partnership with patients (Teasdale, 1987) has to begin with partnership with colleagues and managers. Accepting the holistic approach to patient care may well have to begin by accepting a holistic approach to staff needs. Then perhaps better staff will be recruited and retained for longer and they will give better patient care.

References
Cole, A. (1987) Job sharing – partners in time. *Nursing Times,* **83,** 40.
DHSS (1986) *Mix and match: a review of nursing skill mix.* DHSS, London.
Mallin, H. and Wright-Warren, P. (1987). Review mix and match. *Senior Nurse,* **6, 3.**
Moores, B. (1986) Review mix and match document. *Journal of Advanced Nursing,* **12,** 6.
Teasdale, K. (1987) Partnership with patients. *The Professional Nurse,* **2,** 40, 397-9.
UKCC (1990). *The PREPP Report.* UKCC, London.
West Dorset H.A. (1987) *Standards of Care Quality.* West Dorset Health Authority.

27

Appraisal methods: how do you rate yourself?

Elizabeth S. Wright, SRN, DipN, CHSM
Senior Nurse, Surgical Unit, The Royal London Hospital, Whitechapel, London

Attitudes towards appraisal

A formal system of appraisal is necessary, but which method is most effective? If the whole tactic of appraisal is altered with an aim to improve staff development and career prospects, rather than concentrating solely on criticism of current performance, then the procedure appears much more worthwhile, with long-term planning and objectives designed for the individual's progress, either for her present job or for a different or more senior post.

In the majority of cases within the nursing profession, appraisals are irregular and often serve no constructive purpose for the appraisee. The existence of a staff appraisal interview system compels supervisors to meet with their staff and consult with them on a regular basis, and hence become better informed as to their interests and aspirations (Ansty, 1961). It is insufficient for junior staff nurses to have annual appraisals if they only remain in a junior post for 6 months to a year, and more frequent discussion is necessary to evaluate their progress and needs.

In many professions, including nursing, managers seem reluctant to make any assessment or constructive criticism of their staff. They either avoid doing appraisals or provide ineffective criticisms because they fear to point out weaknesses in performance. This may reflect their inexperience and lack of instruction in methods of appraisal, or possibly their awareness of how difficult it is to make just and accurate assessments, combined with a fear of hostile reactions on confrontation with the appraisee (Fletcher, 1985).

Professional conduct

Being an assessor is a difficult position in which to find yourself, particularly if you work closely with the individual concerned; for instance a sister and a staff nurse working on the same ward. My personal feeling is that one's professional conduct as a senior and therefore a manager, should provide a role model for the staff nurse. The relationship should be friendly and one of approachability and respect, but not familiarity, otherwise the position of assessor loses the credibility necessary for objective criticism to be made. It is to be hoped that the advice will then be received as serious and constructive, and acted upon with intent to improve performance. Managers might find the act of appraisal difficult precisely because they have not maintained a professional relationship with their junior staff.

Current appraisal methods

The most important criterion for a successful method of appraisal is that the manager actually knows the individual concerned, and more importantly her work. Otherwise how can the criticism, good or bad, be justified? How well thought out and personal is the method of appraisal where one person writes a report and another presents it to the individual (commonly a student nurse), often without discussion?

It is preferable that the appraisal is based on first-hand information, but this should include assessment of performance over a substantial period of time, not biased by recent incidents. An overall view of merit is taken into account and should not be marred by personal prejudice.

A common standard by which to assess is difficult to maintain; but in general one should try not to compare to others in a similar post. Assess a person on their own merits in comparison to the standard and experience they should have expected to have attained by that position and after that length of time in the post (Ansty, 1961).

Staff development and career planning

The appraisal may be considered by some managers, and even appraisees, to be an unnecessarily time-consuming process that does not appear to give immediate practical results. An appraisal also involves committing convictions and opinions to paper, which the nurse manager may wish to avoid especially if challenged by the appraisee.

The professional development has long-term implications for clinical practice, but it is not sufficient for the nurse manager to make these assessments and the consequent decisions alone. In order for the most benefit to be gained from the system it is essential that the appraisee is involved in making decisions jointly with the assessor (Pincus, 1982).

I am sure that the fundamental criteria on which to undertake an appraisal, are familiar to all, but they should nevertheless be maintained; such as ensuring a quiet, undisturbed, informal setting, with adequate time set aside. The appraisal needs to be a joint participative exercise between the nurse and her immediate manager in an ambience that is conducive to open discussion, and with strict confidentiality (Stewart, 1978).

The format of the written appraisal form varies greatly between Health Authorities, and the complexity of it depends upon the grade of staff. The actual written evidence of the appraisal is not as important as the two-way discussion. However, it should be completed for reasons of referral and possibly written references at a later date, and as confirmation that the appraisal took place.

Self-appraisal

An increasingly popular and effective method of appraisal which has been implemented in Bloomsbury is self-assessment or self-appraisal. Essentially, the appraisees consider their own ability and skills, and fills out their own appraisal form. The principal advantage of this system is that the appraisees have more opportunity than anyone else to note their own performance and understand their own opinions and conscience, related to weaknesses and strengths within that performance. Self-appraisees are also unlikely to become defensive in response to their own critical analysis of their abilities, although this may prove a natural reaction to another person's criticism. Experience shows that appraisees are more willing to act upon weaknesses or problems that they themselves have identified (Fletcher, 1985).

Although the staff nurse fills out her own appraisal form, it is imperative that her manager discusses each description with her, in order to give an outsider's point of view and assist the nurse's insight with guidance on how to make improvements in each area.

Appraisees seem to be modest in their ratings and realistically a manager needs to guide and help develop the appraisee's skills in self-assessment. The manager may assist in improving not only various practical skills, but also the appraisee's insight into areas of professional development. More importantly, the manager can take the opportunity to give the appraisee credit and praise for work and skills completed with thoroughness and initiative.

How do we meet the many needs of newly qualified staff

A Professional Development Course designed for newly qualified staff nurses is being implemented in Bloomsbury, London. Self-appraisal is incorporated into this course, and is particularly relevant to newly qualified staff who have yet to develop fully the skills of a trained nurse and manager and who require considerable guidance and support in their new role. The project is being undertaken in response to the recognised need for nurses' development in both clinical and professional aspects in the newly qualified staff nurse role, as discussed at the national conference on "Professional Developments in Clinical Nursing – The 1980s", which took place in Harrogate in 1981.

It is the belief of those participating in the professional development course that self-appraisal by the course participants is more appropriate than assessment by examination, because the act of self-appraisal and the personal involvement in setting new targets for achievement serves to take the individual further in their personal development.

Emphasis is therefore placed on self-assessment with related discussion. The format used ultimately provides a detailed descriptive profile of the nurses' strengths and weaknesses in relation to the course objectives, and outlines developmental progress by a comparison of pre-course and post-course assessment profiles. The course members' self-assessment is supplemented by their facilitator's and tutors' comments on their progress.

The course has a six-month programme consisting of supervised and supported practice in a designated training area, involving a facilitator for guidance and practical advice (often the ward sister). The course aims to provide the nurses with the necessary background, awareness, and motivation to pursue a continuous programme of personal development, both clinical and professional. It enables them to develop leadership skills, and prepares them to function as responsible members of the profession. The outline of the course comprises two parts: part one consists of practice under supervision, with emphasis on the clinical role of the registered nurse with a problem-solving context; and part two aims at individual development, which incorporates writing skills, teaching methods, research, and career development as well as leadership skills, within a team and as a practising clinician. Other subjects involving some theoretical tuition are models of nursing and legal and ethical aspects of nursing. The final three study days of the course include seminar presentations by the participants, based on assignment work done during the course, and a concluding debate on professional issues (Smythe, 1984).

I have been facilitator for newly qualified staff nurses who have completed the six-month course. The course has been beneficial to them in providing theoretical support for practical issues and practice. It has encouraged them to seek further education and develop their careers with a confident and inquiring insight into the practice carried out on the wards. The course also allowed me to evaluate the support and needs I was trying to fulfil for my staff nurses. Perhaps other ward sisters should do likewise?

As previously mentioned, this course commenced as a pilot scheme and it was not intended for general implementation until the advantages and disadvantages have been fully assessed and evaluated after 3 years.

I believe that much of the negative feelings that I have expressed regarding staff appraisal result from the fact that so many managers are not taught proper methods of appraisal, and often carry it out ineffectively. There has to be a better way, and I am sure that self-appraisal incorporated into a professional development scheme is a more positive and effective method of identifying the individuals' needs, and of improving and praising their abilities.

References

Anstey, E., (1971) Staff Reporting and Development. George Allen & Unwin Ltd., London.
Fletcher, C., (1985) Means of assessment. *Nursing Times*, **81;27**,24
Filkins, J., (1985) Going round in circles. *Nursing Times*, **81;29**,31
Pincus, J., (1982) Staff appraisal and development. *Nursing Mirror*, **155;21**,47
Smythe, J. E., (1984) Professional development of the newly registered nurse; Guidelines in the Bloomsbury scheme. Unpublished.
Stewart, A. M., (1978) Staff development and peformance review. *Nursing Times*, **74;16**,654.

Bibliography
Dimmock, S., (1985) Starting from scratch. *Nursing Times*, 81;30.
Jessup, G., and Jessup, H., (1975) Selection and Assessment at Work. Methuen & Co. Ltd., London.
Randell, G., Shaw, R., Packard, P., Slater, J. (1972) Staff Appraisal. Institute of Personnel Management, London.
Raybould, E., (1977) Editor. Guide for Nurse Managers. Blackwell Scientific Publications, London.

28

Assessment of a return to nursing course

Stephen O'Connor, MA, BSC, RGN, Cert Ed
Lecturer in Nursing Studies, University of Southampton

The ability of health authorities to attract qualified nursing staff back to practice is critical as it is the quickest measure available to ease the future and, in many areas, current manpower shortages. This chapter reviews the employment outcomes of a return to practice course held in the University of Southampton College of Nursing and Midwifery over a two year period in the late 1980s.

The accepted method of preparing potential recruits is through completion of a return to practice course. Several examples of varying course formats have been published (Warwick, 1988; Morgan and Whitehead, 1988; Green, 1988), all of which would seem proficient for their task. The course run at Southampton University College was similar in format, and the input generally follows the curriculum now set out by the ENB for course 902.

Aims
Following on from previous attempts to evaluate return to practice courses (Donn and Smits, 1988), the aim of this project was to answer four questions about course participants:

1. What are they doing now?
2. What was their reasoning?
3. Did the course influence their decisions?
4. What is the best course of action for nurse managers?

Methodology The 130 participants who completed the course were contacted by postal questionnaire. The respondents were asked structured questions, but were allowed space to explain or add to their answer (Durant, 1988). A questionnaire was designed along these lines and reviewed by the course team. The respondents fell into four categories:

- those who remained unemployed;
- those who returned to employment other than nursing;
- those who returned to private sector nursing;
- those who returned to the NHS.

What are they doing now?

Results Of the 130 questionnaires sent out, 74 were returned in a condition suitable to allow their inclusion in the main study; a usable return rate of 56 per cent was calculated, which, for a postal questionnaire, is a respectable return (Heberiein and Baungarten, 1978).

The results (Table 1) show that 72 per cent of the group are now in nursing employment. To calculate the number that have actually returned to nursing after the course, those already in nursing employment at the beginning of the course must be deducted. At the time of the survey 44 per cent were already in nursing employment (NHS and private) and took the course to update. If these are omitted, the percentage of the sample that returned to nursing after the course was completed was 46 per cent, as opposed to the original 72 per cent.

	Not in employment	Non-nursing employment	Private nursing employment	NHS nursing employment
N=74	12	10	19	33
%	16	14	26	46

Table 1. Employment of participants following the course.

Of primary concern, however, was the percentage of the whole sample who had been encouraged to return to the NHS, as opposed to the private sector. If those who returned to the private sector are omitted, the percentage that returned to NHS was 34 per cent as opposed to the 72 per cent who were in nursing employment at the end of the course.

What was their reasoning?

Those who remained unemployed included not only some of the youngest course members but also some who had been out of practice for a considerable time. They felt significantly less encouraged to return to the NHS or even that they were being obstructed. The staff they encountered seemed less than enthusiastic about their return, and one was told that even though she had been out of nursing for only six years, a newly qualified staff nurse would always be given preference at an interview. Others spoke of an observable low morale on the wards which they found discouraging. The comments most frequently given for non-return stressed lack of flexible hours, which seem to imply they were only offered standard shifts. Significantly, family commitments was the most common stated cause for non-return in this group, explaining why the need for flexible hours and childcare facilities was most frequently expressed in this group (82 per cent). The availability of crêche facilities would help this group most, as was also expressed on several occasions.

Those who returned to employment other than nursing had spent the longest period away from the profession – on average 17 years. They were still actively encouraged to return, however, implying their time out did not adversely affect their attractiveness as potential recruits. Although primarily owing to the lack of flexible working hours, lack of confidence also contributed to their not returning to nursing. Their own comments seem to reflect this, and although several pleas for more flexible hours were recorded, more interestingly, comments on staff attitudes varied; while many felt they were welcomed and that staff were helpful, others noted a degree of indifference. One respondent, who had been out of nursing 16 years, recalled "they said that they did not have time to waste on someone who had been out of acute nursing for so long", this attitude was not expressed as starkly again and much evidence is available to show the opposite view – one nurse, for example, returned to full-time employment within the NHS at the age of 55 after 30 years out of nursing.

Respondents who returned to private sector nursing had the highest average age, which was significantly higher than the sample as a whole. The group was encouraged to return to nursing, but inflexibility was once again a prime concern. Other causes were also raised concerning the morale of nurses in the NHS as well as their own disillusionment with NHS nursing. This group also professed the greatest concern with practical difficulties such as travel to NHS hospitals. The qualitative data from this group raises some interesting issues. Apart for the comments concerning flexible hours, morale and difficulty of travel, one RGN stated she was advised to apply for an auxiliary post by ward staff, another was told "we are flexible but not that flexible", several mentioned they were not given a chance to settle before judgements were made and others stated the only reason they went 'private' was that the nursing homes were quicker off the mark to reply to their enquiries regarding employment.

Did the course influence their decision?

Of those participants who returned to work 64 per cent said the course had no effect upon their decision. Importantly, 70 per cent of these were already employed, and the remaining 30 per cent did not imply that the course had any negative effect. The remaining 36 per cent said that the course had had some effect, of whom a significant proportion (62 per cent) said it had had a positive effect. This would seem positive feedback, but there are some provisions: they may have returned to practice eventually even if the course had not existed (many have done so in the past without such facilities) and it cannot be stated categorically whether the course convinced them to return to nursing or merely reinforced an existing conviction. However, almost all members of the group saw the course as a virtual prerequisite to return to practice. It was seen as a method of raising or gaining confidence, which would occur not just as an outcome of the course itself, but as a result of meeting other women in similar circumstances. Overall the course received no comments of a negative kind, but one respondent did indicate that it reinforced her "worst fears that nursing in the NHS was not for her".

The group that returned to the NHS were concerned with developments in nursing of a practical or clinical nature, and therefore did not find the course a great deal of help in this area. The course itself was not clinically based, and the solution to this problem lies in greater cooperation with the clinical areas.

Evaluation

The overall return rate to NHS nursing following the course was 34 per cent. This figure probably reflects the future picture as people who are already employed by the NHS no longer appear on the courses wishing to update. This may result in smaller courses, a greater percentage return but not necessarily an increase in the overall numbers returning. Many who go on to the private sector should also be attracted to the NHS. Their main demand is for flexible hours similar to those available in other occupations. Of equal importance is the geographical convenience of the private sector in terms of nursing homes and other local facilities. Careful note should be taken of the comments that the private sector was quicker to reply to enquiries. The group that have not yet returned to any employment are a potential source when their family circumstances allow, but crèche facilities, as well as more flexible hours, would hasten their return. The question raised by one respondent: "How flexible is flexible?" would seem to be answered by the fact that as 46 per cent of the respondents were working in the NHS at the time of the survey and of these 85 per cent were working in part-time employment, the hours offered at present are flexible enough to meet the demands of the service in this area.

- A designated person should be responsible for coordinating the course.
- Areas for clinical experience should be carefully chosen.
- All applicants should be replied to promptly with all the necessary information to allow them to make informed decisions.
- A record of all enquiries should be made.
- A live register of all those completing the course should be maintained and kept up-to-date by regular correspondence with those listed.
- Clinical areas should be allowed to be as flexible as necessary in terms of hours and shifts to be able to recruit the staff they require.
- Crèche facilities must be created for those clinical areas that have particular difficulties.
- Standardised recruitment policies would seem to be counterproductive: flexibility must be the key policy.

Table 2. What is the best course of action for nurse managers?

The other causes given for not returning to the NHS lie within the bounds of possible action in the shorter term. The fact that those who were least encouraged did not return may reflect the reality that, at the time, they were not best suited to return given their present circumstances. There was evidence, however, that the more positive the nurse's encounters with full-time staff, the greater the likelihood they would return to the NHS rather than the private sector.

The course would seem to be a positive factor in influencing nurses' final employment decisions, not so much in terms of information, but as a confidence-builder. The group support effect is one that is encouraging and is lost with individual re-entry programmes. The cost of re-entry in terms of individual expenditure seems high at an average of £83, and is almost certainly a conservative estimate (this included the cost of the course, UKCC re-registration and sundry costs such as new shoes and travel). There was no mention of cost as a distinctive disincentive, but this was for a 20 hour course. There may have been some difficulties had the course been 144 hours long, appropriately costed with no possibility of nursing employment until the course was completed; the private sector would therefore be seen as an even more attractive short-term alternative.

Recommendations

Course members return to nursing expecting a shortage and, therefore, plentiful work on their terms. They may be disappointed and dis-illusioned if work is not immediately available and will either retire again or move to the private sector. Given that work may not be immediately available, course graduates should be able to register with the bank, even if no work is available. This would create a live register of nurses having completed the return to practice course as recommended by Gossington (1988).

The idea that all nurses who return need the same degree of re-orientation is not supported by the evidence: confidence is a matter of degree. The concept of a central core course would seem logical for no other reason than to provide group peer support. The clinical practice element must continue to be carefully planned on an individual basis. This would seem to demand that coordination should be a full-time post, that careful selection of wards and mentors must continue, and that, placements should be in the areas most suitable to encourage those returning.

The respondents said they know at least 211 nurses not in employ-ment. However, as some answered this question by saying "several", "quite a few", or "loads", this figure can only be taken as a conservative estimate. This would indicate a pool of untapped resources is available: it is vital the NHS is prepared for the time when these nurses are needed and when their return is actively sought.

References
Donn, M. and Smith, M. (1988) Many happy returns. *Nursing Times*, **84**, 47, 46-47.
Durant, R. (1988) Stepping out. *Nursing Standard*, **3**, 9, 51.
Gossington, D. (1988) Keeping in touch. *Nursing Times*, **84**, 45, 46-47.
Green, W. (1988) Making a comeback. *Nursing Times*, **84**, 32, 50-51.
Herberlein, B. and Baungarten, M. (1978) Factors affecting the response rate to mailed questionnaires. *American Sociological Review*, **43**, 447-62.
Morgan, W. and Whitehead, E. (1988) Back to nursing. *Nursing: The Add on Journal of Clinical Practice*, **3**, 3, 130-31.
Price Waterhouse (1984) Project 2000: report on the costs, benefits and manpower implications of Project 2000. UKCC, London.
Warwick, C. (1988) Return to practice. *Nursing Times*, **84**, 26, 39-40.

29

Teamwork: an equal partnership?

Gill Garrett, BA, SRN, RCNT, DN(Lond), CertEd(FE), RNT, FPCert
Freelance Lecturer, Bristol

From being one of the fundamental tenets in the care of groups such as elderly people and those with mental handicaps, the vital nature of the team approach has become recognised and accepted in all areas of nursing. Many patients have a multiplicity of needs – medical, nursing, therapeutic, social – which no one discipline can hope to meet; only by close collaboration and cooperation can different practitioners bring their skills into concert to attempt to meet them.

Increasingly in recent years, the validity of this contention has been appreciated by both hospital and community workers, and the gospel has been preached. But how effective has the concept been in practice? While no doubt in many parts of the country teams are working efficiently and harmoniously together to the benefit of all concerned, it would seem that in others there are areas of concern which demand urgent consideration and action if the concept is not to prove a meaningless cliché. With this in mind, we shall consider the prerequisites for effective teamwork, point out a few of the common problems which may arise and offer some suggestions as to how these problems may be ameliorated.

Who makes up the team?
One very basic question to ask before considering the work of the team is who makes up the team? On multiple choice papers, students will indicate the doctor, nurse, therapists, dietitians – all the professional partners in the venture. But integral to every team must be the people most meaningful to the individual patient: her family if she has any, her supportive neighbour, or whoever. If our aim is to rehabilitate the patient or to maintain her at her maximum level of functioning, these are people we neglect at our peril – and much more importantly, at the patient's peril. As professionals we must learn that we do not have a monopoly on care, nor do we have a dominant role in an unequal partnership. The contribution of relatives or friends, as agreeable to the patient, is vital – whether discussing assessments, setting goals or reviewing progress; their non-contribution, if excluded from active participation, may indeed frustrate all professional efforts. Although we shall

concentrate on those professionals who are conventionally seen as team members, this point cannot be overstressed.

Why are teams necessary?

Perhaps an even more basic question is, why does the team exist? It is easy to lose sight of the fact that its sole *raison d'être* is the patient and her need. An old adage runs, "The patient is the centre of the medical universe around which all our works revolve, towards which all our efforts trend". In economic terms we are quite used to this concept of 'consumer sovereignty', but in our health and social services management at present, all too often our consumer exists more to be 'done to' rather than canvassed for her opinion, offered options and helped to make choices. A thorny question often raised about the multidisciplinary team is, which professional should lead it? An equally important one not so often posed is, who should be the 'director' of team activity? If we recognise the patient as an autonomous, independent person (albeit with varying degrees of support), surely we must have the humility to acknowledge that this directing role falls inevitably to her. For patients with mental or other serious impairment, of course, the question of advocacy then arises – again an issue subject to much current debate.

Having allocated the role of director to the patient, the team leader then becomes the facilitator of action. It has been said that, "Fundamental to the concept of teamwork is . . . division of labour, coordination and task sharing, each member making a different contribution, but (one) of equal value, towards the common goal of patient care" (Ross, 1986). What do these elements demand? To make for efficient division of labour there has to be an accurate assessment of a situation and the input needed to deal with it, a recognition of who is the best person for which part of the job, and the carrying through of the appropriate allocation. Coordination demands the ability to see the overall, the sum of all the individual parts, and to recognise their relative weightings in various circumstances; it needs effective communication skills and the ability to use feedback to take adjustive action as required. Task-sharing demands that team members have an understanding of different roles and their effect upon one another, that they recognise areas of overlap and are prepared to shoulder one another's problems should the need arise. Such demands are not light; they require considerable training and practice to perfect.

Status and power within the team

Consideration of the second part of the Ross quotation brings us to one of the common problems experienced in multidisciplinary teamwork: ". . . of equal value towards the common goal of patient care". Is that how all team members view their own contribution or that of their partners? Status and power imbalances can make for great difficulties in team functioning; tradition accords high status and consequent power to the medical establishment, for example, with much affection but little standing to nurses. But if nurses have been seen as lacking in power and status, even lower on the rungs of the ladder comes the patient; in general, society grants a very low status to ill and disabled people, and institutional care strips all vestiges of power from inhabitants.

For workers who see themselves as being the juniors in teams, the presence and influence of more powerful members may prove intimidating, and consequently they may make only tentative and limited contributions to discussions and meetings. It is important that they realise that, however 'junior', they have a right to contribute, indeed a duty to do so, if they have what has been described as the "authority of relevance" (Webb and Hobdell, 1975) – if they have knowledge relevant to the patient's own feelings of need or wellbeing which must be brought to the team's attention. So often it is those members who spend more time in close proximity to the patient who possess such authority, rather than the senior medical personnel who may visit her only on a weekly basis.

'Follow my leader'   A second problem may arise out of the power and status imbalance, especially when team members have become used to suppressing their views or do not recognise their authority of relevance – regression into the 'follow my leader' phenomenon. There may be the tendency to leave all the thinking to another group member who is perceived as being more prestigious or simply more articulate, often the consultant. His thinking and directions are seen as definitive, with team members abdicating their own professional responsibility to think and speak for themselves and for their patient from their own vantage points. Except in the unlikely event of the team leader being qualified in a multidisciplinary capacity, this obviously acts to the detriment of patient care – we can none of us prescribe or wholly substitute for each other's contributions. A variation on this 'follow my leader' phenomenon is sometimes seen where two leaders emerge from subgroups in a team, each with his or her own following. In addition to the drawbacks already mentioned, the results in situations like this are invariably divisive too.

'Groupthink'   This is the name that has been given to another possible problem in teamwork; it is generally seen in well-established, long-lived teams whose members over time have grown very used to working with each other. Team meetings are always amicable and 'cosy', there is no bickering or dissension and everyone gets on terribly well with everyone else. The group gives the appearance of having its own internal strength, with a marked sense of loyalty and supportiveness. But this denies that disagreement and conflict are facts of life and often signs of constructive enquiry and growth; all too often such teams ". . . become rigid, committed to the status quo . . . less open to input and feedback.

Hierarchies become established and bureaucratic qualities emerge which resist questioning and change" (Brill, 1976).

Patient confusion   In case this should all seem a little esoteric, consider for a moment one last very basic possible problem in multidisciplinary teamwork – potential confusion for the patient. Unless each member of the team extends to her the courtesy of an introduction to their personal role, with an explanation of how this fits in with the overall individual plan of care, especially in the acute phase of an illness, the patient (particularly if elderly) may well find so many professionals overwhelming and muddling. If she is to feel in any degree in control of the situation and if any confusion is to be lessened, time must be taken to ensure a personal approach, with all care being presented as part of a concerted whole, and with common goals identified towards which all the team are working.

This last problem, then, is usually amenable to a common courtesy and common sense solution. But what about the others? The problems associated with status and 'follow my leader' have a more deep-seated origin and, although rectifiable in the short term in individual teams, in the longer term they demand a close scrutiny of, and changes in, professional education. 'Groupthink' demands flexibility of individuals and a system which encourages and permits a regular turnover of personnel to maintain healthy group dynamics.

Common core training?

If in effective teams there is no room for professional superiorities or jealousies, what is needed is an open, trusting relationship based on knowledge of, and respect for, one another's professional expertise. But this demands in turn an insight into other trainings and backgrounds to understand one another's terms of reference – the differences in emphasis we have in relation to patient care. While individual effort and inservice training programmes can go some way towards this, the difficulties with late attitudinal change are only too well known. Most of our basic feelings about our own profession and those with which we work are formed during our initial training period. Nursing is currently implementing Project 2000, with a common core foundation programme for all nurse practitioners. Is it not time we were much more adventurous, and explored avenues of common core training for all health professionals? Certain knowledge, skills and attitudes are prerequisites whether we are to be doctors, nurses, therapists or social workers – if we learned them together how much easier it would be to practise them together. The intention of such common training would not be to reduce all teaching to the lowest common denominator, but rather to look at areas of mutual concern, highlighting the unique contribution of each professional, and the bearing this has on the work of the other team members.

Value of difference

Educational change may also help us to recognise the value of 'difference' and the constructive use to which conflict may be put, so that 'groupthink' becomes a less likely problem. Better training in interpersonal skills – including assertiveness – should help the creation of a climate in which there is freedom to differ, to look more dispassionately at dissent, while acknowledging the areas of basic trust and agreement that do exist and can be built upon. The need for turnover in team membership has to be balanced, of course, by the need for reasonable stability over a period of time. Change every five minutes for the sake of it helps no one, but there must be recognition that long-term team stagnation (however well camouflaged) is beneficial neither to the group nor to the professionals within it – and certainly not to the patient and her family.

Realism

This chapter provides only a brief overview of a very important area. Readers' personal experiences may differ considerably from the scenarios which have been outlined. It would seem, however, that most experienced nurses have had the experience of needing to temper idealism in striving for effective teamwork with realism, given the situations in which they work. But recognition of this is in itself a step forward; we must have in mind that "under the aegis of teamwork, strange bedfellows are discovering, in time, that they must *learn* to work together before they *can* work together . . . teamwork is not an easy process to understand or to practise" (Brill, 1976).

References
Brill, N.I. (1976) *Teamwork: Working Together in the Human Services*. Lippincott, New York.
Ross, F.M. (1986) Nursing old people in the community. In: Redfern, S. (ed) *Nursing Elderly People*. Churchill Livingstone, Edinburgh.
Webb, A.L. and Hobdell, M. (1975) Coordination between health and personal social services: a question of quality. In: Interaction of social welfare and health personnel in the delivery of services: Implications for training. Eurosound Report No. 4, Vienna.

30
Making the team work!

John Øvretveit, C.Psychol, BSc, MPhil, DPhil
Co-Director, Health Services Centre, Institute of Organisation and Social Studies, Brunel University

Multidisciplinary community teams are often seen as the cornerstone of specialist services in the community for such client groups as people with mental health problems, learning difficulties, addiction problems and elderly people with special needs. It is therefore surprising that, for the most part, little thought and preparation has been given to how they will operate. We shall outline here those features which are essential to the continued success of any team, irrespective of the personalities, aims or organisations involved.

Research method
This chapter draws on a continuing programme of collaborative field research initiated in 1984 with a variety of teams and managers in England and Wales (Øvretveit, 1986) using two types of research:
- Long-term collaboration with individual teams on particular problems of team organisation. The teams are helped to describe features of their current organisation and to clarify alternative future options eg, for referral, case records and crisis services. The team and their managers agree and operate the new arrangement, and the researcher monitors its effectiveness. Two three-year projects of this type were undertaken (Macdonald and Øvretveit, 1987; Macdonald, 1989).
- Other research data comes from problem-centred two-day workshops for teams wishing to improve their organisation or for health and social services managers wishing to develop teams. Two common types of workshops were: to set up new teams in other areas of a district, learning from others already set up, and to help members of a team which is not working well to collaborate more closely.

In a number of cases follow-up workshops were held, to ascertain whether the solutions actually worked. To date 69 of these workshops have been held across the UK, and the research has found that three ingredients are essential to the success of any team: a common base, a team leader and an operational policy. However, we need to be clear why a multidisciplinary team is necessary before we can consider which type of team is most suitable. Given the problems and expense involved in setting up a successful team, both members and managers need to be convinced the advantages are worth the time and effort involved.

Advantages of multiprofessional teams

Why should professional practitioners with different training and perspectives and from different agencies, work closely together in teams? The advantages of multidisciplinary teams are listed below.

Better service   The main function of multidisciplinary teams is to ensure clients get a better service than they would otherwise receive from independent professional and agency help. Although agencies and professionals can agree arrangements for certain professionals to act as case-coordinators, it is usually better if case-coordinators are part of a permanent team. Case-coordinators have an agreed role and are allocated cases through the team. In this way, the team acts as the clear point for all referrals, and clients can rely on one familiar person to help in dealing with the bewildering bureaucracy and range of services they need. By working in a multidisciplinary team, case-coordinators have immediate access to a range of professionals and agencies, and develop a better understanding of the special skills and resources each has to offer, making them better able to meet the needs of clients.

Specialist practitioners working together can identify gaps in local services and formulate proposals for improvements based on understanding and experience of local client needs. It is easier for practitioners to plan and run projects as a team than individually.

Easier workload management   Teams also make it easier to manage workload and to establish common priorities across professions. For teams to work, each profession and agency must agree whether its practitioners will participate part- or full-time. This ensures a stable resource of specialists for the client group. Given the time and skills available, difficult decisions have to be made about priorities, but teams do allow practitioners to share work, with each member undertaking a fair share of unpopular as well as popular work.

Colleague support   Practitioners can often receive vital support and advice from other team members in dealing with complex cases. For example, some community mental handicap nurses are managed by a general community nurse manager, but find a senior social worker in mental handicap understands more than their manager about problems they have with particular clients and their families. Of course, certain types of technical advice can only come from a member of the same profession, and regular contact is necessary to keep up-to-date in profession-specific skills and knowledge. Emotional support is also important in stressful work with clients, and members can be of great help to each other in the team.

The benefits of teamwork do not come about simply because managers and planning groups call a group of practitioners a 'team'. Teams must be planned, funded, nurtured and regularly reviewed. Managers and team members must be clear what type of team they are establishing, and why it is the best arrangement for their client group.

Types of team

Table 1 describes five different types of team. This distinction is the first step in deciding which type of team is necessary. All too often, planning groups recommend a multidisciplinary team be set up without seriously considering which type is most appropriate or whether a team is required at all. Given the time, expense and problems involved in setting up a successful team, managers need to be convinced that such a service is the best way of using scarce resources to meet needs. Unfortunately, there is little objective evidence on the effectiveness of different types of team in different circumstances, and managers need to seek out the experience of others to find what has and has not worked.

The starting point should be an objective and systematic assessment of client needs and the resources available. However, it is usually only after it has been set up that the team begins to look more closely at how it is organised, and develops an accurate assessment of its needs and resources. The five models help clarify how a team is and should be organised.

Clarifying the team leader role

If a decision is made that 'closer' teamwork is required, attention should be given to agreeing common catchment areas for each profession, defining the time allocated by each member to teamwork and establishing a single base. In addition, it is necessary to channel all referrals to this base to establish the identity of the team, to clarify the team leader role and detail an operational policy. The following describes some essentials for establishing accountable service-delivery teams.

The quickest way to establish close and effective teamwork is to start with a clearly defined team leader role. I do not know of any teams which have close teamwork and have survived changes of membership without a clear team leader position. One of the biggest mistakes is to believe that interprofessional and interagency conflicts, rivalries and protectionism can be avoided by not defining a team leader role. Managers cause more conflict and bad feeling in the long run by encouraging the idea that leaving things ambiguous gives them more room to maneouvre in future. It is better to face up to differences and agree the role before problems arise, and recrimination or mistrust result.

Even so-called 'democratic teams' have leaders for different functions, recognising that agreed authority is required to get things done. The main issue is which type of team leader to appoint. This depends on the work they are responsible for, who they are accountable to and the sanctioned authority they have over team members.

A useful way to clarify the division of responsibilities and authority between the team leader and the professional superior is to consider each

Profession-managed informal network   One arrangement, sometimes described as a team, is where each practitioner remains under the management of their professional manager but takes part in regular meetings with other practitioners working with the same client group in the same area. Usually no-one is required to attend or is bound to the 'decisions' made at the meeting, and there is no collective responsibility for providing a combined service. The meetings arise out of the common interests of practitioners in the same area for information exchange, to improve cross-referrals and, on occasion, to arrange shared projects.

Fully-managed multidisciplinary team   Teams with *one* full manager accountable for each practitioner's work and for the service provided by the team. The manager has authority to appoint, assign work, appraise performance and to discipline members. The team usually works on consensus, but with the awareness that final accountability and authority rests with the team manager. In the past, some psychiatric clinics follow this model. The modern variant usually involves a nominated professional advisor outside the team giving advice on aspects of the team members' practice, management, professional training and development.

Coordinated team with shared management   A more common arrangement where each profession (and agency) endorses the role of a team coordinator, who shares responsibilities for managing team members with professional superiors outside the team. The team coordinator is appointed by higher management and is accountable to them for coordinating team members. He or she may, however, be nominated from among the team. Team coordinators rarely have authority to review or override profession-specific case decisions of senior practitioners, but often participate in aspects of management such as appointment and appraisal. Many community mental handicap teams in Wales use this model, with a social services appointee as coordinator.

Core and extended team   This term is used to describe at least two types of team. In one, the core team consists of full-time members (usually nurses and/or social workers), and the extended team of part-time members, usually covering a wider area (such as psychiatrists, clinical psychologists, occupational therapists and speech therapists). In the second type, the core team is directly managed by the team leader who coordinates the extended team which often works elsewhere (for example, a core team of psychiatric nurses based in a day hospital and managed by a community psychiatric nurse manager who also coordinates social workers and other therapists).

'Joint accountability' or 'democratic team'   In these teams, there is no team leader although there may be a team 'secretary' appointed by and accountable to the team. Depending on the task, the team will agree that one member carries out a leadership role for a particular task, with authority delegated by the team meeting. If consensus cannot be reached on a particular issue, the team will use an agreed procedure (usually majority vote) to reach a binding decision. However, majority vote cannot override a member's profession-specific responsibilities.

Table 1. The types of team.

of the areas of personnel management in Table 2 and establish individual or joint responsibility for each task. It is usually possible to define the rights and authority of the two roles by the following three types of authority (Table 3). There are a number of arguments for assigning full responsibility and authority to the team leader, with professional superiors in an 'advisory' role. Members are then challenged to explain the problems which can occur in both the short and long term. Research has found that if the professional superior retains the right to allocate work (management task 3, authority C), this restricts the time a member is available for teamwork and limits the closeness of teamwork possible.

1. Draft job description.
2. Shortlist, interview and appoint.
3. Assign cases and work.
4. Review cases and work.
5. Annual performance appraisal.
6. Training.
7. Disciplinary matters.

Table 2. Areas in which responsibility should be established between the team leader and professional superior.

A The right to be informed or consulted. Should, for example, a community psychiatric nurse manager consult with a team leader (who may be a social worker) about the appointment of a community mental health nurse?
B Joint decision (both team leader and professional superior have the right to veto). Following the above example, should the team leader have the right to veto the appointment?
C The right to decide. Should the nurse manager have the ultimate decision, with or without consulting the team leader?

Table 3. Three types of authority which should be specified between team leader and professional superior.

Operational policy

One of the most important tasks of a team leader is to regularly review the operational policy or to formulate one to propose if management has not provided one. The operational policy is the team leader's main working tool, authorising him or her to call for changes if members do not follow agreed ways of working.

Teams often do not specify the referral procedure to be followed by its members. In one situation, a team leader found that a nurse could not take a priority case referred to the team, which only a nurse could deal with. It emerged that the nurse's caseload was full with cases she had been taking independently from GPs and from a psychiatrist in another area. The team leader assumed all cases went through the team; this was not, however, agreed policy and the team leader had no authority to alter the nurse's practice to ensure the priority case was allocated.

To be a team, is by definition, to have an operational policy: group members need agreements about who will do what in different situations. The only issue is whether the policy is explicit or implicit, in the degree of detail and the areas covered. The advantages of explicit policy are that members are clear about agreed ways of working; it offers guidance; it explains and publicises the purpose and organisation of the team and enables it to monitor and improve its organisation.

A good starting point for a team establishing its policy is to write down their arrangements under certain headings, before discussing and agreeing improvements. The list of headings in Table 4 has proved useful to a number of teams beginning to detail or review their policy.

There are a number of ways of meeting the special needs of people living in the community. It has often been thought necessary to provide more specialist help in the community, and to improve collaboration between professionals. Multidisciplinary community teams have been viewed as the main method of improving services, but usually little thought is given to which type of team is appropriate. If 'close' teamwork is required, a common base which acts as the focal point for referrals is necessary. The role of team leader and team operational policy

---

Aims, priorities, client group and catchment area General purpose of the team, definition of client groups served by the team and those which are not, boundaries of catchment area.

Team philosophy, objectives and priorities General principles informing members of the work and the services offered by the team; specific objectives and current ordering of priorities.

Team membership Name, profession and role, special skills, time available for 'team work' and contact point.

Referrals to and from the team Criteria for accepting assessment and long-term work as a 'team responsibility'; criteria for finishing team involvement; arrangements for informing referrer of actions.

Team meetings   Conduct, agendas and decision-making procedures for team casework decisions, for team management and policy decisions, and for team proposals for service developments.

Case allocation, case-coordination and cross-referrals How cases are allocated for assessment and long-term work; responsibilities of case-coordinator; how cross-referrals and co-working within the team is arranged.

Team leader role Responsibilities; accountability; authority; method of appointment.

Professional superior roles Responsibilities; accountability; authority of each professional superior in and out of the team.

Team systems and procedures General heading eg, for workload statistics and information systems, case records and client access policy, finance and budgets, complaints procedure, staff performance appraisal and development.

Team accountability and performance reporting Group or individual to whom the team is responsible, and their responsibilities to the team; frequency and nature of team reports of workload, achievements and difficulties.

Appendices Proposals for service developments and update plans.

Table 4. Issues to consider in planning or reviewing team policy.

also need to be detailed, agreed and sanctioned. If thought is given to the general framework within which the team is to work, members can concentrate on the details of how they will work together.

References
MacDonald, I. (Ed) (1987) *Managing Change in a Mental Handicap Hospital*. Mental Handicap Services Unit, Brunel University.
MacDonald, I. (Ed) (1989) *The Rhondda Vanguard Community Mental Handicap Service*. Mental Handicap Service Unit, Working Paper, Brunel University.
Øvretveit, J. (1986) *Management and Democratic Teams*. BPS, Clinical Psychology Forum, October.
Øvretveit, J. (1986) *Organising Multidisciplinary Community Teams*. HSC Working Paper, BIOSS, Brunel University.
Øvretveit, J. (1987) Aspects of CMHT Organisation and Management. In: Grant, Humphreys and McGrath (Eds) *Community Mental Handicap Teams: Theory and Practice*. British Institute of Mental Handicap, Kidderminster, Worcs.

31

Shiftwork can seriously damage your health!

Emma Fossey, MA
Research Assistant, Dept. of Psychiatry, Royal Edinburgh Hospital

The concept of shiftwork is by no means new – in early times the extension of working hours into the night was necessary for security. In today's society the growth of industrialisation has rendered these reasons less cogent but has created new ones. Now, economic gain and continuous availability of public services are the main motivational factors behind the persistence of shiftwork. What is recent however, is the recognition that shiftwork has important implications for both the personal wellbeing of the workers and the safety of the general public both in and out of the work place.

Circadian rhythms

Most biological species are equipped with an inherent endogenous pace-making system known as the biological master clock. This is responsible for synchronising the rhythms of our physiological processes with the 24-hour cyclic changes of the earth, such as the cycle of light and dark. The majority of biochemical, physiological and behavioural processes, ranging from plasma concentration of cortisol and body temperature to the sleep-wake cycle and mood, therefore, have cyclic circadian (approximately 24 hour) rhythms. Each individual rhythm has its own unique and very stable temporal relationship with respect to other internal cycles and to the day-night cycle. For example, body temperature rhythm is dependent upon time of day – it reaches a peak during the late afternoon and falls to a trough during the early hours of the morning.

Any form of shiftwork that intrudes into time normally spent asleep will naturally alter these biological rhythms. It also results in numerous physiological and biochemical changes which include increases during the night of serum glucose, uric acid and levels of urinary excretion of catecholamines. In night workers the cycle of sleep and wakefulness is completely reversed and initially is at odds with other rhythms. For example, secretion of the sleep-dependent growth hormone (hGH) coincides with low levels of time-dependent corticosteroids and adrenaline. The abrupt change in sleep times due to night work means that high levels of corticosteroid and adrenaline secretion still occur at the original clock time – during the day when shift workers are trying to sleep, thus reducing the restorative value of sleep. Conversely, low levels of corticosteroids and adrenaline at night when nightworkers must function at their best cause them to be less efficient (Oswald, 1980).

Resynchronisation is a slow process, and in the case of rotating shiftworkers, readjustment is virtually impossible. Studies of transmeridian air travel have shown that it takes a day for the rhythms to adjust to a one hour shift. The process of resynchronisation to the time shift following air travel is facilitated by the social and environmental cues that help us to adjust to the time change. However, in shiftworkers, adapting to the time shift takes longer because the social and environmental time-cues are inappropriate – everyone around is sleeping and it is dark when shiftworkers are awake and trying to work. Even in non-rotating permanent night workers whose rhythms have time to adjust, the social pressure to conform to regular social sleeping times on days off means they too suffer some circadian disruption.

Consequences of circadian disruption

This physiological disruption, plus the psychological strain of shiftwork can have serious detrimental effects on shiftworkers' health and wellbeing.

Sleep Shiftworkers regard sleep as the biggest problem in their day-to-day living. Many have great difficulty falling asleep and/or staying awake at appropriate times. When they do sleep, their sleep pattern is altered and tends to be significantly shorter. There is evidence to suggest that for these reasons there is a high consumption of alcohol, tobacco, sleeping pills and tranquillisers among shiftworkers compared to their day working counterparts.

Eating patterns Eating habits are also upset by irregular sleep-wake hours and the consequences of this are reflected in the high proportion of duodenal ulcers, peptic ulcers and gastroduodenitis in shiftworkers.

Social patterns Studies have shown that shiftworkers often feel isolated from their family and friends and admit they are less able to fulfil their normal domestic roles, such as spouse and/or parent. This interference with normal family life can adversely affect shiftworkers' mental health, manifesting itself in the form of low self-esteem, anxiety and irritability, which in turn can lead to a deterioration of married and family life, and even divorce. Women in shiftwork are faced with these and other domestic problems. For many, their responsibilities to their family take precedence over their own sleep and as a consequence they suffer to a greater extent.

Circulatory and cardiovascular problems A study by Knuttson *et al* (1986) found a relative risk of myocardial infarction (MI) associated with shiftwork. This risk increases with length of time involved in shiftwork up to about 11-15 years, and then drops after over 20 years of exposure, which may be because those workers who are able to cope with shiftwork for such a long period are less susceptible to disease. Another study (Alfredsson *et al*, 1982) found evidence that serum cholesterol is higher in shiftworkers leading in turn to a higher incidence of MI, although this is confounded by the fact that the workers in this particular study were also excessive smokers, which may have been the primary reason behind the high rate of cardiovascular disease.

Psychiatric problems High levels of neurotic disorders and depression have recently been indicated in shiftworkers, and those on permanent night shift and men in general appear to be the more susceptible. While researchers are as yet unsure of the specific cause, it appears to be due to a combination of the physiological and psychological stresses of shiftwork upon the individual.

Whether these adverse effects are serious and lasting has been examined in a number of studies of ex-shiftworkers. Overall, the evidence suggests that former shiftworkers may continue to experience disruption of their sleeping and eating patterns, and that depressive disorders, circulatory, respiratory and cardiovascular complaints may also persist. Their health is also likely to deteriorate with age at a much sharper rate than dayshift workers. Unfortunately, these studies do not give an accurate picture of the general effect of circadian disruption because they are dealing with a sample of the population that is self-selected to a large extent and has already proved more capable of adapting to shiftwork. It is likely, however, that the long-term effect of circadian disruption in the average individual is more serious.

Poor work performance

The quality of work performance over a long period does not decline at an even rate, but fluctuates simultaneously with the peaks and troughs of the rhythms of body temperature and arousal. We experience a greater urge to sleep, a poorer ability to perform and an increased likelihood of making errors or having accidents between the early hours of 02.00 and 07.00, and to a lesser extent in the afternoon between about 14.00 and 17.00, regardless of whether or not we have slept. In terms of general performance, the day shift typically yields higher productivity than either the evening or night shifts, the latter being associated with the lowest performance. Some nurses, however, report that the evening shift is the time of their lowest performance. An important factor in this case is the fact that the division of labour for hospital nurses is such that work stress is distributed differentially over the three shifts according to the type and degree of the stress.

Shift schedules for nurses may vary according to the health board or authority, or from hospital to hospital: there may be a two-shift system in operation with an early shift and late shift and a permanent night staff to cover night duty; or there may be a three-shift schedule, such as morning shift from 07.00 to 15.00, afternoon shift from 14.00 to 22.00, and night shift from 21.30 to 07.30. In studies of the effects of shiftwork on nurses, sleep disturbances are mainly connected with evening shifts and fatigue mainly connected with night shifts. Many nurses find rotating shifts in general the hardest in terms of work performance and job-related stress, followed in turn by the afternoon, the night and day shifts. Indeed in one study nurses on rotating shifts were rated lower than fixed shift nurses by their supervisors in terms of job performance, motivation and patient care (Coffey *et al*, 1988).

A number of studies have also considered the performance of junior doctors suffering from varying degrees of sleep deprivation. They have found that in general, interesting tasks that involve relatively simple motor skills are resistant to the desire to sleep for up to 60 hours. The more mundane and monotonous tasks show a serious decline in concentration and an increase in errors after approximately 18 hours of sleep deprivation. Other studies of performance following sleep deprivation have found evidence of impaired retention, concentration, factual recall and manual dexterity, as well as slowed information processing and problem-solving.

Doctors in their first year also experience more psychiatric problems than any other comparable group of young professionals. Again, sleep disruption or deprivation appears to be the major causative factor rather than for example stress of responsibility, anxiety about personal ability or lack of free time. Studies list hyperirritability, less social affection, depersonalisation, feelings of hostility and an increase in alcohol and substance abuse as major problems for junior doctors. Depressive symptoms and in some cases suicidal thoughts have also been reported, and may be partly attributable to sleep loss.

Generating acceptable schedules

Despite numerous and vociferous complaints by those engaged in shiftwork, there is a paradoxical reluctance among employers to change pre-existing systems. However, between 20 and 30 per cent of workers dislike shiftwork so much that they are forced to abandon it – particularly those aged 45 years or more (Minors, 1988), and more employers are beginning to listen to their employees and to scientists. Some are now trying to implement more acceptable work schedules for their employees.

At present there are three main types of schedule: straight, non-rotating shifts; rapid rotating shifts; slow (weekly) rotating shifts. Chronobiologists agree that the best schedules must take into consideration the natural properties of our circadian rhythms. In this respect, two points must be considered – direction of rotation and the length of interval between phase shifts. Studies have shown that extending the 24 hour day/night cycle is more easily adjusted to than shortening the day/night cycle (Czeisler *et al*, 1982), so night workers are able to accommodate sleep disruption more satisfactorily by going to sleep as soon as they finish their shift – after the normal night-time hours, rather than staying up till around midday and going to sleep before normal sleep time. An improved shiftwork schedule would be one in which the shift changes advance in a clockwise direction – from morning shift to afternoon shift to evening shift and so on. It is necessary to take into account the time for adjustment to a change in shift. In most shiftwork systems this is usually one or two days, but the longer the interval the better.

There is still disagreement as to whether rapid shift rotation or slow rotation is better. Disruption of circadian rhythms caused by transmeridian flight is temporary because the rhythms have enough time to readjust to the new time zone. In rotating shiftwork, the rhythms are continually being disrupted. How well they can resynchronise to a new time schedule depends on the rate of rotation: the slower the rotation the longer the time rhythms have to adapt to the change. In slow rotating shifts, the time interval between each shift is generally only long enough for the rhythms to partially adapt – for example, it takes up to 12 days for the temperature rhythm to adjust to a time shift. This partial resynchronisation is potentially harmful to the rhythms which often do not fully adapt.

Arguments in favour of rapid rotation maintain that it avoids the problem of continual partial synchronisation of rhythms and is therefore a more satisfactory alternative. Although this strategy does avoid partial adaption, scientists are faced with the problem that the cumulative effect of rhythms in a continual state of flux may in the long term cause more harm than any short-term good. More importantly for the workers, rapid rotation causes great disruption to their social and domestic life, and this is why many prefer slow rotation. It may be physiologically more harmful to them, but it does accommodate their more immediate need for time for social and domestic pursuits.

Intervention schemes
At present there is no ideal solution to the problem of shiftwork. There are, however, some compensatory behaviours that can ease the disruption.

Napping Many shiftworkers resort to napping before, during or immediately following their shift to supplement their sleep. Employers in a number of Japanese companies are actively encouraging this and provide rooms in which employees may nap during their shift. However there are both positive and negative aspects to napping. On the positive side, it can lower levels of fatigue, increase performance capacity and diminish reduced alertness. On the negative side, it can cause 'sleep inertia' – the inertia felt immediately following a nap (though this is usually quickly overcome by the restorative benefits of the nap). Napping can also disrupt the subsequent main night's sleep and thus reduces its recuperative quality.

According to Akerstedt *et al* (1989) if you are a 'napper' you can benefit by taking naps at specific times according to your shift schedule. If the next main sleep is going to be taken on the following night, it is better not to take a nap. This ensures the main night's sleep is of good restorative quality. However if the following night is a working night it would be advisable to take an afternoon nap, to reduce the inevitable fatigue that accompanies night work.

Exercise   A number of studies on women have found that physical exercise can temper some ill effects of shiftwork. Their results have shown that regular, moderate physical training increases physical fitness and subsequently can reduce fatigue and musculoskeletal symptoms. There is also an increase in efficiency on memory-loaded tasks and subjective alertness. Further evidence indicates that the physiological effects of the exercise can speed up the process of resynchronisation of disrupted circadian rhythms, so that adapting to new shiftwork schedules can occur more quickly.

Changing practices for the future

At present, shiftwork is in some respects self-defeating. Instead of benefiting from higher turnover, employers are losing money through increased errors, accidents, sick leave, slower productivity and staff turnover. Employees too are beginning to realise the detrimental effect of shiftwork on their health by far overshadows any pecuniary benefit it may have. By its very nature, shiftwork will always entail physiological and psychological disruption, but the degree of disruption and the resulting threat to the health and safety of both the workers and the public can be tempered. In America, in particular, attempts are being made to achieve this: departments of chronobiology (the study of circadian rhythms) have been established and many concerned employers including the Philadelphia Police Force, the Federal Aviation Administration and various chemical plants are turning to the chronobiologists for advice about improving their shiftwork schedules. In Germany too, companies are beginning to recognise the gravity of the situation and offer their workers general check-ups and the opportunity to normalise their rhythms at regular two or three year intervals at special hospitals. Britain, unfortunately, has been rather slow to follow their example, but changes are beginning to be made. Altering the structure of long-established shiftwork schedules is likely to meet with resistance, but those who have already done so are aware of an increase in productivity and in addition often have a more content work force. While the concept of shiftwork in our society remains necessary, it need no longer be to the detriment of the health and safety of those involved, if only employers take these factors into account when planning their shifts.

References
Akerstedt, T., Torsvall, L., Gillberg, M. (1989) Sleep and Alertness – Chronobiological, Behavioural, and Medical Aspects of Napping. Raven, Press New York.
Alfredsson, L., Karasek, R., Theorell, T. (1982) Myocardial infarction risk and psychosocial work environment: an analysis of the male swedish working force. *Social Science Medicine*, **16**, 463–647.
Coffey, L.C., Skipper, J.K., Jung, F.D. (1988) Nurses and shiftwork: effects on job performance and job-related stress. *Journal of Advanced Nursing*, **13**, 245–54.
Czeisler, C.A., Moore-Ede, M.C., Coleman, R.M. (9182) Rotating shiftwork schedules that disrupt sleep are improved by applying circadian principles. *Science*, **217**, 460–63.
Knuttson, A., Akerstedt, T., Jonsson, B.G., Orth-Gormer, K. (1986) Increased risk of ischaemic heart disease in shift workers. *Lancet*, **2**, 89–91.
Minors, D.S. (1988) Practical applications of circadian rhythms to shiftwork. The Biological Clock – Current Approaches. Inprint (Litho) Ltd, Southampton.
Osald, I. (1980) Sleep as a restorative process: human clues. *Progress in Brain Research*, **54**, 279–88.
Reinberg, A., Vieux, N., Andlauer, P., Guillet, P., Nicolai, A. (9181) Tolerance of shiftwork, amplitude of circadian rhythms and ageing. Night and shiftwork: Biological and Social Aspects. Pergamon Press, Oxford.

Bibliography
Haider, M., Koller, M. Cervinka, R. (18) Night and Shiftwork: Long-Term Effects and their Prevention. Verlag Peter Lang, Frankfurt, Germany.
Monk, T..H. and Folkard, S. (Eds) (1985) Hours of Work. John Wiley, Chichester.
Reinberg, A., Vieux, N., Andlaver, P. (1981) Night and Shiftwork: Biological and Social Aspects. Pergamon Press, Oxford.
These books give a comprehensive account of the negative effects of shiftwork and current ideas on preventative techniques.

Acknowledgements
Thanks to Dr Colin M. Shapiro for his advice. Emma Fossey is currently supported by a grant from the Asthma Research Council. Further financial support was provided by the Edinburgh Sleep Research Trust.

Your Teaching Role

32

Building confidence: a development programme for newly qualified staff nurses

Sue Thame, BA

Independent Management Trainer, Pinner, Middlesex

When you first qualified as a staff nurse, would you have welcomed yet more training? The findings of a review conducted by Hillingdon Health Authority (1986) clearly showed that one of the major causes of dissatisfaction among nurses was the lack of training and education immediately after qualification. The authority therefore made it a priority to pioneer a development programme for newly qualified staff nurses.

Setting up the programme

In June 1987 Barbara Baker, an experienced nursing tutor, was appointed Senior Nurse Professional Development, with a remit to create a programme for newly qualified staff nurses. The key purpose was to prepare a more confident and skilled staff nurse for the future, and help with retention and recruitment.

The programme outline suggested a two year course (later amended to 14 months) and newly qualified staff nurses would be recruited both internally and nationally. They would be offered an attractive package: five days off-the-job training in management and interpersonal skills; three-monthly study days in their own selected subject areas; on-the-job support and counselling from a full-time nursing tutor; on-going written assignments; and planned four-monthly rotations between different wards. The nurses' individual development would be based on their own assessments of their areas of greatest need, drawn from a broad spectrum of learning objectives. Their choices would be made in consultation with the nurse tutor and their nurse managers. The heart of the programme was to be the on-the-job counselling and support. This programme outline has been fully implemented.

My involvement in this project came about by invitation from Barbara Baker. I was already working with Hillingdon on an extended programme for nurses to improve their communication skills. Mounting such a major project within tight deadlines could have been more than just a headache – it could have spelt disaster. The coordination and communication required was extensive – not least finding, within a year,

30 nurse managers who would enthusiastically accept and train a revolving nursing staff. The Authority, however, organised itself efficiently by establishing a steering group that could be effective across the district, co-opting people who were enthusiastic, believed in the basic concept and could communicate across the hospital complex. The steering group had to influence people with hard facts and persuasive argument to obtain the resources and commitments required.

Since the new programme was to be based on findings of Rogers and Lawrence (1987) it was essential that all those involved agreed the basic rationale behind it. There were also all the politics of organisational life that must be attended to, in order to manage an innovation like this successfully. Too often, the power games for managing innovation are dealt with *sotto voce*, as if it is not quite 'naice' to speak and think the politics of a situation through clearly. The steering group's composition ensured the delicacies of diplomacy would be addressed. Each hospital and the community was represented on the group by a senior nursing manager. There was a senior representative from the nurse planning committee, a tutor from post basic education and Barbara Baker herself.

The first programme

The first programme began in February 1988 and we have some measure of the impact on the initial five participants, all of whom have found the programme a positive experience. Perhaps the most noticeable strength of the programme is its clear learning objectives. For the first time there is a full picture of what kinds of development a newly qualified staff nurse requires, with real support in attaining those aims.

At the start of the course the nurses are given a 20 page document on guidelines and objectives of the course (Baker, 1987). Daunting? Perhaps – until they see and understand the treasures it offers. It is their route to learner-centred development, and to taking charge of their own development. There is a comprehensive description of the aims and structure of the course and a full listing of the range of learning objectives they can choose to pursue for themselves (Table 1). Later they receive a profiling instrument to help them assess their starting point across all the learning objectives – to select their priorities for development. The evaluation forms, which enable the nurses to monitor their own progress, are used at the end of their ward allocations.

This comprehensive documentation ensouls the philosophy being pioneered at Hillingdon, and if my reading of the literature is correct, they are pioneers within the NHS as a whole too. At the core of their approach is the belief, from their own experience, that an effective hospital service must be based on a workforce constantly aware of the need to learn and change. Responsibility of this kind must be shared between employer and employee, because neither, alone, can know what is best. Both sides must interact to identify individual and group learning needs and to meet those needs. Nurses have traditionally been spoon-fed their basic

---

Six Key Aims

1. Interpersonal skills

At the end of the course the nurse will have an appreciation of the factors involved in good communications and an increased awareness of self and others.

Four specific objectives are listed

eg, use a problem solving approach

: thinking skills

: transactional analysis

2. Management of patient care

At the end of the course the nurse will understand the principles of clinical management and the role and responsibility of the staff nurse.

The nurse will be able to draw up and administer the individual nursing care plans based on the nursing process following the pattern of assessing needs, planning nursing care programmes, delivery of the care and evaluation.

Seven specific objectives are listed

eg, identify features of stress and anxiety in patients and relatives

: signs of stress

: symptoms of stress

: stress in hospitals

3. Teaching and assessing

The nurses will have an understanding of the learning process and a basic knowledge and skill in teaching and assessing.

Fourteen specific objectives are listed

eg, identify the factors which stimulate and sustain motivation in learners

: needs, drives, motives

: need to achieve and fear of failure

: rewards and punishment

: nature and necessity of feedback

And so on with   Aim Four – Ward Management

Aim Five – Personnel Management

Aim Six – Nursing Research

Table 1. Staff nurse development aims and learning objectives.

training in an authoritarian teaching environment that ill-prepares them for the dynamic responsibilities they have to face on the ward. Their further education has been conspicuously neglected. Now, when their demands for more training are being heard, the time is also right for them to collaborate in shaping their own further development.

Shifting into this mode of joint-responsibility requires a bit of a helping hand from those who have more experience and the will to show the way. Practical tools are also needed, like the guidelines given to participants, which show nurses how to start assessing themselves, start discussing their progress with other more senior people and making judgements for themselves on what to pursue for their own development.

The Hillingdon programme of self-development is supported by an off-the-job programme in which the nurses attend a five-day course with an emphasis on raising their self-awareness. This involves profiles, questionnaires and exercises which introduce them to different models and languages for understanding their thinking style and behavioural styles (Table 2). The nurses find the introduction to this approach exciting because for most of them psychology is a new world – and this approach involves the psychology of health and self-confidence through self-awareness, rather than the psychology of illness.

The 'B' Model (O'Neill, unpublished).
The Colours Model (Rhodes and Thame, 1988).
Transactional Analysis (Harris, 1973).
Temperaments Model for Stress (Thame, unpublished).
Maslow's Hierarchy of Needs (1954).
Theory X and Y (McGregor, 1960)
Hygiene and Motivation Factors (McGregor, 1960).

Table 2. Models used in the staff development programme.

Underlying the variety of approaches is a common thread – the unravelling of the processes of management and communication. The key to development, as we see it, is systems learning; recognising patterns within different kinds of data, so that knowledge from one situation can be transferred to the next. Although this is central to the nursing process, many nurses find it difficult to understand and apply. This is a special field of research and study by our consultancy (Rhodes and Thame, 1988), so our knowhow fitted well with the aims set out in the staff development programme.

Self-confidence
The first week of the programme devotes a lot of time to issues of self-confidence. On the fourth day there is a major exercise originally devised for salesmen, which involves a brain-storm in which the nurses generate lists of adjectives to describe their personalities to one another. They sort and categorise the listings into positive and negative attributes, based on observed behaviours during the course, then identify how each individual can work to capitalise on their strengths and improve on their weaknesses. Handling this kind of exercise must be done skillfully to

ensure the individuals can work together honestly and supportively – its successful completion gives the nurses a real insight into the subtleties of self-assessment and leads to self-evaluation later in this programme.

The final day of the first week focuses on identifying key objectives for each nurse to work on. Although this is a detailed piece of work which involves considering many learning objectives, it is rewarding for the nurses because it sets the path for the kinds of tasks each must keep in the forefront of their mind. The week finishes with a visit to their new wards.

On-job learning

During their first months on the job the nurses are asked to keep a personal diary to encourage them in the processes of inner reflection. It is suggested that they write notes on their thoughts and feelings, what upsets them, what gives them pleasure, who they learn from, who makes difficulties, and so on. They are then asked to complete written assignments from the diaries, applying the behavioural models to real life happenings on the ward. This encourages them to look more objectively at situations which may have upset them at the time.

Throughout these weeks on the ward the nurses are visited and encouraged by the programme's nurse tutor, David Richards. Since this is David's first tutoring post, he has had to find his way, like the young nurses in the wards. This is especially exciting because it demonstrates the best qualities of joint development. David understands the ward situation, and his caring approach means the nurses have someone to turn to who knows the difficulties they face. At the same time, he can view their development not as their direct manager but indirectly, working with managers to enhance the nurses' learning opportunities.

Review and preparation for assignments

Our first study day, held in May 1988, produced encouraging developments. We began by reviewing the nurses' assignments, and heard some moving accounts of how they had tackled difficult situations using the behaviour models to help them analyse other people's intentions and shape their own responses. One particularly moving account told how one of the nurses encountered a desperately ill female patient who appeared to be showing aggression. Other nurses were struggling to restrain her, and the scene was violent and distressing. The nurse looked beyond the appearances, and recognised that the woman was terrified. A loving and calming hand was stretched out to her, soothed her and she became peaceful. A short while later she died. The nurse felt glad to have brought peace at the end.

The next activity was a series of role-plays through which the nurses could prepare for their next assignments. This involved their interviewing a senior member of staff to obtain information about a subject area they particularly wanted to investigate, linked to one of their learning objectives. For example, if they wished to extend their understanding of manpower management, they would interview a senior personnel officer. The nurses' first reactions were fear – they do not have much contact with senior people's roles, but after we had finished the role-plays they felt confident and excited at the prospects.

These assignments began in May 1988, and the first few months' progress caused great enthusiasm among the nurses. Later they attended the ENB 998 Teaching and Assessing course, and did a variety of assignments based around their six weekly off-the-job study days.

Developments since the programme's introduction

The nurses who joined the first programme have now graduated, and all plan to pursue their professional development through the Diploma in Nursing. The reports of their work have all been excellent and they have developed their confidence and skills in both practical nursing and communications.

This programme which commenced in March 1988 has run successfully, enabling 45 staff nurses to gain further development. However, due to the many changes in the NHS, our Health Authority and the education division, it has been necessary to discontinue the course in its present form with effect from March 1991.

All is not lost, though. Due to the noticeable benefits, the service side were very keen to continue with staff nurse development. Therefore a three month course commenced in September 1990 for Hillingdon Health Authority staff only. They are seconded from their area of appointment. We have maintained the same philosophy, aims and structure of the previous course. The course commences with a five day foundation and then five study days covering the same topics as in the previous course. The ENB 998 Teaching and Assessing in Clinical Practice has now been omitted.

References

Baker, B. (1987) *Guidelines of Course and Objectives*. Hillingdon Health Authority, London.
Harris, T. (1973) *I'm OK, Your OK*. Pan, London.
Herzberg, F. (1966) *Working and the Nature of Man*. World Publishing, Cleveland, Ohio.
McGregor, D. (1960) *The Human Side of Enterprise*. McGraw-Hill, New York.
Maslow, A.H. (1954) *Motivation and Personality*. Harper and Row, New York.
O'Neill, H. (Unpublished) *The 'B' Model*. Research for London Borough of Hillingdon.
Rhodes, J. and Thame, S. (1988) *The Colours of Your Mind*. Collins, London.
Rogers, J. and Lawrence, J. (1987) *Continuing Professional Education for Qualified Nurses, Midwives and Health Visitors*. Ashdale Press and Austen Cornish Publishers, London.
Thame, S. (Unpublished) Temperament Model For Stress.

Sue Thame, can be contacted at:
Sue Thame, Joint Development Resources,
24 Cecil Park, Pinner, Middx HA5 5HH.
Tel: 081-866 1262.

33

From text book to reality: student nurse training needs in stoma care

Teresa M.D. Finlay, RGN, OncNC
Ward Sister, John Radcliffe Hospital

Undergoing surgery and the formation of a stoma is a drastic life event for the patient concerned, no matter why the stoma is necessary. Numerous problems, both physical and psychological are encountered, including altered body image, lowering of self-esteem and self-concept, denial and psychosexual neuroses and changes in excretion habits, dietary habits, and day-to-day physical and social activities. While the stoma therapist provides a continuing service of care and support for patients and their families, nurses working in areas specialising in gut surgery are the patients' first line teachers, counsellors and advisers, preparing them for and helping them begin a new phase of their life. "Teaching is of paramount importance if the . . . nurse is to . . . improve the care of the stoma patients" (Elcoat, 1986).

Nursing students allocated to these areas will be unable to gain the skills of an experienced stoma therapist, and indeed they do not need to. They do, however, need to gain some insight into the difficulties encountered by these patients, and to learn how to effectively establish 'continence' of newly formed stomas for inexperienced patients, or how to maintain it for ostomists debilitated by further disease or surgery.

Almost all nursing students new to surgical nursing have never seen a stoma other than in text books, and have many preconceived ideas based on myth, rumour and fantasy. Their own fears and self-image concepts tend to influence their ideas and approach to ostomists initially, and these need to be considered so that they can begin to effectively consider their patients' needs. "The aim for learners in the clinical environment is to be able to meet patients' needs competently and independently" (Ewan and White, 1984).

Preparation
Theory Before acquiring the practical and psychological skills involved, it is vital that students have a working knowledge of the anatomy and physiology of the digestive and urinary tracts. They also need to understand the diseases predisposing people to the formation of a stoma, and the siting and type formed in consequence, if they are to

have some concept of the implications for patients. Diagrammatic representation of anatomy and expected anatomical changes with the stoma's formation are useful tools and should be available for repeated easy reference by the students, both independently and in teaching situations.

The practical aspects of how each type of stoma works need to be considered – students must understand that a urostomy is a diversion of the urinary flow from the bladder via a small section of the ileum, isolated from the remaining small bowel, with continuous flow of urine. An ileostomy diverts the faecal stream from the remaining ileum or colon, passing liquid faeces almost continuously, while a colostomy will pass more formed stool less frequently – depending on which area of the colon is diverted to the skin. These considerations all affect the choice of appliance for patients, and management of their stomas.

Psychology   It is now widely recognised and understood that the psychological implications of having a stoma are severe. New ostomists' body-image is altered drastically, and they experience anger, grieving and loss of self-esteem. Students must be aware that these emotions are common among new ostomists, though not usually until they have recovered from the immediate postoperative period (usually two to three days). So that students may begin to consider patients' psychological care, they must develop thinking, listening and responding skills with consideration of their own self-awareness. This process can be extremely threatening and is in itself an enormous area to tackle – these skills are attained with years of experience, but the foundations are often laid for students in this area of experience. Informal group sessions on self-esteem and perception, progressing to altered body image, either with the stoma therapist or an experienced nurse, will encourage students to think about themselves – "how would I feel if . . .". Where appropriate, after discussing individual feelings and perceptions, mini role-play could be used, such as getting students to wear an appliance for a time to see what it feels like, thus heightening their awareness. In these areas, the leader of the teaching session must be aware of individual learners and have respect for them. "Psychological safety is essential for learners if they are to function at their best . . . this implies lack of threat and the ability to react honestly without fear of humiliation" (Quinn, 1980). There is a wealth of literature on stoma care to which students may be referred (see Bibliography).

Learning
Practical skills   As it is recognised that newly formed stomas cause patients a great deal of anxiety, the first practical experience students encounter needs to be considered carefully. While they may be eager to see and tackle the 'real thing' as regards emptying or changing an appliance, the patient's needs are paramount. In the first days and weeks

following surgery, patients are becoming acquainted with many new and painful emotions, and need to learn to deal with their stoma themselves. If an inexperienced nurse either chooses naively, or is sent unwittingly, to care for a patient, including removing and refitting a stoma appliance, there is a great potential for the situation to become disastrous. Possible difficulties abound, such as inability to fit a new appliance, causing trauma to the stoma or skin; confusing patients with a poor or different method which they will undoubtedly pick up; and most traumatic, causing distressing leakage and/or soiling either immediately or some time later, only reinforcing the patient's feelings of being dirty, a lesser person, no longer 'normal' or socially acceptable. Patients may also express many emotions and need psychological support and reassurance, signs of which inexperienced nurses will not necessarily recognise or be able to respond to.

It is vital that each student accompanies an experienced nurse as an observer initially. The nurse should consider which patients are more or less likely to be able to cope with the presence of an observer, and discriminate accordingly: in assessing patients' needs, involvement of partners, carers and/or families must be considered. While some individuals may strive for independence, others may wish or need to involve those close to them in learning to deal with and accept their stoma from the beginning. This must be pointed out to students, so that in planning patients' care, times for teaching techniques and demonstrating, as well as interviews with their nurse and/or stoma therapist can be arranged so as to accommodate partners or carers.

Having explained the procedure to suitable patients and confirmed with them that they are happy for a student to observe, the nurse should state the objective, run through a sequence of 'part skills' and then demonstrate the skills of actually emptying and/or changing the appliance, step by step. This provides valuable information both for the student and the patient present.

When the student has watched the nurse performing these skills and concurrently interacting with the patient – ideally on several occasions – she or he should then be ready to try the sequence. An experienced ostomist who can talk the student through the process is a boon, as they have usually dealt with many of the psychological problems and are adept at handling their stoma. Ideal situations seldom present themselves, however, and again nurses must take care in allocating patients to students. A patient with whom a student has been able to develop a rapport and with whom the nurse has previously demonstrated should be allocated where possible. "It is important to be sensitive to the patient's feelings in a teaching situation and provide ways in which he can opt out without feeling uncooperative" (Quinn, 1980).

In performing the procedure students will naturally be anxious and cling to the 'step-by-step' sequence demonstrated previously. It is useful for patients to have a supply of appliances selected for them in their own locker, as this minimises confusion for them and their carers, and students will not have as much anxiety in selecting the appropriate appliance. During the procedure the teacher must "give verbal rather than physical guidance as the student must learn control of their own muscles" (Quinn, 1980). After it is completed, feedback must be given in a friendly, non-threatening way, using praise and encouragement, and away from the patient environment.

Supervision must be continued until students both demonstrate and express confidence in changing and emptying appliances. They need to be encouraged to continue seeking advice and guidance without feeling they have failed, if they encounter a new problem. As both student and patient grow in experience and confidence, the student will be able to adapt the newly acquired skill to different situations with less need for supervision. It must be stressed, however, that praise and encouragement are vital to back up and reinforce confidence and dexterity.

Counselling skills   In addition to the anxiety of learning the practical aspects of stoma care, students are often heard to recount, "I just didn't know what to say . . .". While it is hoped that some awareness will be gained, there will undoubtedly be situations that arise when students caring for patients with new stomas are confronted with an emotional situation they feel uneasy about and unable to handle. It is useful for students to either accompany an experienced nurse when admitting a patient, and/or the stoma therapist on a preoperative visit. The experienced practitioner's skills in counselling and preparing a patient for surgery and the formation of a stoma can then be observed. In the initial interview the nurse will enquire of the patient what his or her understanding of the forthcoming surgery is, and then discuss the procedures and likely outcome of the expected operation. This allows the student to gain some insight into how potentially painful or embarrassing subjects are approached and dealt with in the immediate situation. Students should be assured that they will not be able to deal with every patient's anxieties personally, and that they should know when and where to seek help. Patients' continuing need for counselling after their stay in hospital should be pointed out, and information and resources detailed. Where possible, it is helpful for students to meet patients with whom they have been involved after discharge from hospital, either in follow-up clinics or with the stoma therapist, possibly at home in the community.

A cumulative process

Learning the skills involved in stoma care is a cumulative process, occurring over a long period of time and many encounters. It is difficult to achieve skill in this area and even impossible to teach to students effectively during a few weeks' specific nursing experience. Caring for and teaching patients in itself is a difficult undertaking, with so many fragile emotions and needs involved, so how much more are the problems compounded by trying to meet students' learning needs as well? It is difficult to find suitable conditions, but provided that nurses realise that there will never be a perfect time, setting or patient, and available resources are used to their full potential, students can and do manage to "develop cognitive strategies which will enable them to 'think on the job', to create innovative solutions to unusual problems which arise, and to generalise their professional and personal experiences to responsive nursing practice" (Ewan and White, 1984).

References
Elcoat, C. (1986) Stoma Care Nursing. Balliere Tindall, London.
Ewan, C. and White, R. (9186) Teaching Nursing. Croom Helm, Beckenham.
Open Technology Project (1986) Interpersonal Skills. Continuing Nurse Education Programme, London and Manchester.
Quinn, F.M. (1980) Principles and Practice of Nurse Education. Croom Helm, Beckenham.

Bibliography
Alterescu, V., Watt, R.C., Smith, D.B. (1985) The ostomy. *American Journal of Nursing*, **85**, 11, 1242–53.
    An excellent all round guide to stoma care.
Dyer, S. (1988) Development of stoma care. *Professional Nurse*, **3**, 7, 226–30.
    A useful reference source for students.
Dyer, S. (1988) Stoma care: choosing the right appliance. *Professional Nurse*, **3**, 8, 278–83.
    A good product guide.
Kennedy, J. (1984) Students and cancer. *Nursing Mirror*, **159**, 2, 27.
    A useful analysis of student attitudes and their effects on patient care.
Medicine Group UK (1987) Ostomy and Ostomy Patients. Medicine Group UK, Oxford.
    A useful book to recommend to students.
North, K.L. (1987) Stoma care. *Nursing,*, 3, 21, 308.
    A useful reference guide.
Sundeen, S.J. *et al* (1985) Nurse-Client Interaction: Implementing the Nursing Process. Mosby, St. Louis.
    A valuable guide to the use of the nursing process in stoma care.

34

The age gap: teaching students about health education for the elderly

Beverley Holloway, MA, RGN, RNT, Cert Ed
Staff Development Facilitator, BUPA Hospital, Portsmouth

Evidence shows that the average age of the UK's population is increasing (Phillipson, 1985). With continuing general improvements in healthcare helping people to live longer, the elderly are an increasingly large group of the hospital population. Student nurses will therefore be exposed to large numbers of elderly people throughout their training and future careers, so it is important that aspects of caring for the elderly well, rather than simply the elderly sick are considered.

When teaching student nurses about the health education needs of the elderly, the teacher is confronted with the same problems that have made the appropriate and effective provision of health education for elderly people so difficult. This in itself can provide a powerful experiential tool with which to examine the issues surrounding this area of health promotion. These problems include ageism, stereotyping and a difference between normative and expressed needs.

The students reach their care of the elderly module at the end of the first year. At this stage, each has experienced three clinical placements: a basic care ward – which may be medical, surgical, or elderly nursing, – followed by medical and surgical placements. Consequently, some will have already come into contact with elderly people.

Students' attitudes
A useful starting point when teaching student nurses about health promotion in elderly people is to encourage exploration of their own attitudes to them. Despite the fact that many are familiar with elderly people on a personal level, or have worked in nursing and rest homes, and claim an affection for them, accurate analysis of perceptions often reveals issues which need to be discussed and clarified. Skeet (1985), claims that: "Looming over all these major issues is ageism – the deeply rooted discrimination against the elderly . . . one source of this prejudice is the fear among young and middle-aged people of joining the ranks of the ignored and the dispensable. . ." To allow student nurses to function with elderly people they must be given the opportunity, through

discussion, to free themselves from the constraints of an ageist approach. This does not detract from the effect of the attitudes of the elderly themselves, and students need to be made aware of the often fatalistic view adopted by the elderly: Muir-Gray (1983) found that some elderly patients felt they should avoid exercise as 'the body will wear out'.

Students are asked to write down their feelings about being old, and how they imagine they will be when they reach old age. Responses vary; some students openly admit they are frightened by the prospect of being old and alone; others feel they would be frustrated by not being able to do things they wanted. Overwhelmingly however, students find it almost impossible to imagine what it is like to be elderly, and it is generally found enlightening to discuss what effects this inability to imagine has on the care given to the elderly.

A further productive exercise is to ask students to describe elderly stereotypes; these frequently resemble those cited by Brearley (1975) "the rigid, inflexible, dogmatic elder or the charitable, loyal, upright figure." A recent addition to this list was described by one student nurse as "a cantankerous old so-and-so". The effects of stereotyping can then be discussed, for as Brearley points out "it is a small step from the acceptance of the stereotype to the adoption of it personally."

Thus, attitudes and images, particularly in the negative sense with ageism and stereotyping, can be raised as important influences in health promotion for the elderly. Comparing different perceptions of needs of the elderly appears to generate interest and concern for them in the students. They are asked to determine what they see as the health education needs of the elderly. They are then asked to examine either normative needs or felt and expressed needs. Various methods of data collection are used, as the students feel appropriate, and this will usually include interviews with professionals and elderly people, literature reviews, and amassing available health education or promotion material.

Role play

An alternative method, depending on time availability, involves dividing the students into small groups, and asking them to imagine that they are either a group of elderly people or nurses working in a care of the elderly unit. They are then asked what they feel the health education needs of the elderly might be. Each group can be carefully selected depending on their responses to how they feel about becoming old themselves. The exercise appears to work well in that each group tends to identify different aspects of health education.

Students are usually surprised to discover a gulf between normative needs and expressed needs of the elderly. Their own beliefs are frequently similar to those of health professionals, such as emphasis on hypothermia or the need for mobility. The greatest impact, however, occurs when the students analyse the responses of the well elderly people they have interviewed (where possible), and discover the elderly themselves are less concerned with physical or even specific aspects of health, but see social and psychological health as most important. Overwhelmingly the elderly articulate their problems in financial terms, expressing particular needs such as assistance with telephone installation and bills. The lack of awareness regarding the services and schemes that are available to assist them financially enforces the sometimes inadequate or inappropriate provision of health education or promotion. To simply criticise existing provision would not only be a negative exercise, but would also deny the valuable contribution made by many groups, organisations and individuals concerned with caring and providing for the health of the elderly.

The next activity requires the students to find out what exists in terms of health education, and who is making the provision. They are asked to find examples from each tier of the national framework which exists to meet the needs of the elderly. At central government level they can explore provision made by the Department of Health, and that of Social Security, at a local level how the NHS and local authorities provide for their elderly, and – importantly – the work of the voluntary organisations.

Purpose-made materials

Apart from a global view of how organisations work, students are encouraged to examine specifically produced materials for the elderly, such as 'Helping Yourself to Health', a resource pack produced as part of the Pensioners' Link Health Education Project (1987). Our district health authority's education department is extremely helpful in allowing students to explore the resources they have on offer for groups and individuals within the district. With this information, the students can identify and piece together a picture of what material is available locally for health professionals to use when providing elderly people with health education. At this point it is useful to look at the disciplines involved, and it is important to air feelings about other professional groups, as this may uncover negative attitudes. An understanding and acceptance of contributions made by all the different groups and individuals encountering the elderly is desirable to maximise and coordinate efforts. Nurses, working in a variety of settings, form one of the many groups, and the student nurses are asked to think about their possible contribution, before going on to list other groups whom they believe contribute to the health education of the elderly.

Planning to meet needs

As a final exercise the students are divided into groups of three or four and asked to draw up a plan to meet the health education needs of the elderly. They are asked to look at what provision is required nationally, locally and individually and to say how they feel this could be best achieved. The students are also asked to think about how they could provide health education for those already in hospital. It is encouraging that by this stage they usually state the importance of listening to what the patient says. Having shared their ideas, the session closes with a look at the work of Brocklehurst (1976) and Phillipson (1985) whose contributions to this field have been significant.

While these exercises have been designed to be carried out in the classroom-based setting, they are readily adaptable for use in clinical placements, be it in hospital or the community. Caring for the elderly has historically been seen as lacking both appeal and glamour. However, more recently there has been a thrust towards promoting interest and a positive image in this field. It is hoped that by teaching today's students about this vital area and by facilitating their confrontation of the issues surrounding the elderly, they will be able to competently make useful contributions to an already committed team.

References
Brearley, C.P. (1975) Social Work, Ageing and Society. Routledge and Kegan Paul Ltd., London.
Brocklehurst, J.C. (1976) Health education in the elderly. *Journal of the Institute of Health Education,* **14,** 4, 115–20.
Muir-Gray, J. (1983) Beliefs and attitudes – the ageing process (2), August 17, *Nursing Mirror,* 36–37.
Pensioners' Link Health Education Project (1987) 'Helping Yourself To Health'. Pensioners Link.
Phillipson, C. (1985) Developing a health education strategy with older people. *Journal of the Institute of Education,* **23,** 3, 184–87.
Skeet, M. (1985) 'Some international concepts of old age'. *Nursing,* **41.**

Bibliography
The following sources of information are recommended to those wishing to further explore this subject.
Garrett, G. (1987) Health Needs of the Elderly, Macmillan, London.
   An extremely readable book, this would be an excellent place to start for anyone wanting to gain an overview of the health needs of the elderly.
McClymont, M., Thomas, S., Denham, M. (1986) Health Visiting and the Elderly. Churchill Livingstone, Edinburgh.
   A useful book, not only for health visitors, but for any health professional wanting to understand more about the application of health education theory to practice with the elderly.
Muir-Gray, J. and McKenzie, H. (1986) Caring For Older People. Penguin, Harmondsworth.
   A comprehensive, practical book, focusing clearly on the health needs of the elderly. The information is useful to professionals, families with elderly members, and the elderly themselves.
Tinker, A. (1986) The Elderly in Modern Society, Longman, Harlow.
   A background of how the elderly have come to be in their present position in society. The book not only presents information clearly, but looks at existing literature and relevant research.
   For further resources, or specific information the reader is advised to contact their local Health Education Department, local voluntary organisations such as Age Concern or the Health Education Authority.

35

A step in the right direction: providing supernumerary placements for nursing students

Peter Savage, BSc (Hons) RMN, RGN, PGCEA, DPSN
Nurse Tutor, Southampton University College of Nursing, Southampton

Despite the upheaval and misunderstandings surrounding Project 2000, it could be argued these proposals merely place nurse education on a par with higher and professional educational systems. Concepts which appear revolutionary to nurses, such as supernumerary status, educationally directed experience, research consideration in educational input and clinical practice are traditional practices for many of our professional colleagues. One unmistakable conclusion is that 'traditional' preparation of learner nurses is antiquated – the present three year apprentice system can be traced (cynics may say unchanged) to Nightingale in the 1860s.

The life of a student nurse

The world of the student nurse has been well researched. Melia's (1982) famed 'tell it as it is' suggests much student time is spent as part of the labour force 'getting the job done', but with inadequate information and while trying to learn the social rules of the ward. In the psychiatric sector Bissell (1984) identified a high incidence of student burn-out due to loss of ideals and "a personal surrender to the external realities of the job". Interestingly, events which students perceive as most stressful are employee- not educationally-related, such as understaffing and being shown up by other staff (Birch, 1983). Most of a student's time is clinically based and Davis (1983) cites ward sisters as important role-models for learners. If the crux of psychiatric nursing is interpersonal skills (Peplau, 1962), considerable research evidence suggests sisters/charge nurses offer poor role-models (Altschul, 1972; Cormack, 1976; MacIlwaine, 1983). Uptake of nursing literature and research by senior nurses may be at an embarrassingly low level (Wells, 1983).

The scheme described in this article was developed in the elderly care unit of Knowle hospital, a large, closing down psychiatric hospital with the common problems of staff shortages and low morale. Students had been allocated for 12 weeks to a long-stay psychogeriatric ward, and used as a 'pair of hands' in a task-orientated care system. With the cooperation of the unit clinical manager it was agreed only one learner at a time need be rostered to the ward. Thus, if three learners are allocated to the ward, each spends four weeks on rostered service; the remaining eight weeks are supernumerary, when the students are allocated to the clinical unit and do not appear on the off-duty of any ward. To compensate the ward for this loss of person hours, extra nursing assistant time is allocated. Some managers have argued that increased permanent staff time is easier to manage than the often erratic flowthrough of student nurses. This supernumerary period is called 'the programme'.

The programme

Each learner is allocated a clinical supervisor/mentor - initially, six supervisors were selected from the unit, and their preparation was largely through individual discussion with the author, though all had previously completed the local assessors course. Six supervisors were considered adequate, as a maximum of three students are allocated to the programme, and it is also relatively easy to maintain communications with a small group. With hindsight however, six is too small a number, and has been seriously depleted by staff movement, holidays and sickness. Thus, eight to 10 supervisors are required to ensure personal supervisorship to three students at the same time. Unfortunately this means supervisors may spend lengthy periods without a student, which may mean they get out of touch with students and the programme. An alternative would be to allocate two students per supervisor, which decreases the need for supervisors but increases their workload. Northcott (1989) has described a structured mentor preparation course which would be more cost-effective.

Learning objectives: care of the elderly programme

• Demonstrate how nurses can promote an aspect(s) of health of a patient(s) within this clinical area.

Table 1. Example of an objective for the programme.

Learners, in personal interview with a tutor, are given objectives for the programme based on the nursing competencies (Table 1) and a menu of people, places and skill resources relevant to elderly care. To help students meet their objectives, they are expected to meet their tutor and supervisor, separately, at least once a week and to hold a weekly seminar with other programme students. Each student also completes a learning diary based on the learning cycle described by Honey (1988; Table 2).

During the weekly tutorials the diary provides an opportunity for students, with their tutor or supervisor, to reflect on learning experiences and, with guidance and supervision, contract future learning experiences. The diary can also be used to stimulate discussion during the tutorials: Table 2 shows sample entries. In the first example the student had attended a lecture about caring from the carers of elderly people, and considered it an important learning event. The tutor was able to help the student to reflect upon that learning, encouraging understanding, as well as direct the student to the relevant literature.

Date	Event	Conclusions	Learning objectives	Action plan
	A descriptive account of what happened during the activity	What did you learn from the event?	What learning objectives relate to your conclusions?	What will you do with this information?
	Lecture on caring for the carer. Discussion with tutor about the subject.	Aware of stressors on carer. Important to support carer. Important to consider family/ social factors not just patient's condition. Need to meet needs of family.	1 & 2	Read notes from tutor, obtain references from library. Discuss topic with CPN. Arrange to visit self-help group and discuss with organiser.
	Visit and discussion with sister on long-stay ward about breakfast routine ie, one nurse stays in dining room to serve meal to patients as they arrive for meal. Other nurses help patients from bed to dining room.	Patients have meal when they are ready, not when staff are. Breakfast time is pleasant and quieter. Takes less time to get patients prepared for the day.	8	As a staff nurse on similar ward I'd introduce a breakfast routine like this one.

Table 2. The learning diary.

The student was also able to visit a local self-help group and discuss that experience with a group organiser. In this example the 'action plan' led to the next 'event', but this does not need to be the case, indeed students have included long-term plans, such as things they intend to do when qualified or on their next ward (second entry, Table 2). The contract between student and supervisor or tutor is effectively a verbal one and is in keeping with the design elements of andragogy proposed by Knowles (1984; Table 3).

Improvement in care

The programme has been running since January 1989, and while student-client contact has clearly reduced, the quality of the contact has increased. There are many examples of this qualitative improvement in care, including the instigation of validation therapy. This occurred when one student read about the subject in the nursing press, then contacted nurse researchers in another hospital to gather more information. Later, while allocated to an elderly care ward, she educated ward staff about validation therapy, and with their support its techniques were implemented into the care of selected clients. Students have also been involved in the setting up and running of reality orientation (RO) groups. The students, under direction of the tutor and supervised by clinical staff, using published assessment procedures such as Rimmer (1984), assess clients' suitability for the groups then participate in and lead the groups. Finally, at the end of the 12 week placement, the students evaluate client behaviour and the effectiveness of the group and the RO techniques.

The condition of the contract between student and supervisor/tutor.	
Elements	**Requirements**
Climate	Mutuality, respectful collaborative, informal
Planning	Mechanism for mutual planning
Diagnosis of needs	Mutual self-diagnosis
Formulation of objectives	Mutual negotiation
Design	Sequenced in terms of readiness. Problem units
Activities	Experiential techniques (inquiry)
Evaluation	Mutual re-diagnosis of needs and measurement of programme

Table 3. The design elements of andragogy, from Knowles (1984).

Students on the programme have learned how to utilise and discuss nursing research reports, as in the case of validation therapy, and have presented prècis of research reports in the unit teaching sessions. It is anticipated that research critiques will be a more common part of these sessions now a research appreciation component has been introduced into our post-qualified RMN courses. Instead of students' energy, time and morale being devoted to 'getting the job done' it is now devoted to learning nursing. One other potential benefit of the programme, particularly for the unit manager, is that many of the students have said they would like to return to nursing elderly people when qualified. Learner evaluation of the programme has mainly been positive.

Problems

There are, of course, problems with such a programme, such as supervisors expecting students to spend too much time in a particular area. Nursing is essentially practical, and students must have an opportunity to practise their skills. Such problems may be overcome by supervisors and students establishing specific outcome criteria for each competency, so both know the standard required from the student; Table 4 shows one such performance criteria for the health promotion competency.

Learning objectives
Demonstrate how nurses can promote an aspect(s) of health of a patient(s) within this clinical area.

Performance criteria
Assist and encourage allocated patients to participate in mobility activities eg, dancing, ball throwing, keep fit, during afternoon sessions.

Table 4. Examples of objectives for programme and possible performance criteria.

A recent addition to the programme has been client allocation, which was a response to uncertainty in both students and supervisors as to exactly what was expected from students. The student is allocated two clients within the clinical responsibility of the supervisor for the duration of the programme, enabling the supervisor to directly supervise the student who has ample time to design and implement care plans.

Again the emphasis is on quality not quantity as the student is expected to use a nursing model and published assessment procedures. Additionally, nursing goals and actions are expected to follow the guidelines given by Binnie *et al* (1984). Another possible development to increase students' and supervisors' awareness of learning could be the use of a process recording device (Open Tech Project, 1986). This would supplement the learning diary, while qualitative aspects of student-client interactions could be analysed in tutorials and seminars.

The menu has altered considerably since the programme began and is now more multidisciplinary and community orientated. Most of these changes have been generated by the students and supervisors. This type of 'grounded theory' curriculum development has the advantage of giving some 'ownership' to the participants, but could get out of hand if resources are not audited for their educational value. Additionally, the assessment and feedback of the students' performance are requirements of good educational practice. Initially, pre-existing ward reports were used for this purpose, but are manifestly irrelevant to the programme. A replacement document based on Steinaker and Bell's (1979) experiential taxonomy (Table 5) has now been introduced. The anchor statements for the five levels of competency are based on the experiential taxonomy levels of "exposure, participation, identification, internalisation and dissemination". Students' attainment levels can be plotted by their supervisor, producing an attainment profile for each student. This emphasises a role conflict, in that the supervisor is also assessor, but pragmatism dictates this is the only option, although it does illuminate a need for supervisor support, update and discussion time.

Unit 2 programme - care of the elderly mentally infirm							
Student's name........................			Assessor's name..................				
Competency	**Performance criteria**	**Level of competency**					
	Statement of behaviour (to be) demonstrated	1. Observed by learner	2. Performed under maximum supervision	3. Performed under minimum supervision	5. Able to disseminate information or teach others about competency	Assessor's initials	Learner's initials / Date
1. Demonstrate how nurses can promote aspect(s) of health for a patient within this clinical area.							

Table 5. Assessment profile documentation.

A transition towards Project 2000

In general terms, the selection and preparation of supervisors for Project 2000 will need to be highly specific and extensive. Ideally, only those who can demonstrate clinical competence and evidence of professional update should be considered for supervisorship. In psychiatric nursing we should consider developing new and externally accredited courses in subjects such as counselling skills, to demonstrate our academic and practical usefulness, and nurse teachers should demonstrate use of and/or participation in nursing research as evidence of competency to facilitate courses in professional education. This supernumerary programme is a transition from traditional nurse training towards the preparation required by Project 2000. As with all transitions, the process is dynamic, at times racing forward with good ideas, at others falling back due to poorly thought out ideas. A lengthy period of trying out, understanding and developing such schemes is required for tutors and clinical staff prior to the demands of studentship under Project 2000.

References
Altschul, A.T. (1972) Nurse Patient Interactions. Churchill-Livingstone, Edinburgh.
Binnie, A. *et al* (1984) Systematic Approach to Nursing Care - Course. Open University Press, Milton Keynes.
Birch, J.A. (1983) Anxiety and conflict in nurse education. In: Davis, B.D. below.
Bissell, B.P. *et al* (1984) Helping students survive institutionalised patients and burn-out in staff in chronic psychiatric care facilities. *Perspectives in Psychiatric Care*, **22**, 3, 108-14.
Cormack, D. (1976) Psychiatric Nursing Observed. RCN, London.
Davis, B.D. (1983) Student nurses' perceptions of their significant others. In: Davis, B.D. (Ed) Research into Nurse Education. Croom Helm, London.
Honey, P. (1988) You are what you learn. *Nursing Times*, **84**, 36, 34-35.

Knowles, M.S. (1984) The Adult Learner - a Neglected Species. Gulf, Houston.

MacIlwaine, H. (1983) The communication patterns of female neurotic patients with nursing staff in psychiatric units of general hospitals. In: Wilson-Barnett, J. (Ed) (1983) Nursing Research. John Wiley, Chichester.

Melia, K.M. (1982) Tell it as it is - qualitative methodology and nursing research: understanding the student nurse's world. *Journal of Advanced Nursing*, **7**, 4, 327-35.

Northcott, N. (1989) Mentorship in nurse education. *Nursing Standard*, **3**, 24, 25-28.

Open Tech Project (1986) Interpersonal Skills. HMSO, London.

Peplau, H.E. (1962) Interpersonal technique: the crux of psychiatric nursing. *American Journal of Nursing*, **62**, 6, 50-54.

Rimmer, L. (1984) Reality Orientation - Principles and Practice. Winslow Press, Bicester.

Steinaker, N. and Bell, R. (1979) The Experiential Taxonomy: a new approach to teaching and learning. Academic Press, London.

Wells, J. (1983) A survey of uptake by senior nursing staff of nursing literature on research and effects of nursing practice. In: Davis, B.D. (Ibid).

Acknowledgement

With many thanks to the students who participated on the programme and to the clinical staff who supervised the students, without whom the programme could not exist.

36

Not just another pair of hands: developing a learning environment on the ward

Monica C. Coates, RGN
Staff Development Sister, Elderly Care Unit, Southampton General Hospital

'Just another pair of hands', 'no priority given to learning during allocation on ward areas'. These are common complaints of pre-registration nursing students and their tutors. The elderly care unit at Southampton General Hospital decided to try to overcome this problem and promote a positive approach to learning, and to identify it as a priority within the unit. This had to be achieved without compromising the philosophy of the unit:

* patients will receive a high standard of individualised care;
* patients and carers will be directly involved in planning and evaluating their care;
* the unit is recognised as a centre of excellence;
* a multidisciplinary approach to care is used by all the team.

The unit

The elderly care unit consists of 112 beds, divided into three acute assessment and two rehabilitation wards. Average bed occupancy ranges from 71-96 per cent. The unit has the whole time equivalents of 110 nurses, 75 per cent of whom are trained nurses and 25 per cent are untrained. The staff mix is shown in Figure 1.

The unit also has an assistant clinical service manager, one senior clinical nurse, a rehabilitation specialist, one sister per ward and a clinical tutor. Learners are allocated for 11 weeks in the middle of their second year of preregistration study, with each intake averaging 12.

How are learners assessed?

The learners are continually assessed for practical skills, and are linked to a trained staff member who is responsible for teaching, supervision and assessment. Assessment is formative, concerned with identifying learning problems and providing learning opportunities. On completion of the module, the final level of performance of the learner is identified (continuing assessment of nursing practice guidelines – Southampton University Hospitals Combined School of Nursing, 1986).

As well as being allocated to a named assessor, learners also have a named link nurse, who acts as a back-up to the assessor, and would act as assessor if the named assessor was absent. The learner must work with their assessor a minimum of twice a week, and both assessor and link nurse are involved in assessing the learner's allocation.

At the preliminary interview (held during the first week of allocation) learning needs are identified by the learner and an action plan compiled by learner and assessor. Learners are encouraged to self-assess their performance and discuss their strengths and weaknessess. An intermediate interview is held during the sixth week of allocations, at which learners' performance is discussed and the action plan reviewed. A final interview is held during the twelfth or thirteenth week, when the allocation is assessed overall.

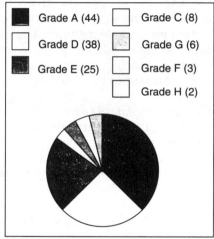

Figure 1. Number of staff per grade on the unit.

Aims for learner allocation

Our prime aim is that learners will enjoy their allocation and develop a positive attitude towards the care of elderly people, and this is achieved through the following objectives:

- to develop and extend the specialised skills required for caring forelderly people;
- to become aware of the ageing process, the multiply pathology of elderly people and how it affects their care;
- to work with a questioning and supportive multidisciplinary team;
- to participate in an holistic approach to care;
- to recognise and develop rehabilitation skills;
- to participate in and understand self-medication theory and practice;
- to extend pharmacology knowledge;
- to understand the theory and participate in ward management.

Plan and content of learning

If these objectives were to be achieved, we had first to recognise our own weaknesses as a unit, by critically analysing previous learners' evaluations of their allocation. Staff from the school of nursing were also involved in discussions regarding learners' needs within the curriculum.

Following these consultations the unit introduced an orientation day, to take place on the first working day of the allocation. The day commences with a chance get to know the staff and their respective roles, then the individual ward aims and objectives are discussed. Learners are encouraged to discuss their own positive and negative attitudes towards the care of the elderly allocation. This is achieved by watching a video depicting a woman who appears to be demented, which follows the events leading to her finally regaining her independence. This highlights the conflict the patient and her family face and how they are treated by the multidisciplinary team. The group then discuss their possible roles within this scenario.

In the next session learners are asked to record their feelings – positive and negative – towards the allocation, and discuss these feelings as a group if they wish. A list of individual and group needs is produced from this exercise, and is circulated to the wards and evaluated by the assessor and learner at each interview.

The afternoon of the orientation day is taken up in meeting ward sisters and discussing unit policies regarding fire, lifting and resuscitation. Finally, the learners have a 'walkabout' of the unit, and are given a written information package to keep and refer to for reference.

'Rehabilitation week' was introduced for learners to develop a wider appreciation of the roles and involvement of the multidisciplinary team. During their visits to the community, they develop their knowledge of the facilities available, and come to appreciate the importance of good communication between hospital and community staff. Becoming supernumerary for one week of their allocation, they work directly with individual members of the multidisciplinary team, such as the physiotherapist, occupational therapist, social worker, speech therapist and dietitian. During this week they also discuss the wider aspects of rehabilitation with the rehabilitation specialist sister, and visit a residential home. This improves their understanding of the role of residential care and enables them to discuss their attitudes to it.

One of the most beneficial developments from the learners' point of view was the introduction of compulsory attendance at the weekly afternoon tutorials. In these two hour sessions, subjects previously agreed by the learners are presented and discussed by internal and external speakers. Subjects range from counselling skills to the role of the dietitian. Fifteen minutes are spent on agreed revision topics of anatomy and physiology and how to relate them to the care of elderly people. This was introduced after learners highlighted it as a particularly weak area of knowledge.

The role of the clinical teacher and involvement with the learners is a high priority within the unit. On average the clinical teacher works with learners twice during their allocation, and is always present at the weekly tutorials to develop continuity and deal with any personal or professional problems.

The support of and the involvement with the school of nursing is a priority, and a named link tutor from the school works closely with the clinical tutor. The link tutor has a 'walkabout' the unit once a week on a named day, which is well advertised, and all staff are encouraged to discuss any problems, enabling direct feedback from the wards. The link tutor also regularly meets the senior clinical nurse regarding any general nurse management issues which may affect the learners. To enable the clinical tutor and link tutor to support and advise the assessors, a two monthly support meeting is held for mutual support and general discussion on areas highlighted by continual assessment.

Have we achieved our objectives?

Staff on the unit would be the first to acknowledge that to progress we must always question our methods and approach and be prepared to accept new ideas. To facilitate this, every learner completes an evaluation form, in which they assess all aspects of their allocation. These are critically reviewed and a summary sent to all wards, the school of nursing, management, and the senior nurse advisor. A meeting is then held with the clinical tutor, link tutor, all the learners, representatives from the individual wards and the unit manager. Learners are encouraged to highlight areas of strength and weakness within the unit and these are discussed and plans of action initiated.

Prior to the introduction of the orientation day, evaluations generally included comments such as "I felt thrown in at the deep end" and "I was unaware of the other wards on the unit and their roles". The learners felt their allocations were not well structured and that their roles within the unit were not defined. They were also unsure of the unit's aims and objectives. Following the introduction of the orientation day, they felt welcomed to the unit, and found it useful to meet the sisters and be aware of unit policies and philosophies prior to commencing work. They particularly enjoyed considering and developing their own ideas of care of elderly people and their development needs.

Before compulsory attendance to the tutorials, learners felt guilty about having to ask to leave the wards, and the ward staff did not always feel happy to release all learners. It was felt that no continuity developed between the learners and the clinical tutor. After compulsory attendance, sisters felt able to organise off-duty more effectively, as managers were aware of and accepted the development, while learners felt they were seen as a priority, and found tutorials useful to develop group support and discuss areas of concern.

The rehabilitation week was praised, as learners felt under no pressure from the ward workload. They enjoyed being able to work directly with the multidisciplinary team and discuss their own ideas about care with them, and found it beneficial to compare working on an acute area with a rehabilitation area within the unit. During their allocation learners can attend weekly case conferences, medical ward rounds and accompany the consultants on domiciliary visits. They are also given the opportunity – under close supervision – to develop their managerial skills, and, when appropriate, escort patients on outside visits.

Medical staff are supportive of the learners and are involved in regular formal and one-to-one teaching on the unit. Involvement and contact with the clinical teacher was felt to be of great value. It was reassuring for learners to know they could meet the clinical teacher at the weekly tutorial to discuss any problems.

Before the 'walkabout' by the link tutor, staff felt unsure what this role entailed, and there appeared to be little direct contact with the school of nursing. After its introduction, however, staff felt more supported, and became more aware of how to relate theory to practice. They also enjoyed being able to question their own career plans with the link tutor, particularly related to education.

Staff development
The evaluations from the allocation in general are extremely positive. A large proportion of learners apply to the unit for first time posts and remain for an average of one to two years. They particularly enjoy being seen as a priority and not just a pair of hands. Since all staff on the unit participate in continuing education, the learners find them a great source of knowledge and reference. Staff development is achieved by:
- individual development programmes;
- monthly meetings of senior ward staff discussing a research-based approach to care;
- orientation programmes – two weeks for trained staff, one week for untrained staff;
- monthly sisters' meeting and two monthly sisters' study days;
- monthly ward meetings.

The way forward
Within the last four to five years the unit has developed many interesting and rewarding ideas, such as primary nursing and self-medication. Primary nursing is practised on all wards in the unit, and learners have become more aware of their own accountability and developed their own philosophy of patient care. Self-medication is in progress on one ward and we would like to extend this to the whole unit, so the nurses become more actively involved with their patients in discussing compliance and patient understanding: a well researched and recognised problem in elderly people.

We are currently setting up a trained staff forum – a monthly meeting at which trained staff from all wards discuss and research a previously agreed topic. The long-term aim is to audit district standards within the forum and to tackle specific problems identified as a result of this. A structured staff development programme has been implemented with a staff development sister in post, and the nurses have set their own nursing standards.

Learners on the elderly are unit are valued members of the team with recognised learning needs which we are continually trying to meet. This is reflected not only in their positive evaluation, but also in the number who return to us as trained staff. We welcome the supernumerary status of the learner with Project 2000 and have already gone some way towards meeting this with our present learners. Over the next two years, while we still have learners in the traditional training system, we would look to do even more to prepare for the inevitable changes and ensure that at no time could learners in care of the elderly be 'just another pair of hands'.

References
Southampton University Hospitals Combined School of Nursing (1986) Continuing Assessment of Practice Guidelines.

Acknowledgement
Thanks to all the staff on the elderly care unit for their help and support with this chapter.

37

A means to a long-term goal: helping colleagues become rational career planners

Kevin Teasdale, MA, Cert Ed, RMN
Director of In-service Training, Pilgrim Hospital, Boston

Good quality career counselling is hard to find. Too many people allow their career direction to follow a random pattern, hoping that all will turn out for the best in the end. Even though at the beginning of their careers many nurses may feel compelled to accept the first opportunities that come along, it pays to remember that career options decline as we grow older and that choices made in the past may restrict the freedom to choose in the future. It is an important part of the role of experienced nurses to offer career counselling to more junior staff, to help them to mature not only as nurses but also as rational career planners. To offer this help, it is essential to have a clear model of counselling in mind, and to understand that the process involves much more than simply helping nurses gather information about job vacancies.

- Self-awareness
- Opportunity awareness
- Decision-making
- Handling transition

Table 1. Four key elements of rational career planning.

Rational career planning

Rational career planning involves knowing both oneself and the job market, matching the two, and handling the stress which always comes with change (Teasdale, 1991). All four elements are linked, and a counsellor should help colleagues ('clients') through a cyclical process of exploration and feedback around them. It is important this is a continuing process: as individuals we may move *towards* maturity in rational career planning, but can never fully attain it, since our values, beliefs, abilities and circumstances will change over time, as will the job market. In the past, it was assumed all that was required was opportunity awareness - career counsellors would provide information on jobs which nurses could then act on. This approach is much in need of an update.

John Malkin, Senior Lecturer in Vocational Guidance at Nottingham Polytechnic, has developed a model of career counselling which is a valuable introduction to anyone new to this specialist area. Since many nurses may already be familiar with Egan's model based on exploration, understanding and action (Egan, 1982), this chapter integrates it with Malkin's ideas in order to explain the basics clearly. The integrated model (Table 2) is presented from the counsellor's viewpoint.

Essential preconditions
Pay attention to rights
Develop an equal and adult relationship

Exploration
Agree an explicit contract
Help the client to review his or her career

Understanding
Present a diagnosis
Check out the diagnosis with the client
Proceed only when diagnosis is mutually agreed

Action
Agree the areas the client will work on
Help client to make an action plan

Table 2. The integrated model.

Clients' rights

Whether career counselling occurs at a single interview or as a longer-term counselling contract, certain essential preconditions are necessary for the process to be both safe and helpful. These can be addressed by being open about the rights of both client and counsellor. As a counsellor, you should consider where you stand on the ideas described below, tailoring them to your own views as you think fit.

Confidentiality This concept needs attention since it often creates profound dilemmas. What if the client tells the counsellor he or she has broken the law or is a drug user? There are limits to confidentiality - it is not an absolute - and the client should be told what these are at the start.

Respect Try to establish an adult relationship based on mutual respect, while being aware of the potential complications of a relationship in which the counsellor has a position of power in the hierarchy of the organisation. For example, a ward sister might have a vested interest in getting a talented young staff nurse to work in her area, but would be abusing her power position if she used her skills to direct the staff nurse in this way. The ward sister should therefore either let someone else offer counselling, or put her cards on the table right at the start and allow the staff nurse to decide whether or not to discuss career plans with her.

Competence in the counsellor   Competence in this context is often misinterpreted to mean being an expert on the job market or on the availability of postbasic courses, whereas the collection of information is generally best left to the client. A counsellor needs to be competent in the counselling process, of which attention to rights is the cornerstone.

Autonomy   This means clients are capable of making decisions for themselves, and that their right to do so is upheld by the counsellor at all times. Notice that clients' expectations can get in the way of this: they may press you to tell them what they should do, perhaps as a way of avoiding responsibility for the outcome.

Environmental factors   Clients have a right to the things which make counselling interviews possible such as time, punctuality and privacy.

Having an outcome   Counselling is more than listening, and involves helping someone to move in a goal-directed way towards a plan of action. Counselling is not a ritual to be gone through: it leads somewhere, and clients have a right to leave if they are not satisfied with either the process or the direction in which it leads.

Counsellors' rights
Respect   Involves clients appearing at the agreed time, being honest and not just going through the motions of a counselling interview.

To confront clients if they are not being honest   This may mean ending the consultation, but a counsellor should first give the client a chance to explore why he or she is not being honest. It may be because the client is *sent* for the interview (this can occur in tutor/student situations), so check out the client's assumptions about the process first.

Environmental ground rules   Counsellors have a right to be angry if clients are not punctual etc.

To use a counselling model   Within limits, this means the counsellor can direct the sequence of events of the counselling process in line with the model adopted, but the model and sequence must be open and negotiable from the start. A counsellor has a right to explain the process and the client to challenge it at any stage.

To offer a referral   Knowing the limits of your competence, being able to say, "I don't know", and a right not to take on a client.

The integrated model
The counsellor tries to help clients explore factors which are influencing their approach to career development. The counsellor spells out his or her view of the essential preconditions for useful career counselling and clients are encouraged to respond.

Establish a relationship   Develop a mutual dialogue and set the client at ease, taking time for this. Aim for a positive relationship which works at a pace and in a style with which the client is comfortable.

Identify the client's expectations   Ask questions such as: "How can I be helpful to you?" and "Can you begin by telling me what you expect from me?" Very often nurses will expect definite things such as information about a particular course or a specialist career path.

Respond to clients' expectations   Set out the limits of what you are able or prepared to do. Are you willing simply to give information or are you prepared to offer a wider discussion? Explain your agenda as a counsellor in terms of the rights listed above. For example, you might say: "I see my role as helping you to help yourself. I would really like to help you to check out how you are planning and organising your career at present. If you are doing it okay, that's fine, but if not, we will address any problem ahead, and only then take on the specific information issues which you raised. Is that something you are prepared to accept from me, or would you prefer not to go into that depth at the moment?"

Make a contract   If the client wishes to proceed, explain the integrated counselling model and agree how you will operate within it. Spell out your mutual rights in this process, and check agreement. For example, you will help your clients explore the extent to which they are acting as rational career planners by inviting them to talk about their career to date and their values and ambitions for the future. When you feel this has been completed in sufficient depth, explain your diagnosis - stating which areas of career planning you believe they would benefit from working on. Invite them then to discuss this diagnosis with you, and when you are agreed, help them to make their action plan. Check clients actually understand and are willing to accept this process, particularly the formulation and presentation of a diagnosis, and proceed only when you have reached mutual understanding and agreement on this.

Review past and present

Invite clients to explore with you their track record as rational career planners. Clients will explain their career path in their own way, but the counsellor needs to help them review it using the four elements of the rational model.

• **Self-awareness**   Invite exploration along the lines of: "What are you looking for in your proposed career move? Which of your needs do you hope it will satisfy?" "Describe your career to date...start off with when you left school, and at each transition, describe what led up to the move, what you were hoping for from it, and what the outcome was." "What would you say you have learned about yourself so far? What are you particularly good at doing? What are your weaknesses?"

• **Opportunity awareness**   Aim to review how broad a grasp clients have of the range of opportunities open to them. Ask questions such as: "You are thinking of applying for this particular job, were there any alternatives you considered?" "You are thinking of becoming (say) an infection control nurse, what do you know about what an infection control nurse does? What qualifications and experience do panels look for when selecting infection control nurses?"

• **Decision-making**   In terms of matching self to opportunities, aim to assess the level of sophistication in the way the person makes decisions. For example, ask: "Are you someone who plans things out, or do your career moves just happen?" "How much do *you* feel in control of your decisions, and how influential are other people?" "What is your plan of action for moving your career in the direction you want it to go?"

• **Handling transition**   Any change in career path is likely to result in stress, either for the individual or his or her immediate family and friends. It is helpful to encourage clients to explore their previous experience of handling similar transitions. For example: "How do you feel about change, is it something you welcome or fear?" "Thinking about when you first took up your present job, what was the most stressful thing about it?" "How did you handle that stress?" "Do you envisage any problems with your planned move?"

Understanding
Making a diagnosis is an intellectual skill, and demands real concentration. A counsellor must listen carefully to what clients are saying, amassing clues about their strengths and weaknesses as rational career planners. Is a client in charge of his or her own career direction? Is there a pattern of growing self-awareness in career planning? Does the person's career track record show if his or her job expectations were met by their outcomes or not? Is the person aware of the full range of opportunities available? Does the client's assessment of his or her strengths and weaknesses tally with career evidence? Is the client thinking short- or long-term? Can he or she cope with the pressures of change? What are the client's favoured coping styles?

As a counsellor, your knowledge of the particular work area does not have to be high. You are trying to form a judgement on your clients' capacity to take rational action concerning their careers, and to present it to them in an honest yet supportive way. To make such a judgement demands intellectual honesty, especially when trying to help a friend.

Explaining a diagnosis is challenging, demanding both honesty and caring. If the contract was carefully discussed and agreed at the start, the diagnosis is more likely to be given fair consideration by the client. For example the counsellor might say "I think you might benefit from being clearer about what you want from your career, not only now, but over the next five to 10 years. From what you have told, you seem to have made some spontaneous career decisions in the past, which have not always worked out as you wanted. Also you seem to have set your sights too high for what you were able to cope with at the time. How do you feel about what I am saying so far?"

Many counsellors who were trained in a non-directive style of counselling will initially find this approach quite alien. Notice however that the counsellor is *not* saying "I don't think this is the right job for you", but is addressing the planning **process**, not its content. Provided the contract was understood and the interview process made open, the client continues to retain control throughout.

Finally, the counsellor must aim to establish mutual agreement. Diagnosis must, again, be mutually agreed, with the counsellor working within limits the client can accept. If the client accepts only part of the diagnosis, it may still be possible to work usefully on the area of agreement. Only in extreme cases of wide disagreement should the counsellor consider offering a referral. If the groundwork was done and the counsellor made the whole process open to the client, a reasonable level of mutual agreement will generally be possible.

Action

Begin by agreeing a plan of action This involves problem-solving in the areas identified for further work. Try to help clients to summarise for themselves which aspects of the rational model they feel they need to work on in greater depth. Self-awareness issues will lend themselves to further analysis of values and wants. Opportunity awareness means seeking information in a systematic way. Matching the two will usually involve detailed consideration of alternatives, and explicit explanation of the reasons for accepting or rejecting them. Transition issues are directly related to the field of stress management. The actual techniques employed at the problem-solving stage will depend on the preferences of the client and the outlook of the counsellor. The bibliography gives some references and contacts which may be helpful at this stage.

References
Egan, G. (1982) The Skilled Helper. Brooks/Cole, California.
Teasdale, K. (1991) A structured way to fulfil ambition. How to make rational career plans. *Professional Nurse*, **6**, 11, 644-48.

Bibliography
Priestley, P. *et al* (1978) Social Skills and Personal Problem Solving. Tavistock, London.
    A valuable source book on problem-solving.
Teasdale, K. (1991) A structured way to fulfil ambition. How to make rational career plans. *Professional Nurse*, **6**, 11, 644-48.
    Self-help ideas which can be adapted to the counsellor-client context.

Useful address
ENB Resource and Career Services, Woodseats House, 764 Chesterfield Road, Sheffield S8 0SE. Tel: 0742 551064.
This is a confidential information and careers advisory service available to nurses.

Managing Stress and Handling Aggression

38

What about the carers? The need for staff support in healthcare

Jan Long, SRN, SCM
Staff Support Service Facilitator, Swindon Health Authority

Stress is a normal and necessary part of working in healthcare settings. However, the rising costs of good healthcare are increasing the pressure on all staff to provide the quality of care expected by an informed public.

The issue of who cares for the carers has been disregarded for too long, but the threat of falling recruitment in the 1990s is beginning to occupy the minds of managers. To adequately staff departments in the future, the nursing profession will have to employ at least 50 per cent of all female school leavers with the minimum qualifications of five GCSEs, or their equivalents! The need to conserve staff is, therefore, essential.

Carers' inability

The other major hurdle to looking after the carers is their own inability to accept the need for it. This is particularly true among more senior people, brought up to believe that to be unable to cope is to be a 'failure'.

Many nurses see their role as carer only and that making demands for themselves is a selfish and unnecessary luxury. I consider this to be a 'cop-out', and challenge those who pay lip-service only to both their own needs and those of their staff. Many carers will give defensive answers to the question of staff need:

- "My staff can come and see me any time I am not busy."
- "I don't need support, I can cope."
- "It's not worth it, I'm leaving anyway."
- "We don't have the money."

In response to these and other excuses, many carers have learnt negative, defensive, coping mechanisms to protect themselves. Some use alcohol, smoking, food or even drugs to escape from unacknowledged feelings. Some opt out, become sick, absent themselves on feeble excuses or leave the profession altogether, causing further loss of resources.

What is burnout?

Cherniss (1980) describes burnout as "A process in which a previously committed professional disengages from his/her work in response to the stress and strain experienced in the job." He lists some of the signs and symptoms of job stress and burnout (Table 1).

Sense of failure.
Absenteeism.
Clockwatching.
Sleep disorders.
Discouragement.
Indifference.
Increased physical illness, coughs, colds, flu etc.
Inability to concentrate and increased marital and family conflict.

Table 1. Symptoms of burnout.

Cherniss explains burnout as being in three stages:
1. Imbalance between demand and resources.
2. Immediate short-term effects – anxiety, tension, fatigue and exhaustion.
3. Changes in attitude and behaviour; becoming detached and cynical – defensive coping.

By becoming cynical and pessimistic carers reduce the guilt and frustration associated with stressful work. Detachment from their patients helps carers psychologically, but the negative effects of staff detachment cause patients to feel more vulnerable and isolated in a situation which for them is already stressful. This can delay their recovery and ultimate release from medical care.

Much research has been undertaken into the measurement of burnout, but little into the effectiveness of interventions. In 1988, I was sponsored by the Artemis Trust to research support services in the USA, to look at models of support and to try to find statistical evidence of their effectiveness. Although our health systems are different, there were many areas where the stresses and strains were identical.

Research

Hare (1988a) compared 10 hospitals, both acute and long-term, to measure the effects of burnout in various settings. During this research only two of the 10 institutions showed any real interest in the results of the study. Those two who did were actively concerned with improving staff morale and awaited the results with interest. They were long-term units, and out of all 10, had the highest level of staff job satisfaction and lowest burnout scores. They also had no staff vacancies.

In another study, Hare compared the needs of trained and untrained nursing staff (Hare, 1988b). On the whole, those who had most direct patient care were the less qualified or junior members of staff. These staff were not expected to deal with the complex emotional needs of their patients, yet were most likely to be faced with these needs. This left them feeling helpless and inadequate.

Hare also noted that those least qualified are much more likely to use negative coping strategies – alcohol, cigarettes or avoidance (sickness, absenteeism) – than to try and deal more effectively with their dilemma, such as by talking, relaxation, using interventions.

Norbeck has completed several studies to measure the effects of burnout using her own measurement tool (Norbeck, 1981; 1982; 1985). She spoke of a short-term study in one coronary care unit which showed that where nurses attended regular support groups, patients made a significantly quicker recovery. This particular survey was too small for publication, but is continued by Dubovsky, in another study of staff at a coronary care unit, where a psychiatrist was employed for both staff and patient support (Dubovsky, 1977). There was a significant drop in patient mortality rate compared to a control unit.

Dubovsky suggests that as staff are less caught up with interpersonal difficulties and distractions, they may be more alert to small changes in their patients. They may also spend more time with the patients, effectively supporting and calming them. The direct result was a shorter hospital stay for patients in this expensive, high-powered unit.

Support models

The American experience offered various support models from support groups, one-to-one counselling, relaxation, self-awareness, professional development and management training, all of which are known to have a direct effect on morale and job satisfaction. From a financial point of view, however, a more effective argument will be that of reducing staff turnover, sickness, absenteeism and the possible effects on patients, thereby reducing mortality and length of stay. When nurses and other health professionals exhibit manifestations of burnout it is not only they who are likely to suffer. Their behaviour plays a major role in affecting the quality of care delivered and the attainment of services by people in need of them.

No-one is a bottomless well of resources. We all need time out, space, rest and recuperation, and we all need to be cared for. If these needs are not satisfied, we become anaesthetised. How can we give of ourselves when we are not in contact with the needs within ourselves? If we continue to try and function without refilling ourselves we will be empty and artificial, mechanically acting out a role and not really caring.

At a national conference of professionals concerned with this issue, held in 1989, it was agreed that a wider network of support was required to encourage the development of services. Accordingly, The National Association of Staff Support (NASS) was launched with the support and sponsorship of The Artemis Trust. We were also made aware of people in the UK who were trying to set up support services in isolation.

One of the first aims of this organisation was to research 'best practices' within the UK to provide information for those districts and hospitals and individuals who are forward thinking enough to want to provide support for all levels of staff. This has already begun. Another major aim was to set up regional groups to provide support and encouragement and to enable a sharing of experiences in the field.

Within three years of its birth, NASS has brought together progressive general managers, tutors, doctors, nurses, qualified counsellors and other healthcare professionals and has shown that successful management can go hand in hand with humanity. Many areas are not so enlightened, however. Some have no positive support programme at all and some have concerned, knowledgeable people thwarted by complacency.

What can we do?

It is time we all made positive moves, not only to be aware of the needs of our patients, but to be more aware of our own! It is time to put our own house in order, to stop expecting a mythical 'them' to come to a mythical 'rescue'. We must realise that *we* are them. We are the health service and we can affect what happens to us.

The following are personal suggestions for a professional action plan:
- Acknowledge your own need for support. Show by example that we do not 'fail' if we find the pressure of caring stressful. Rather, we prove our humanity, the failure is in the accusation.
- Learn to communicate effectively. Attend courses and seminars, and **practise**.
- Do not confuse counselling with support. It is a much abused and overused word and there are other ways of supporting. Skilled counselling is only one way. Counselling is not: advice giving; disciplining; telling; manipulating.
- Learn to love and respect yourself, follow your own self-development and become self-aware.
- Read – anything and everything, know yourself but develop a sound foundation of knowledge too.
- Find like-minded people within your area – they are there. Talk to anyone who will listen. Make a case of need to managers and personnel departments for trained support facilitators.
- If you are trying to set up a service or a group and would like support, get in touch with NASS at the address given left.

You are as valuable and important as any of your patients. Valuing yourself will teach you to value others, colleagues, family or patients.

References

Cherniss, C. (1980) Staff Burnout: Job Stress in The Human Services. Sage, London.

Dubovski, S.L., Getto, C.J., Adams, G.S., Palisy, J.A. (1977) Impact on nursing care and mortality. *Psychiatrist on The Coronary Care Unit, Psychosomatics*, **3**, 18–27.

Hare, J., Pratt, C.C., Andrews, D., (1998a) Predictors of burnout in professional and paraprofessional nurses working in hospitals and nursing homes. *International Journal of Study*, **25**, 105–15.

Hare, J. and Pratt, C.C. (1988b) Burnout: differences between professional and paraprofessional nursing staff in acute care and long-term facilities. *Journal of Applied Gerontology,* **7,** 1, 60–72.

Norbeck, J.S., Lindsay, A.M., Carrieri, V.L. (1981) The development of an instrument to measure social support. *Nursing Research,* **30,** 5, 264–69.

Norbeck, J.S. (1982) The use of social suport in clinicial practice. *Journal of Psychosocial Nursing and Mental Health Services,* **20,** 12, 22–29.

Norbeck, J.S. (1985) Perceived job stress, job satisfacion and psychological symptoms in critical care nursing. *Resesarch in Nursing and Health,,* 8, 253–95.

For further information about NASS, contact: Grace Owen, NASS Secretary, 9 Caradon Close, Woking, Surrey GU21 3DU. NASS has regional groups running throughout the UK.

39

A strategy for managing change and stress: developing staff support groups

Emrys Jenkins, RMN, RGN, RNMH, RCNT, Cert Ed (FE), RNT, DipN, BEd (Hons)
Senior Tutor, Cefn Coed Hospital, West Glamorgan College of Nursing and Midwifery

Ian Stevenson, RMN, RGN
Ward Manager, Cefn Coed Hospital, District Services Unit, Swansea

Nursing is a highly stressful occupation at the best of times (Bond, 1986). In times of change, stress is exacerbated, and currently a number of forces are at work which all radically affect the character of the profession. These include Project 2000 and all associated changes - support workers (and their training); 'supernumerary' students; links with higher education and branch programmes; continuing changes associated with general management philosophies; the Griffiths (1988) proposals for community service developments, and political, sociological and demographic influences, such as Working for People (DoH, 1990).

In such a climate it is probably more important than ever before that nurses consider their individual and collective responses (rather than just reactions) to stress and change. Several authors have suggested methods of recognising, reducing and responding to stress in ways which promote optimum health (eg, Holland, 1987). The English National Board has acknowledged the need to help nurses accommodate change positively, and has produced learning packages aimed at effecting this process (ENB, 1988; 1989), while the development of support networks has been repeatedly shown to be effective in stress management (Cobbs, 1976), and is one method which lends itself to teams of nurses providing mutual help. In essence, this is carers caring for each other.

Formal mechanism
The issue of staff support has been actively pursued by the team of psychiatric nurses working on Afan ward at Cefn Coed Hospital, Swansea. Staff feel their experiences have contributed to enhanced communication and work performance, as well as providing a network of social support.

Afan opened in June 1985, and by November 1986 many staff had identified an increasing breakdown in communication and morale. The nurses recognised the need for a formal mechanism to reverse these unhelpful and stressful events, and to achieve some support for staff. A regular group meeting was established, facilitated by the unit's psychologist. After 10 months, the psychologist moved jobs, and the group temporarily ceased to meet, until a nurse tutor was asked to fulfil the facilitating role. Over the past two years the group has continued to meet regularly.

To provide an opportunity for staff to:

1. Describe and discuss ideas and feelings considered relevant to the work of the team.

2. Confront each other in ways which help recognition and resolution of problems or potential problems.

3. Achieve aims 1 and 2 in an atmosphere characterised by equality, acceptance and responsibility for self, and therefore:-

4. Improve communication and reduce work stress.

Table 1. Aims of the group.

Meetings are scheduled for alternate weeks, but in practice this is variable, taking account of clinical demands, staff commitments and holidays. The original aims of the group have remained, however, and can be seen in Table 1. Team members collectively constructed their own ground rules, and the facilitator was charged with keeping to them. These were both simple and crucial (Table 2).

---

1. Members will speak in the first person, saying 'I' rather than 'we', or 'one'.

2. Transactions will operate on an adult-to-adult basis, with no 'game playing'. Members are regarded as equals.

3. Sessions will last for a maximum of 45 minutes.

4. All nurses working on the ward (including the senior nurse) will be eligible to attend.

5. Contributions will be characterised by honesty, sensitivity and confidentiality.

Table 2. Ground rules of the group.

Group process issues

Feelings have been a prominent feature of group sessions: individuals have cried, and have been encouraged to describe their feelings rather than having them denied or negated; anger has been expressed both towards colleagues and self; frustration, uncertainty, disappointment, pride-fulfilment and happiness have all been verbalised, accepted and explained by participants. The group has served a 'cathartic' function, which is helpful (Heron, 1977), while the group's supportive stance has always provided people with positive feedback about their worth, based on readily identified behaviours, contributing to mutual support and esteem boosting. Individuals have been helped to consider themselves in terms of the balance between their strengths and weaknesses - something which may often prove difficult for an individual alone, receiving no feedback from others.

The events, experiences and circumstances which have figured in generating these feelings have obviously been wide-ranging, but typical examples have included staff changes (particularly when highly respected people have moved on) and day-to-day communication breakdowns. Often, this has been a simple oversight or lack of thought, and the group has provided a useful venue for clarification. Some stressors have related to the nature of the patient population, such as when people with suicide problems or aggressive behaviours have been nursed. Yet others concern pressures 'external' to the ward - staff being repeatedly moved to other units, or changes advocated by local and national policies. The latter have included new demands made in relation to clinical grading, major service changes (community services developments) as well as the backdrop of the NHS reforms.

These 'organisational' and 'personal' stressors are constantly being differentiated by the group. Ultimately, stress and responses to stress are dependent upon individual perception and coping ability. Stress does not exist 'outside' people; the crucial issue is how they respond to stressors. The support group has had a positive influence in relation to both types of stressor. Most significantly, problem-solving strategies (brain-storming options and consequences) have been adopted to help individuals and the team as a whole. The following comments on the value of the group have been made by participants:

"It's so useful to be able to speak up without feeling constrained by status."

"I really do need this group - this week especially!"

"The group has made me feel that I am appreciated by others, and it's an opportunity for me to give back some affirmations."

"Part of the reason why we work so well as a team is because we do speak up and we do support one-another."

In terms of process, sessions are constructed around beginning, developing and ending, with the facilitator clarifying, confronting and supporting. Involvement by all participants takes place, sometimes through the use of 'rounds' of each person in turn. Crucially, sessions end on a positive note, even in times of perceived adversity.

Qualitative impressions of results

There is a strong impression that the aims of the group are being met consistently. It enhances communication, teamwork and morale, while stress is reduced (or at least coped with more effectively), and links with and between teachers and clinicians are established, and continue to improve. In relation to staff retention, we offer no empirical data that the group has helped, but several nurses who have left the unit have been instrumental in instigating similar groups in their new work environments. Sessions are perceived as being necessary and meeting a need. The teacher has learned that groupwork principles are essentially the same, whether the group is made up of students, clinicians or patients/clients, and students have been helped to relate theoretical principles to meaningful practice. Similar groups have been requested by clinicians working throughout the district, and are now facilitated by tutors in many wards and day units.

A conscious effort

Developing social support at work needs conscious attention. The support group is one way of identifying need, providing support and encouraging teamwork. By paying attention to the process during meetings, self-awareness is developed, as is acknowledgement of personal responsibility for feelings, actions and ideas, which help in problem solving. The open sharing of feelings has led to peer support and better stress management; to quote Seashore and Barnowe (1972) "When work cohesiveness is high, work stress is decreased".

Of course, social support may be useful, but it does not provide a 'perfect answer' to stress-related problems. Well-supported people can still experience negative effects of stress. "Social support is not now, nor will it ever be, a panacea for all problems of occupational stress and health, both physical and mental" (House, 1981). The group has, however, formed a 'vehicle' for enabling personal decision-making, and acceptance of responsibility.

Stress is exacerbated by such factors as pain, aggression, and staff shortages, but these have less impact than the absence of positive conditions such as good relationships, challenge, appreciation (Pines and Kanner, 1982) and a sense of control over life and work (Dayley, 1979; Pines and Maslach, 1978). The support group has helped to create an awareness of these positive conditions, occasionally during times when negative conditions abound. Also, while individuals, particularly newly qualified staff, have been working at accommodating role changes, the group has helped counter the phenomenon of 'reality shock' (Kramer, 1974). The effects and results of the staff support group seem to strongly reflect the conclusions of a variety of writers whose work shows that social support can and does reduce work stresses, promote teamwork, communication and retention of staff. At a time when nursing is approaching increasing competition in the labour market, these factors surely require action, and setting up staff support groups is one effective method which is relatively easy to adopt.

References

Bond, M. (1986) Stress and Self-Awareness: A guide for nurses. Heinemann, London.
Cobbs, S. (1976) Social support as a moderator of life stress. *Psychosomatic Medicine*, **38**, 300-14.
Dayley, M.R. (1979) Preventing worker burnout in child welfare. *Child Welfare*, **58**, 7, 443-50.
English National Board (1988; 1989) Managing Change in Nursing Education. Work Packs 1 &2. ENB, London.
Griffiths, R. (1988) Community Care: An Agenda for Action. HMSO, London.
Heron, J. (1977) Catharsis in Human Development. Human Potential Research Project. University of Surrey, Guildford.
Holland, S. (Ed.) (1987) Managing Nursing: Stress in Nursing Workbook. Heinemann, London.
House, J.S. (1981) Work Stress and Social Support. Addison-Wesley, USA.
Kramer, M. (1974) Reality Shock: Why Nurses leave nursing. Mosby-Year Book, St. Louis.
Pines, A.M. and Kanner, A.D. (1982) Burnout: lack of positive conditions and presence of negative conditions as two independent sources of stress. *Psychiatric Nursing Mental Health Service*, **20**, 8, 30.
Pines, A. and Maslach, C. (1978) Characteristics of staff burnout in mental health settings. *Hospital and Community Psychiatry*, **29**, 4, 233.
Seashore, S.E. and Barnowe, J.T. (1972) Collar colour doesn't count. *Psychology Today*, **6**, 53-54.

Bibliography

Caplan, G. (1981) Mastery of stress: psychosocial aspects. *Am. J. of Psychiatry*, **138**, 413-20.
Cassell, J. (1976) The contribution of the social environment to host resistance. *Am. J. of Epidemiology*, **102**, 107-23.
  Both examine stress in relation to social contexts.
Kashoff, S. (1976) Nursing your stress. *Journal of Emergency Nursing*, **2**, 2, 12-20.
  Recognition of potential stressors in emergency nursing, and ways of coping.
Michenbaum, D. (1985) Stress Innocculation Training. Pergamon Press, Oxford.
  A specific approach to improve coping.
Price, B. (1985) Moving wards - how do student nurses cope? *Nursing Times*, **81**, 9, 32.
  Illustrates direct, indirect and palliative coping strategies.
Selye, H. (1974) Stress Without Distress. McGraw-Hill, New York.
  Outlines 'healthy' response to stress.
Smythe, E.M. (1984) Surviving Nursing. Addison-Wesley, Menlo Park, USA.
  A comprehensive analysis of the concept of stress, from the American perspective.
Wycherley, R. (Ed.) (1987) Living Skills. Outset Publishing, Bexhill-on-Sea.
  A manual of interpersonal and relationship skills which examines stress using three models - physiological, transactional and environmental.

40

Can grief be turned into growth? Staff grief in palliative care

Maggie Fisher, RGN, Dip LSN, RCNT, Dip. Couns
Nursing Director, St Catherine's Hospice, Crawley

Grief is a natural response to loss. Nurses who work with people who are dying and those close to them are exposed to experiences which demand a grief response: whenever we lose something or someone in whom we have invested ourselves emotionally, we have a need to grieve. Formal and informal staff support structures for nurses working in palliative care can help them to come to terms with this grief, and in doing so help facilitate a healing process. This chapter was written from a palliative care perspective, but is applicable to any of the environments in which dying people are nursed.

What influences grief?
The most important determinants of grief have been defined as falling into six categories (Parkes, 1972a).

Who the person was What was the relationship between the grieving person and the one who has died?

The nature of the attachment This includes the strength and security of the relationship, and whether there was any ambivalence in it. Often the grief will increase in severity proportionate to the intensity of the relationship. In a highly ambivalent relationship, guilt is often expressed as 'Did I do enough?', along with anger at being left alone.

The mode of death How did the person die? Dimensions associated with the mode of death include whether there was advanced warning or whether it was unexpected. A number of studies suggest that people grieving for someone who has died suddenly have greater difficulty coming to terms with the death than those who received advanced warning (Parkes, 1972b; Parkes and Brown, 1972).

Historical antecedents To predict how someone is going to grieve, an awareness of how he or she has coped with previous losses is required. An individual's previous mental health history is important, particularly in people with a history of depression, as they often have greater difficulty coming to terms with loss.

People with a large number of crises prior to bereavement tend to have more difficulty coping with their grief. It is also important, however, to assess how people perceive these crises.

Personal variables These include the individual's developmental stage, age, sex, conflict issues, ability to cope with feelings and stress.

Social variables The social subculture to which the person belongs provides the individual with rituals and guidelines for grieving.

In terms of 'who the person was' to the nurse, a patient's death may not initially be considered a loss, but a strong attachment may have formed between nurse and patient and his or her family. Nurses may become attached to patients through involvement with their psychosocial or spiritual care and therefore make an emotional investment. This can also happen as a result of involvement in the physical aspects of patient care, although sadly, this is sometimes underestimated. Nurses, for example, may make a considerable emotional investment when dressing a patient's fungating wound over a period of time, but dressing a wound of this kind which will not heal and can only be made comfortable, may lead them to question their investment, and ask: "Did I do enough?"

Responses to death

How did the patient die? Did he or she die 'well'? Palliative care involves relief of suffering, promoting quality of life, and ultimately a 'peaceful' death. In a recent paper, Stedeford (1987) posed the question: 'Hospice: a safe place to suffer?' Nurses involved in palliative care tend to expect to relieve *all* suffering. As a specialty, palliative care has developed expertise in relieving physical symptoms of disease to such an extent that nurses can expect patients to be pain free. In turn, we tend to feel we have failed them if they endure distressing symptoms for any period of time – we can also even expect to relieve emotional anguish.

Nurses frequently join palliative care teams because they feel dying and bereavement has been, in their view, managed 'badly' in other environments, and consequently, often join with high ideals. Having some warning of the loss may enable staff to 'cope' with a patient's death: often, nurses in palliative care find the sudden death of a patient more difficult to cope with than the expected one. An example would be the patient who has a sudden haemorrhage and dies sooner than was anticipated; most people deteriorate gradually over a fairly predictable period of time and die 'peacefully', so an acute event within a chronic scenario can be stressful for staff because it was unexpected.

Many nurses enter the profession because they want 'to save' people from distress and suffering, and those in palliative care may set themselves up to 'rescue' dying people from distress and suffering. The nature of the attachment, the mode of dying and the mode of death will all influence the ways in which patients and those close to them, including staff, deal with their painful feelings. Anger about impending death may even be projected onto staff, who may be accused of negligence. A patient who is unable to tolerate the knowledge that he or she is dying may project it onto others symbolically by saying things like, "you are stealing my money", or more directly "you are killing me with these drugs". Nurses may also, of course, displace and project their own feelings on to patients or their families *and* on to each other.

It is important to ask nurses applying to work in palliative care how they perceive they have dealt with their past personal and professional losses, and how they cope with their emotions. Their personal coping strategies will influence their ability to work effectively in palliative care.

Social variables include nurses' social subculture, and also possibly their professional culture and subculture. Nursing tends to foster and reinforce the concept of the nurse in the role of the strong one who is 'in control'. The subculture an individual comes from influences their ability to 'cope' with palliative care, as does whether or not their grief is legitimised and given opportunity for expression.

Does the palliative care team facilitate the grief of its members informally and/or formally? Does the team have guidelines and rituals for staff grief and take into account staff members' life change events?

Working with grief and bereavement touches us personally in at least three ways. It may:

• make us painfully aware of our own losses;

• contribute to our apprehension regarding our own potential or feared losses;

• arouse existential anxiety in our personal death awareness (Worden 1983).

Working with people who are terminally ill may also touch us in these ways. Raphael (1980) expands on this, and considers that working with dying and bereaved people heightens "mutual empathy and identification", as the loss experience is universal. This makes it difficult for nurses in the palliative care team *not* to over-identify.

Patients who are dying are a threat to our sense of power, mastery and control. We can feel our actions have no impact upon the experience, regardless of what we do – ultimately our patients die. Seligman (1975) noted that 'learned helplessness' can lead to debilitation and depression, which dovetails with recent writings on professional burnout; Maslock and Jackson (1979), for example, describe burnout as: "A syndrome of emotional, physical and occupational exhaustion and cynicism frequently occurring among individuals who do 'people work' and spend considerable time in close encounters with others under conditions of chronic tension and stress." Nurses in palliative care are vulnerable to professional burnout.

Bowlby (1980) touched on the problems encountered by being in close, prolonged contact with people who are dying or bereaved: "The loss of a loved person is one of the most intensely painful experiences any human can suffer and not only is it painful to experience but also painful to witness, if only because we're so impotent to help." Parkes (1972b) echoed this sentiment when he said: "Pain is inevitable in such a case and cannot be avoided. It stems from an awareness of both parties that neither can provide the other with what he wants. The helper cannot bring back the person who is dead and the bereaved person cannot gratify the helper by seeming helped."

The adjustment process

If accumulated grief is not worked through, palliative care nurses are every bit as vulnerable to experiencing unresolved grief as other individuals who cannot grieve. How then can and do nursing staff adapt to becoming 'comfortable' with working with dying and bereaved people? Harper (1977) developed 'The Schematic Growth and Development Scale in Coping with Professional Anxieties in Terminal Care' from social work experience. It outlines the possible emotional and psychological process adjustment of people who work in palliative care.

Stage one (intellectualisation) During the initial experience, practitioners focus on professional knowledge and factual or philosophical issues. This stage is marked by periods of brisk activity as though the practitioners try to manage their anxieties by understanding their working environment, its policies and procedures. Conversations with patients, families and other members of staff are superficial and impersonal, and at this point, death is 'unacceptable'.

Stage two (trauma) Practitioners feel guilty and frustrated as they confront the reality of their patients' impending deaths, and also face the prospect of their own. They feel uncomfortable with the contrast between their own health and that of their patients. Realising that their patients' suffering and deaths *are* inevitable, they move from intellectualising to becoming emotionally involved.

Stage three (depression) The most crucial of all the stages is 'the grow or go' stage: the practitioner either accepts the process of dying and the inevitability of death or leaves. Acceptance, however, comes through a period of grieving.

Stage four (emotional arrival) This is marked by a sense of freedom as practitioners are depressed or preoccupied by either their own health or death. This does not mean they feel *no* pain when working with dying people, but can be empathetic rather than sympathetic, now able to see the patient's world through his or her eyes without making it their own.

Stage five (deep compassion) The culmination of previous growth and development, this stage sees the practitioner able to relate compassionately to the dying person in the full acceptance of his or her impending death. Deep compassion requires self-realisation, self-awareness and self-actualisation, and concern at this stage is channelled towards 'humane professional assessment of need'.

Grief as an ongoing process

Harper's model parallels, in many respects, my own adjustment to working with dying and bereaved people, together with my observations of other people working in palliative care. However, everyone works through the model at a different pace. Harper presents this model as one of 'developmental stages' but, on reflection, it may be more of an ongoing process. Stage five is presented as a culmination point, which can appear rather static, but as a model of initial adjustment to palliative care, it provides a helpful developmental model. After an initial adjustment period, an ongoing process of adjustment occurs which is specific to individual relationships, and is reflected by the fact that nurses react differently at each meeting with a new patient and his or her family. The stages can therefore coexist; for example, a nurse may feel 'deep compassion' for one individual, but can equally be in stage two ('trauma') with another, perhaps particularly someone with whom she or he identifies in some way, whether at a conscious or unconscious level. I tend to feel I get into the 'deep compassion' stage but not through it – I am never self-actualised. From time to time, for example, when I make an emotional investment in a particular patient I may move from stage four ('emotional arrival') or five ('deep compassion') into two ('trauma') or three ('depression').

Harper sees stage three in terms of staying in the specialist field or leaving it. This stage can also be viewed, however, as one in which nurses may use distancing tactics to defend themselves from making emotional investments, and their decision can be seen as the result of a stage two ('trauma') experience. Some people may try to avoid emotional investment altogether as a result of their personal or professional training. Our defenses are there for a reason and need to be respected, but if a team member is constantly emotionally defended, this will inevitably affect the psychosocial and spiritual care she or he can offer.

Harper's model is helpful for assessing staff adjustment and need for support. It is particularly important to be aware of staff who become enmeshed in *any* of the stages. Initially, when perusing this model, I thought I needed to be particularly aware of people who got stuck in one of the first three stages, but I now increasingly question the ability of staff to stay in stage five, as sometimes they can slip from stage five into stage one. Stage five can probably never be fully worked through, as it is impossible to always feel deeply compassionate.

"You cannot prevent the birds of sorrow from flying overhead; but you can prevent them from building nests in your hair" Chinese proverb.

Formalised support

In palliative care, grief is an ongoing process to varying degrees, at different times and for individual people. Worden (1983) considers there are 10 principles to be followed which enable people to work through their grief (Table 1). Reviewing these 10 principles in the context of palliative care, nurses have many potential ways of 'actualising' their loss. If they are present when a patient dies, they are confronting the person's death and may also confirm their death to the family. They may also carry out the washing and preparing of the body with the family or a colleague, or go to see the body at the patient's home (if appropriate), in the mortuary or at the undertaker. Nurses may also be involved in enabling the family to express their feelings. Involvement in these aspects may, however, block their own expression of grief.

---

1. To help the survivor actualise the loss: the person needs to accept that the loss has occurred so he or she can deal with its emotional impact. Acceptance comes through talking about the loss.
2. To help the survivor identify and express feelings.
3. To assist the survivor to live without the deceased.
4. To facilitate emotional withdrawal from the deceased.
5. To provide time to grieve.
6. To interpret 'normal behaviour': Worden considers this to be the understanding of normal grief behaviours because, after a significant loss, many people feel they are going a little crazy, as they may experience hallucinations and a heightened sense of distractability.
7. To allow for individual difference.
8. To provide continuing support.
9. To examine defenses and coping style.
10. To identify pathology and refer.

Table 1. The 10 principles of grief (Worden, 1983).

Gray-Toft and Anderson (1986) underlined the importance of a sense of 'closure' for nurses when a patient dies; this consists of nurses' desire to be present when a patient dies, sharing the loss and the grief with the family, assisting in the preparation and transportation of the body to the mortuary and attending the funeral. They also noted, however, that these practices were stressful, and that stress arose when nurses, for whatever reason, were denied a sense of closure. This is certainly true of my own personal experience and observations, and for other members of the palliative care team. Non-nurse team members may, in fact, have less opportunity for closure than nurses.

Worden's fifth principle of 'providing time to grieve' is central, together with his eighth, 'the provision of continuing support'. By giving 'specific opportunity' for staff to grieve and 'continuing support', nurses' grief, coping styles and difficulties can be worked through, their individuality acknowledged, 'bereavement overload' (Kastenbaum, 1969) and 'professional burnout' prevented or identified and worked through.

Many palliative care nursing teams have no formalised 'specific opportunity' or 'continuing support' for staff, but frequently have a formalised support system for patients, those close to them, and volunteer bereavement visitors. Should 'those close to them' not include professional staff who make an emotional investment? If patients, those close to them, and volunteers need structured support, surely then palliative care staff also grieve and need support?

Three philosophical approaches underline bereavement counselling:

- bereavement counselling should be offered to everyone on the basis that it is a traumatic event;

- some people will need help to come to terms with their bereavement, but will wait until they get into difficulty before recognising their own need for help and, hopefully, seeking it;

- it can be predicted who is likely to have difficulty, and early counselling will prevent unresolved grief reaction (Worden, 1983); this approach was used in the Harvard Bereavement Study (Parkes 1972)

These philosophical approaches can be applied to the support of palliative care staff. The balance between bereavement and job satisfaction can be a fine one. Some studies of stress in palliative care demonstrate that emotional investment in patients who are dying is both stressful *and* a major source of job satisfaction (eg, Wilkinson, 1987). Some staff at particular times may encounter difficulties and may or may not recognise their need for help and seek it, so it is necessary to ensure structured as well as informal staff support is on offer.

Some grief theorists, notably Kubler-Ross (1975), Parkes (1972) and Morris (1986), see the growth potential in grief. Morris, in fact, sees grief as "a healing process if the circumstances are facilitative". We need to ensure that environments in which nurses care for dying people facilitate staff grief and provide an environment in which staff can develop.

References

Gray-Toft, P.A. and Anderson, T.G. (1986) Sources of stress in nursing terminal patients in a hospice. *Omega*, **17**, 27-39.

Harper, B.C. (1977) Death: the coping mechanism of the health professional. South Eastern University Press, Greenville.

Kastenbaum, R.J. (1969) Death and bereavement in later life. In: Kutscher, A.H. (Ed) Death and Bereavement. Springfield, Illinois.

Kubler-Ross, E. (1975) Death: the final stage of growth. Prentice Hall, London.

Maslock, C. and Jackson, S. (1979) Burned out cops and their families. *Psychology Today*, **79**, 59.

Morris, P. (1986) Loss and Change. Routledge and Kegan Paul, London.

Parkes, C.M. (1972a) Determinents of outcome following bereavement. *Omega*, **6**, 1975, 303-23.

Parkes, C.M. (1972b) Studies of Grief in Adult Life. International Universities Press, New York.

Parkes, C.M. and Brown, R.J. (1972) Health after bereavement: a controlled study of young Boston widows and widowers. *Journal of Psychosomatic Medicine*, **34**, 449-61.

Raphael, B. (1980) A psychiatric model for bereavement counselling? In: Shloenberg, B.M. (Ed) Bereavement Counselling, a Multi-disciplinary Handbook. Greenwood Press, Conneticut.

Seligmen, M.P. (1975) Helplessness: on depression, development and death. Freeman, Oxford.

Stedeford, A. (1987) Hospice: a safe place to suffer? *Palliative Medicine*, 1, 1, 73-74.

Wilkinson, S.M. (1987) Nursing patients with cancer: satisfaction and stresses. In: Faulkner, A. (Ed) Ballière's Practice and Research in Nursing the Patient With Cancer. Ballière Tindall, London.

Worden, J.W. (1983) Grief Counselling and Grief Therapy. Tavistock Publications, London.

41

A terminal case? Burnout in palliative care

Ann Nash, MN, SRN, DipN, RCNT
Nurse Consultant, the Macmillan Education Centre, Dorothy House Foundation, Bath

Working alongside patients and families coping with the problems of advanced disease is a stressful field for healthcare professionals, yet the specialty attracts large numbers of nurses and other professionals. This chapter reviews the significant literature, attempting to throw light on the incidence of burnout in palliative carers.

Stress

The concept of burnout is not new. Florence Nightingale was aware of the strain and pain of caring, and acknowledged carers' responses and reactions to that stress. The term 'stress' was first used in this context by Cannon in 1925. He coined the word 'homoeostasis', suggesting that the body would normally return to a steady state after such disturbance within the system.

Selye (1956) defined stress as a state of wear and tear, experienced as fatigue, uneasiness or illness, and described a basic biochemical model of adaptation to stress. There is no doubt that this biological reaction is significant, and can be observed. Mind, body and behaviour are closely intertwined, and this leads to a potentially healthy adjustment to the demands of daily living. Appropriate responses to stressful situations enable us to function usefully (Schafer, 1987).

Caring for dying people

Hingley (1985) observes that the public image of stress is generally negative, and explores what elements of nursing give rise to negative feelings of being under stress. In Hingley's work, nurses identified dealing with death and dying as a specific stressor, and this was linked to the expectations that patients will be cured and restored to health by the medical profession. Dying is a normal activity, yet these expectations of cure and health can lead to feelings of inadequacy and, where dying is accepted as inevitable, nurses may also feel unable to cope with the special demands of that specialist role.

The activity of dying, however, is not limited to patients. Nurses who work with the dying and bereaved are brought face to face with their own mortality. This self-awareness can lead to a higher level of stress than the nurse can cope with (Bond, 1986). On starting to work in terminal care, most nurses have high ideals. Idealistic nurses can be exciting, innovative and enthusiastic (Swaffield, 1988), but some of their ideals are unattainable and unrealistic. Standards are not always achievable due to financial, environmental or personal constraints and limitations, and the burnout response in idealistic nurses in such situations may be infectious, affecting a whole group of carers.

Significant stressors

Ward (1985) and Lunt and Yardley (1986) investigated the working patterns of specialist home care nurses in palliative care and observed that, while the stressors involved in caring for the dying and bereaved are undeniable, the major stressors identified as leading to burnout were to do with relationships with other professionals. Those professionals were identified as managers who did not understand or support the aims and objectives of the service and members of the primary health care teams, notably GPs and district nurses, who sometimes blocked the way to good care by their ignorance or in their response to a perceived professional threat. The inability to achieve good pain control and family support led to overwhelming stress in nurses, causing them to question whether the effort was worthwhile.

Vachon (1987) identified the stressors for caregivers in several areas. She was able to establish that dying patients are not the real problem, and observed stressors within the work environment which were significant.

In her investigation of nurse training for terminal care, Simms (1984) identified the specific stressors for this group, which are lack of specific boundaries leading to overwork, and the inability to limit caseloads and workloads due to an ever increasing demand for specialist input. So these nurses appear to be subject to two major areas of over-stress – lack of useful management of time and objectives, and specific relationships with powerful colleagues who might influence outcomes negatively.

Need for support

Managers and educators involved in developing specialist roles have a specific responsibility to prevent burnout in these nurses, and having recognised the signals of distress, must develop useful interventions (Wilkinson, 1987). Supportive interventions may form a useful basis for the development of coping strategies (Heron, 1986), but the concept of nurses needing personal and professional support is still not widely accepted. Most nurses turn to colleagues informally for such support, but Adey (1987) suggested that it was lacking from teams and managers, and that most nurses felt inadequate in accessing appropriate support when needed. If it is to be effective, this support is needed before this stage, and to enable nurses to deal with the dilemma of reality vs. idealism, it must be available formally and regularly (Nash, 1985).

The implications for nurses of this development of self-awareness of death and dying, when caring for patients in a cancer ward was explored by Baider and Porath (1981). Using the group process, the nurses were able, in a formal setting, to reveal and share their feelings of frustration, anger and sadness. Such team support can be catalytic and cathartic, but can lead to a certain anxiety and wariness about the depth of shared feeling. This group was, in fact, abandoned as a consequence.

Personal involvement
The combination of high technology areas with extremely vulnerable patient groups, as in paediatric oncology units (Waters, 1985) and bone marrow transplant units (Pot-Mees, 1987), demands an acknowledgement of the need for prevention, awareness and early treatment of burnout. Nurses are, therefore, encouraged towards self-help, self-awareness and self-knowledge (Bleazard, 1984).

This development of knowledge of self, acknowledgement of personal reactions and awareness of own needs is essential to useful helping. Such personal work enables a level of involvement and helping which has more to offer the patient, but requires built-in supportive/supervisory intervention. Bailey, Burnard and Smith (1985) organised a workshop for managers involved in supporting staff, to examine methods of preventing and dealing with burnout. They used experiential exercises to raise awareness of the potential effects of burnout. Their concept of 'degrees' of burnout could enable managers to interrupt this process. The group was able to plan preventive measures.

Such workshops allow professionals to acknowledge that stress exists, that over-stress can be dangerous, and that we must learn to recognise the early stages ot burnout in colleagues and, hopefully, in ourselves. Only when stress is accepted as an inevitable consequence of striving for high standards in a climate of severe constraints will we plan and be ready to tackle consequences effectively.

Growth
As we have seen, if such stressors did not exist, there would be little impetus towards improving standards of care. The starting point is the acknowledgement that nurses are people too (Holland, 1987), and that they are reacting to life and death both within and without the work environment; growing and learning about themselves among others. Caring for the dying and bereaved provides an opportunity for personal growth, working alongside professionals who also struggle with the problems of growth and change. While the stressors are huge, the rewards and satisfactions (both personal and professional) in palliative care are enormous.

References
Adey, C. (1987) Stress: who cares?. *Nursing Times*, **83**, 4, 52-53.
Baider, L. and Porath, S. (1981) Uncovering fear: group experience of nurse in a cancer ward. International *Journal of Nursing Studies*, **18**, 47-52.

Bailey, C., Burnard, P., Smith, R., (1985) Breaking the ice. *Nursing Mirror*, **160**, 1, 26-28.

Bleazard, R. (1984) Knowing oneself. *Nursing Times*, **80**, 10, 44-46.

Bond, M. (1986) Stress and Self-Awareness: A Guide for Nurses. Heinemann, London.

Cannon, W.B. (1935) Stresses and strains of homeostasis. *American Journal of Medical Science*, **189**, 1.

Heron, J. 1986 Six Category Intervention Analysis. Human Potential Research Project, University of Surrey.

Hingley, P. (1985) Stress in nurse managers. Royal College of Nursing Research Society, June.

Holland, S. (1987) Stress in Nursing. *Nursing Times*, **83**, 21, 59-61.

Lunt, B. and Yardley and Hospital Support Teams for the Terminally Ill. Cancer Care Research Unit, Southampton (unpublished).

Nash, A. (1985) Bereavement: staff support. *Nursing*, **2**, 43, 1288.

Pot-Mees, C. (1987) Beating the burn-out. *Nursing Times*, **83**, 30, 33-35.

Schafer, W. (1987) Stress Management for Wellness. Holt Reinhart and Winston, New York.

Selye, H. (1956) The Stress of Life. McGraw Hill, New York.

Simms, M. (1984) Nurse training for terminal care. *Senior Nurse*, **1**, 34, 21-22.

Swaffield, L. (1988) Burn-out. *Nursing Standard*, 14, 2, 24-25.

Vachon, M.L.S. (1987) Occupational Stress in the Care of the Critically Ill, the Dying and The Bereaved. Holt Reinhart and Winston, New York.

Ward, A.W.M. (1985) Home Care Services for the Terminally Ill: A Report for the Nuffield Foundation. University of Sheffield Medical School.

Waters, A.L. (1985) Support for staff in a Paediatric oncology unit. *Nursing*, **2**, 43, 1275-77.

Wilkinson, S. (1987) The reality of nursing cancer patients. *Lampada*, **12**, 12-19.

Primary Nursing

42

What is primary nursing?

Liz Tutton, BSc, SRN

Liz Tutton wrote this chapter whilst she was Nurse Practitioner, Nursing Development Unit, Oxford

The concept of primary nursing emerged from the University of Minnesota hospitals in the late 1960s (Manthey et al, 1970). In her book on primary nursing, Manthey indicates that in her work area there was general dissatisfaction with the existing system of team nursing, where a group of nurses had a generalised responsibility for a group of patients (Manthey, 1980). Nurses felt that care was fragmented, communication channels were extremely complex and no one was totally responsible for patient care. This chapter discusses the Oxford Nursing Development Unit, which was closed on 5th April 1989. It is hoped that this regrettable decision by the Health Authority will not inhibit the continuing development of primary nursing in Oxfordshire and elsewhere.

"Primary nursing is a system for delivering nursing service that consists of four design elements: allocation and acceptance of individual responsibility for decision making to one individual; individual assignment of daily care; direct communication channels; one person responsible for the quality of care administered to patients on a unit 24 hours a day, seven days a week" (Manthey, 1980). These four elements could be seen as responsibility, patient allocation, communication and care giver as care planner.

Responsibility

The primary nurse takes full responsibility for decision making in patient care, with an 'associate' nurse taking responsibility for carrying out the care planned for the patient when the primary nurse is off duty. An associate nurse is a qualified member of staff who is developing the skills to become a primary nurse. He or she is responsible to the primary nurse, who can be contacted, if necessary, when off duty. In some settings using primary nursing, all nurses act as primary nurses for a small number of patients and also work as associate nurses with other patients for whom another colleague is the primary nurse.

The primary nurse accepts three major responsibilities. She collects all the information, including research findings, needed to care for her patients and makes it available to her colleagues. She also assesses the patient and produces a written plan of action and criterion for evaluation. Finally the primary nurse accepts responsibility for planning and co-ordinating the patient's discharge.

Patient allocation

The patient is allocated to one primary nurse who has a group of associate nurses working for her when she is off duty, and when on duty has the responsibility of administering total care to her patients. An important aim of this is to eliminate the performance of isolated technical tasks which lead to patient centred nursing.

One of the purposes of primary nursing is to simplify the system for communication between all professionals concerned with each patient. The primary nurse communicates directly with everyone involved in her patients' treatment, including the doctor, pharmacist, dietitian, physiotherapist and also patients themselves, and takes responsibility for obtaining and disseminating information to relevant members of the health care team. Communication at hand over periods is simplified by the primary nurse handing over directly to the associate nurse caring for her patients. Continuity of care leads to nurse and patient becoming more knowledgeable about each other, which allows for improved relationships. This gives the nurse more chance of therapeutically using her skills of teaching, guiding and helping and allows the patient to become more actively involved in his or her care and make more informed decisions.

It would seem logical that the care plan would be most useful and practical if the person who formulates it actually gives the care. In this way the patient's real needs are more likely to be stated in it.

Oxford Nursing Development Unit

The Oxford Nursing Development Unit (ONDU) at the Radcliffe Infirmary was closed following a funding decision by Oxfordshire Health Authority in 1989. It was a unique example of primary nursing. The beds were designated as nursing beds rather than as 'medical' beds, so the nurse carried full autonomy and responsibility for patient care.

Based on the principles and philosophies of the Loeb Center in New York, ONDU was a unit run for patients needing intensive nursing care as opposed to 'doctoring'. The concept of nursing as a therapy is relatively new, and the idea that nursing has a positive outcome for patients is of increasing importance to nurses (McMahon, 1986). Patients were admitted to the unit as soon as they are medically stable, and stayed until they were fit for discharge. Priority was given to expansion rather than extension of the nurse's role: building up nurse- patient relationships: using communication and counselling skills, education and teaching to allow patients to make informed choices, and making use of nurses' unique position to give physical care. Patients were involved in planning their own care if they so wish, and make their own decisions about daily activities. There were no routines to be followed, visiting hours were open and family participation encouraged.

Primary Nursing is a system for delivering nursing care (Manthey, 1980) and it provides an ideal environment for the use of the nursing process and nursing conceptual models. ONDU used primary nursing in conjunction with the Roper, Logan and Tierney (1980) model of nursing based on the use of 12 activities of daily living. The unit had four types of staff, in common with other primary nursing centres:

Primary nurse   Primary nurses take a case load of eight patients each, carrying full responsibility and accountability for their care. They assess, plan, implement and evaluate this care, leaving a written plan for associate nurses to implement in their absence. If a change in this plan of care is needed, the nurse practitioner is contacted and will either give a verbal instruction or visit the unit.

Associate nurse   These are trained nurses, often part-time, who carry out the care planned by the primary nurse, under whom they are divided into teams. They have a case load of eight patients.

Ward orderlies or care assistants   Ward orderlies help with domestic or non-nursing tasks so that the nurse can remain at the bedside with the patient. They help with bathing, kitchen work and general domestic duties and are directly accountable to the primary nurse.

Ward coordinators   These are clerical assistants who perform duties such as filing, ordering stores, arranging patient appointments, typing and general telephone duties. 'Walkie-talkies' facilitate quick communication between nurse practitioners and ward coordinator, which again frees the nurse to be with the patients.

ONDU showed that patient centred nursing within the framework of primary nursing improves patient satisfaction, quality of nursing care and leads to shorter stays in hospital for patients. The closure of the unit to 'save money' was a regretable short-term decision.

References
McMahon. R. (1986) Nursing as a Therapy. *The Professional Nurse*, **1**, 10, 270-272.
Manthey, M. (1970) Primary Nursing, *Nursing Forum*, **IX**, 1, 65-83.
Manthey M. (1980) The Practice of Primary Nursing. Blackwell.

Bibliography
Bowes Ferres, S. (1975) Loeb Center and its Philosophy of Nursing. *American Journal of Nursing*, **75**, 5.
   Describes the setting up, running and philosophy of the Loeb Center.
Lee, M.E. (1979) Towards better care 'Primary Nursing' *Nursing Times*, Occasional Paper, **75**, 33.
   Lee suggests that the clinical nurse should take responsibility for good quality nursing care. She discusses primary nursing as a means of making this responsibility explicit.
Marram, G.D. et al (1974) Primary nursing: a model for individualised care. Mosby.
   An in-depth study of nursing organisational systems, including some studies on the effects of primary nursing.
Roper, N., Logan W. and Tierney, A. (1986) The elements of Nursing (Second Edition) Churchill Livingstone, Edinburgh.
   A description of the nursing model based on activities of living which can be used as a basis for assessing and planning nursing care.

43

The role of the associate nurse

Sarah Burns, RGN
Lecturer/Practitioner, John Radcliffe Hospital, Oxford

Since primary nursing was implemented at the John Radcliffe Hospital, much attention has been focused on the primary nurse role (Tutton, 1986; MacMahon 1987). Primary nursing is the system whereby all patients and clients are allocated to a primary nurse on entering care. This nurse is then responsible for their nursing round-the-clock as long as it is needed. She is both responsible and accountable for the care she plans and gives. However, the primary nurse can rarely be the sole provider of this care and is therefore assisted by associate nurses. It is important to examine the role of the associate nurse, as without a clear understanding, it may be interpreted as having low status, which we at the John Radcliffe have found not to be true.

Throughout the period of nursing development those nurses who function exclusively as associate nurses have coped extremely well with the perceived threat to their own role, which was caused by uncertainty and inexperience making it difficult to see the eventual role clearly. Now we can review some of the changes to our fundamental thinking.

Who should be an associate nurse?
Experience of the associate nurse role is almost a prerequisite to becoming a primary nurse. The potential for personal and professional development is great and, I feel, vital in preparing a primary nurse.

Most of our associate nurses are newly registered or part-time qualified nurses, but student nurses may fill this role as long as they have appropriate supervision. It should also be remembered that the associate nurse may be another primary nurse in the team who is providing cover during a colleague's absence.

Hierarchy
The hierarchical structures which supported our traditional nursing practice have had to be dismantled where they were found to be inhibiting us. For example, our communication network previously meant that the associate nurses discussed nursing care issues with the sister or nurse in charge, who would then decide whether to take the issue to the nurse specialist, doctor or other professional. This inhibited

the development of the associate nurses' confidence and creativity. To combat this all had to work hard to promote and support direct communication, so the associate nurses can initiate discussion with any professionals. We have found the role of sister has become one of advisor on clinical issues rather than major decision-maker.

We have tried to transfer the values and beliefs about the relationship with clients to our relationships with each other. These hinge on the nature of the relationship between the nurse and client – it must be a close partnership, with each party able to identify the other – the notion of 'my nurse' or 'my patient' as Manthey (1970) puts it.

The freedom and comfort required to develop the partnership can be inhibited by an hierarchical nursing team, but an open atmosphere of mutual trust and respect helps partnerships to flourish. It is important to recognise, however, that this is not the whole answer – individual nurses must want to develop these relationships. For many nurses this is uncharted territory and can be perceived as very threatening.

Part of the willingness to participate comes from each member feeling valued as part of the team, a feeling which is very much influenced by the ward sister. Manthey (1970) suggests that the ability of the ward sister to change her role and allow open and free staff relationships to develop is crucial to the overall implementation of a primary nursing system. Regular ward meetings, sometimes with the ward sister disclosing her own fears, worries and triumphs encourage an atmosphere in which other nurses feel able to disclose and share feelings. This open interest in and care of each other is new for many nurses. It is important that all members of the team work to develop an atmosphere in which individuals feel comfortable disclosing their feelings without fear of ridicule or retribution.

Smaller teams

One way of promoting this working relationship is to break the large nursing team into smaller teams. Headed by one or more primary nurses, the rest of the small team is composed of associate nurses. These teams look after a small group of patients within the ward or department, allowing all staff continuity of care – that is looking after the same patients each time they are on duty. Without a team approach, an associate nurse who acts exclusively in that role can find herself looking after one primary nurse's patients one day and another's the next, so she herself does not experience continuity of care.

One associate nurse described this as feeling like a foster mother. Having worked hard at developing a good relationship with one group of clients she had to hand them back to the primary nurse feeling very much as a foster mother might feel when returning a child to its natural mother. Using a team approach means the associate nurse looks after the same group of patients whenever she is on duty.

The diagrams illustrate examples of team membership. In Figure 1, meeting clients' nursing care needs is the responsibility of the primary nurse. The associate nurses assist in carrying out this care, especially when the primary nurse is off duty. Clarification of care can be elicited from the care plan, but as the associate nurses can have as much continuous contact with the clients as the primary nurse, communication is generally easier, more effective and less open to error or breakdown. Figure 2 illustrates that where there is more than one primary nurse in a team each will 'associate' for the other when she or he is off duty, thus acting in both roles on one shift. The associate nurse will 'associate' for both primary nurses in their joint absence.

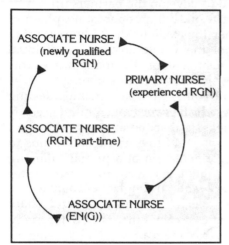

Figure 1. The primary nurse is responsible for nursing care in this team, helped by the associate nurses.

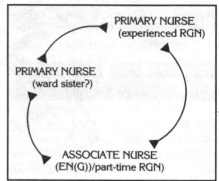

Figure 2. When the team has more than one primary nurse, they will 'associate' for each other, both helped by the associate nurse.

The feeling of belonging gained from the team approach, of contributing to the care of a group of clients, of receiving acknowledgement of one's endeavours all reflect Maslow's hierarchy of needs. The stage is then set for the creative contributions of the associate nurse in giving highly personalised nursing care.

Guidelines

For individual nurses to reach this point, some guidelines are necessary. Up-to-date job descriptions and standards help clarify what is and what is not expected, but it is important that individual nurses feel that acknowledgement is made of past experience and special abilities. Setting personal targets from job performance reviews is helpful in this area, which is ripe for development by ward sisters.

Associate nurses are essential members of the nursing team within a primary nursing system. They are accountable for their own practices, and their contribution to clients' care is active rather than passive. They are trained to use professional judgement in their clients' interests, and to evaluate their own practice. The level of decision-making expected from associate nurses can vary, but all team members should be clear about it. They, and nurse managers, must also acknowledge that some associate nurses may have extensive experience and expertise.

If the associate nurse role is to emerge as a positive and valued role within a primary nursing system, all members of the team need to examine all aspects of their behaviour which might inhibit freedom of speech and action in other team members. Otherwise the associate nurse will merely be the primary nurses' handmaiden.

References

Manthey, M. (1970) A return to the concept of my nurse and my patient. *Nursing Forum,* **9,** 1, 65-83.

Manthey, M. (1980) *The Practice of Primary Nursing.* Blackwell Scientific, New York.

Maslow, A. (1970) *Motivation and Personality* (2nd Ed.) Harper Row, New York.

44

A change worth the making: implementing primary nursing

Susan Waterworth, MSc, RGN, DipN (London), RNT, DANS, ICU Cert
Clinical Nurse Specialist, Royal Liverpool Hospital

Primary nursing is an approach whereby each patient has their own primary and associate nurse, facilitating continuity and consistency of patient care. Primary nurses have 24-hour accountability for the care they plan, and implementing a primary nursing system involves a critical rethink of the traditional way nursing is practised, which can be a difficult process. This chapter describes how this rethink occurred on one unit and how the change was implemented.

Assessing our approach to care

Primary nursing was adopted on an extremely busy haematology and bone marrow transplant unit, where the previous approach to patient care was first assessed. This was done in several ways, but the overall framework was an examination of the structure, process and outcome of nursing care on the ward (Donabedian, 1969).

Structure refers to the resources available, such as staffing levels and skill mix. It also includes support services, equipment and the presence of policies and a philosophy of care. Process refers to the method of organising care such as patient allocation and task allocation, and includes the assessment, planning, implementation and evaluation of care. Nurses' communication and patient teaching skills as well as research-based practices would also be included in this category. Outcome refers to the effects of the care on patients and patient satisfaction. Nursing staff satisfaction and their development are also included in the outcome category.

As a clinical nurse specialist, part of my role involved working on the ward assessing, planning, implementing and evaluating patient care. This enabled me to work closely with my nursing colleagues, acting as a participant/observer - a role used by researchers in qualitative research studies. The management part of my role included monitoring standards of patient care. Observation and discussion took place with both patients and staff; each member of staff was interviewed, and asked how they felt about their present role and for suggestions on improvements to patient care. Meetings also took place with members of the multidisciplinary team, who identified problem areas from their perspective.

In relation to process, two other tools were used as indicators of our approach to promoting individualised patient care: Miller's (1985) Ward Practice Profile 'Are you using the Nursing Process?' and Brooking's (1986) Nursing Process Measurement Tool. Miller's profile enables a systematic assessment of the method of organising nursing care in relation to care planning, nursing organisation, coordination of care, integration of care and specific work organisation. Brooking's tool includes a ward nurse's self-rating scale, consisting of 37 nursing process items, which allows an assessment of all stages of the nursing process, such as patient involvement in care planning.

The assessment revealed, overall, a highly committed nursing team who were trying to adopt a patient centred approach to care. From the structural assessment, no formal nursing philosophy existed. There were inconsistencies in care planning, care giving, under-utilisation of trained nurses' skill, and some dissatisfaction with the RGN's role, particularly in relation to management skills. The approach to organising care inhibited the nurses' accountability for care, while there was also a lack of planned patient teaching and some shortcomings in discharge planning. Discussions with staff often revealed that reasons for doing something were based on "that is the way we do it here" or "we have always done it that way", but staff were aware of the limitations of this reasoning.

The literature (Ciske, 1979; Manthey, 1980; Sparrow, 1986) on primary nursing *suggests* it can promote accountability, authority, responsibility and autonomy. Primary nursing can also be used to develop staff and promote consistency and continuity of care. The care planner mostly provides the care, which is important for evaluation of care.

Since the initial assessment and planning for primary nursing were carried out on the unit, it is interesting to note that the document 'A Strategy for Nursing' (1989) supports the development and evaluation of primary nursing.

An answer to all our problems?
Primary nursing was not viewed as the means by which all our problems would be solved, but was implemented as part of an overall strategy to promote the unit as a centre for excellence. It took nine months of planning and preparation before the actual implementation of this major change took place. The assessment, however, made it possible to determine 'where we were at' as far as primary nursing was, reflecting on the extent to which we had adopted its key concepts of accountability and responsibility. The unit's staff were highly motivated to promote individualised patient care, yet the structure and method of organising patient care did not facilitate this. The RGNs' accountability for care was not recognised within the present structure, and they were not responsible for specific patients apart from on a daily basis. There was no continuity of care by specific nurses, and this affected the

consistency of care delivered.

Many strategies exist for implementing change, and it was essential that one was adopted. Kotter and Schlesinger (1979) have identified reasons for resistance to change, such as parochial self-interest, where staff may fear losing something of value - this applies not only to enrolled nurses, but also to ward sisters. Misunderstanding and different perceptions may also cause resistance.

Kotter and Schlesinger (1979) also discuss how resistance can be dealt with, citing education, communication, participation, involvement, facilitation and support. All of these were incorporated into the change plan for our unit, and are ongoing to maintain and further promote the change to primary nursing. Change itself is stressful, particularly if it creates uncertainty. Adopting a management style that alleviates stress has been identified as important (Bailey and Sproston, 1987), particularly in highly stressful areas such as oncology (Wilkinson, 1987).

Lewin's Force Field Analysis (1951; Table 1) was used to identify both the driving and restraining forces and proved useful for increasing awareness. The driving forces could be harnessed and the restraining forces limited.

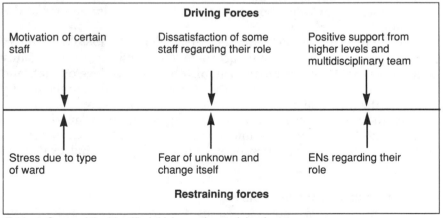

Table 1. Some of the identified driving and restraining forces.

Ottoway (1976) stresses the need to adopt a bottom-up approach to change, and it was important that all staff in the unit felt involved and able to contribute to the implementation of primary nursing. Ottoway (1976) also points out that support from the top is required, and this was provided by senior nurse managers. A 'timetable of events' was planned, and this included meetings, courses and visits. Meetings were arranged, initially, to explore the prospective changes, and aimed to:

• discuss why change may be needed;

• explore why primary nursing is a way forward;

- discuss the principles of primary nursing;

- provide opportunity for staff to express their views and make suggestions.

Staff attitudes

Quite naturally, the meetings uncovered some negative attitudes among staff to implementing primary nursing, and comments included, "we're too busy, we've not enough staff"; "What about sickness?"; "What about the stress of nursing patients for longer periods, particularly if they have been coming to the unit for several years?". These concerns needed to be discussed freely, so that staff could see the possible benefits of primary nursing for both patients and themselves.

Visits to other units already using primary nursing were arranged so that staff could see and discuss it with nurses using this approach to care; this proved useful in reducing some areas of concern. Two ward sisters went on separate visits to these units, giving them the freedom to talk about changes in their own role, which they may not have voiced had their own staff been present.

The skills, knowledge and attitudes that staff needed were identified so that adequate preparation could be given. Although Rule 18 and the trained nurses' competencies state that nurses should be able to assess, plan, implement and evaluate care, as well as teach patients, it is evident that these skills need further development post-registration. At a Primary Nursing Network meeting (1989), Gerry Bowman, Nurse Manager at Leicester presented a paper on preparing primary nurses, based on 10 years' experience of primary nursing in a medical unit which identified staff development as vital if primary nursing is to succeed.

Nursing process workshops were already being held for trained staff at the hospital and most were able to attend these. Further discussions were also held in the clinical area. Counselling workshops were organised with our in-service training officer, and several nurses are attending counselling courses in their own time. Information has been provided on patient teaching, which has been given a higher profile. A senior staff nurse attended a primary nursing conference, and was able to give the rest of the unit positive feedback and encouragement. The King's Fund Primary Nursing Network has been a valuable source of support, while regional meetings have provided a forum for discussion with other nurses using primary nursing or who are thinking about this approach to care.

Primary nursing information sheets were formulated for all day and night staff, to update them on progress. Communication with other people coming to the unit was vital, and letters were distributed and informal discussions took place. Further meetings with staff were held to examine the practicalities of the system, such as how many patients each primary nurse would have, and the implications of completing off-duty.

A way forward

In comparison to other units, our approach to practising primary nursing is still in its early days. Continual ongoing development and support of staff have been arranged, study days organised, and distance learning packages on topics such as assertiveness, patient teaching, individualised patient care and stress management obtained. Senior members of the nursing team act as facilitators to other staff, while newly appointed associate nurses have a primary nurse as their mentor.

Hunt (1988) notes the need for appropriate evaluation of primary nursing, but, what constitutes an appropriate method is highly debatable - reflecting the complexities of evaluating nursing. Our evaluation will be ongoing and will form a case study approach, and an assessment of structure, process and outcome will continue to be used.

To provide further information and act as a baseline, Monitor (Goldstone *et al*, 1983) is used as part of the evaluation process. This tool was developed to provide an objective assessment of certain aspects of patient care. It involves interviews with patients and nurses, observation of nursing documentation and examination of resources. One of its major drawbacks is its focus on nursing documentation (Barnett and Wainwright, 1987) while assessment of the process of care is severely limited. For example, in evaluating a patient's nursing assessment, the nursing documentation is referred to; how well the nurse carried out the assessment from the nurse-patient relationship and communication skills perspective is not evaluated. In considering the evaluation of primary nursing, the limitations of the tools used need to be considered.

To maintain the change and further develop a primary nursing approach, all new staff in the unit are taken on with the understanding that this is our approach to care. The roles of the primary nurse, associate nurse and ward coordinator have been drawn up by the nursing team, and job descriptions for both primary and associate nurses formulated. Regular meetings are held to ensure staff continue to voice their con-cerns, resolve problems and make suggestions for further developments.

Despite meetings and information sheets the permanent night staff did not feel as involved in primary care as staff on day duty. There do seem to be genuine difficulties for night staff (Remington, 1989), particularly where bank nurses are used. However, the introduction of internal rotation and the reduced use of bank staff has helped to address this problem.

Primary nursing appears to act as a catalyst for other changes, and one of the difficulties has been that hospital policies have slowed down or prevented certain further developements from taking place. For example, our hospital policy still required two nurses to carry out the drug administration round, so attempts to introduce more flexibility for the primary and associate nurses are proceeding more slowly than we would wish.

Patients' responses

Although we have only been practising primary nursing since July 1989, staff are more accountable and patients have made positive comments about the new system. Patients who have experienced care in the unit both before and after primary nursing was introduced have stated their preference for it, saying they now know who their nurses are and have greater trust and confidence in them because of their indepth understanding of their problems. As one patient put it: "you're not constantly having to make new relationships with the nurses and explain everything again". A checklist of 'how well are we practising primary nursing' has been devised, and consists of questions relating to the key concepts. A question related to responsibility for example, would ask "Do primary nurses have responsibility? How is this in evidence?" whereas a question on accountability would ask "Are primary nurses accepting their accountability?".

The staff are working hard to deal with problems in a constructive way. As a team, they have been willing to reflect on their practices - no easy task - as a way of developing themselves and the care they give. As nurses, we must continually strive to improve patient care, and one of our starting points has been to adopt a primary nursing approach as one of our strategies.

References

Bailey, D. and Sproston, C. (1987) Understanding Stress: Part 1. HMSO, London.

Barnett, D. and Wainwright, P. (1987) Between two tools. *Senior Nurse*, **6**, 4, 40-42.

Bowman, G. (1989) Preparing Primary Nurses. Paper presented at the Primary Nursing Network Meeting, London.

Brooking, J. (1986) Patient and Family Participation in Nursing Care: The Development of a Nursing Process Measuring Scale. PhD Thesis, University of London, King's College.

Ciske, K.J. (1979) Accountability - The essence of primary nursing. *Am. J. Nursing,*, **9**, 892-94.

Department of Health Nursing Division (1989) A strategy for Nursing. DoH, London.

Donabedian, A. (1969) Some issues in evaluating the quality of nursing care. *Am. Journal of Public Health*, **59**, 1833-36.

Goldstone, L.A., Ball, J.A, Collier, M.M. (1983) Monitor: An Index of the Quality of Nursing Care for Acute Medical and Surgical Wards. Newcastle-upon-Tyne Polytechnic Products Ltd.

Hunt, J. (1988) The next challenge. *Nursing Times*, **84**, 49, 36-38.

Kotter, J.P. and Schlesinger, L.A. (1979) Choosing Strategies for Change. *Harvard Business Review*, March-April, 106-115.

Lewin, K. (1951) Field Theory in Social Science. Harper and Row, London.

Macdonald, M. (1988) Primary nursing: is it worth it? *J. Adv. Nursing*, **13**, 797-806.

Manthey, M. (1980) The Practice of Primary Nursing. Blackwell, Oxford.

Miller, A. (1985) Are you using the nursing process? *Nursing Times*, **81**, 50, 36-39.

Ottoway, R.M. (1975) A change strategy to implement new norms, new styles and new environment in the work organisation. *Personnel Review*, **5**, 1.

Remington, J. (1989) Night Rites. *Nursing Times*, **85**, 1, 30-31.

Sparrow, S. (1986) Primary Nursing. *Nursing Practice*, **1**, 142-48.

Wilkinson, S.M. (1986) The Satisfactions and Stresses of Nursing Patients with Cancer. Unpublished MSc Thesis, University of Manchester.

Legal and Ethical Issues

45
Confidentiality

Elizabeth M. Horne, MA
Managing Director, Professional Nurse

The Code of Professional Conduct (UKCC, 1984) states that: registered nurses, midwives and health visitors shall: "Respect confidential information obtained in the course of professional practice and refrain from disclosing such information without the consent of the patient/client, or a person entitled to act on his/her behalf, except where disclosure is required by law or by the order of a court, or is necessary in the public interest."

Conflicts in practice
Isolated from practice, this statement may seem reasonable, but practitioners are daily faced with decisions based on the application of these principles in situations which may contain inherent conflicts of interest. They need confident, working definitions of the elements involved, and to establish clear priorities between the expectations of their patients and those of a wider public. Not so easy when, for example, a sister in a psychiatric day hospital finds a patient in possession of large quantities of controlled drugs that he cannot have obtained legally, or an occupational health nurse is asked by her manager for information about an employee. These examples are cited by the UKCC in an advisory paper on confidentiality (UKCC, 1987), which suggests that the most difficult problem for practitioners is identifying and establishing the boundary between clients' expectations that information will not be disclosed, and the expectations of the public that they will not be unreasonably put at risk.

Confidentiality is important for effective communication
The knowledge that confidentiality will be respected is important for effective communication. There is much information people would not discuss with anyone unless they knew the recipient was completely trustworthy in their offer of confidentiality. Without this trust they may choose to keep quiet, which could affect their health.

Standards of confidentiality should be made clear to clients
It is not practicable to obtain clients' consent every time information needs to be shared with other health professionals, so it should be made known to all clients what standards of confidentiality are maintained.

The practitioner who holds the information must ensure, as far as possible, that it is imparted in strict professional confidence and for a specific purpose serving interests of the client. An individual practitioner is responsible for deciding when it is necessary to obtain the explicit consent of a patient or client.

Practitioners must be familiar with how record systems are used, who has access to them and what are the risks to confidentiality associated with their use. Where students, or those involved in research, require access to records, the same principles of confidentiality apply, and the patient's consent must be sought where appropriate, and the use of the records closely supervised.

Breaches of confidentiality

The principle of confidentiality must be the rule, and breaches of it exceptional; the practitioner must be sure that the best interests of theclient, or thoseof confidential information. The interests of the community may, occasionally, take precedence over those of an individual.

The withholding or disclosing of confidential information may have serious consequences, and the practitioner's decision can be extremely difficult. However, the responsibility cannot be delegated. The individual practitioner must make the decision, and must be able to justify it. It may be helpful to make a written note of the decision and reasons for it on the file for future reference. Situations of this nature can be very stressful, and if other practitioners are aware of them, it may be helpful to discuss the problems. However it is still the responsibility of the individual practitioner, and he or she must ultimately make their own decision.

The UKCC Advisory Paper on Confidentiality is available from: UKCC, 23 Portland Place, London W1N 3AF (send a S.A.E.). It discusses the responsibility of individual practitioners for confidentiality, and the everyday implications for practice, the ownership and care of information, and some of the issues which arise when confidentiality is deliberately breached.

References

United Kingdom Central Council for Nursing, Midwifery and Health Visiting, (1984). Code of Professional Conduct for the Nurse, Midwife and Health Visitor. Second Edition. UKCC, London.

United Kingdom Central Council for Nursing, Midwifery and Health Visiting, (1987). Confidentiality: A UKCC Advisory Paper, UKCC, London.

46

Informed consent: a patient's right?

Alison Kennett, RGN, Cert. Onc
Research Sister, Royal Marsden Hospital, Surrey

Nurses involved in patient education all face the decision of what information should and should not be disclosed. The boundaries of patient advocacy are unclear and nursing ethics must play a part in providing guidelines for what is divulged. In areas such as oncology nursing, the issue of informed consent is particularly important and should be discussed.

Research has shown that the more knowledge patients have about their disease and its subsequent treatment, the more they are able to participate in their own care and the better they feel, both mentally and physically (Hayward, 1973). This research is related specifically to postoperative patients but from my experience in oncology this statement is still most relevant. Indeed it is used on the inside cover of the Royal Marsden Hospital patient education booklet series on all subjects relating to cancer. But the problems arise when we consider who should tell patients, what they should be told, when it should be told and also where it should be told.

Before a patient receives any care it is essential to obtain an informed consent. Failure to do so can give rise to both civil and criminal proceedings (Martin, 1977).

What is informed consent?
A doctrine of informed consent has evolved and patients' rights, as established in the doctrine, have direct implications for the nursing profession collectively and individually. By law, no diagnostic or therapeutic procedure can be performed on a patient without him having been told the risks of the procedure and the alternatives to it prior to giving his consent (Bucklin, 1975). As far back as 1914 Judge Cardozo declared that "every human being of adult years and sound mind has a right to determine what should be done with his or her own body". The principle of informed consent is derived from Anglo-American law which holds that an individual is master over his own body and, if mentally competent, may choose to refuse even life-saving treatment. The United States has much published material on the whole issue of informed consent, whereas English sources are much less abundant. No doubt this is due to the fact

that America has substantial legislation in this area, particularly the Patients' Bill of Rights which includes many of the elements listed below.

Elements of informed consent   The essential elements of informed consent should include:
- a full explanation of the proposed treatment involving important incidental procedures;
- information in a manner intelligible to the patient involving as little jargon as possible;
- explanation of inherent risks and benefits;
- alternatives to proposed treatment;
- adequate time to allow the patient to question the proposals, to ensure the patient realises he has the option to withdraw consent from the treatment or procedure whenever he likes — indeed he has the right to refuse any treatment initially.

Obtaining informed consent
There appear three difficult areas in obtaining a meaningful consent:
  i)who should give the information?
  ii)what information should be disclosed?
  iii)where should the information be given?
  Both Miller (1980) and Bucklin (1975) state that it is the doctor's responsibility to provide enough information to his patients so that an intelligent decision about the procedure can be made. Barkes (1978) also says that disclosure for consent should be regarded as the doctor's prerogative as he is the one to perform the procedure and his is the ultimate responsibility for the communication of facts. In most cases it is the doctor who obtains the consent but in some incidences it may be the senior nurse who obtains the signature on the form after the doctor has explained the procedure.
  Besch (1979) in investigating the possible barriers to obtaining a meaningful consent, found that the doctor-patient relationship appeared to interfere with patient autonomy. The patient tended to trust the doctor's recommendation completely and many did not understand that it was a choice that was being asked of them and not complete compliance. Comments such as these illustrate this: "I guess the doctor knows best." "I wasn't going to argue with him, he knows what he is doing." "If that's what you think I should do, doctor."
  Surely, by virtue of this authoritative role, the physician may, inadvertently, introduce an element of coercion into the consent procedure, thus preventing the patient from making a voluntary decision. "Coercion nullifies consent" (Meissel, 1977).

Effective communication
"Doctors often find it difficult to relax with patients who have incurable cancer and this impairs their ability to communicate effectively with them"

(Hanks, 1983). It must be here that the creation of a patient advocate position would be enormously beneficial to ensure the patient's comprehension of the medical information before making a decision. The nurse can amplify, clarify and encourage questioning if the doctor has used jargon-laden phrases and shrouded the true message sufficiently to render a patient unclear as to what the doctor is actually explaining. I feel that it is the nurse who may be more skilled and more aware of non-verbal cues and other communication techniques. She is constantly at hand to answer any subsequent questions that may be posed by the patient, whereas the doctor is likely to be off the ward most of the time and only contactable by going through the time consuming bleep system.

The nurse herself has to be well informed and perceptive in order to assess the extent of the patient's comprehension. This will only come as a result of an established rapport with the patient with whom the nurse has had most contact and who, I suggest, has the patient's wishes foremost in her mind.

What to disclose
Wells (1979) stated that "In the treatment of malignant disease it is often at diagnosis that a catalogue of deceit and half-truths begins, when those whose responsibility it is fail to be honest with the patient and the members of the health care team become entangled with the complicated task of keeping information from the patient."

This makes a mockery of obtaining subsequent informed consent for necessary procedures. Another problem is that explanation is time consuming and some physicians would argue that full explanations produce unwarranted anxiety. It is known, however, that explicit information prior to a procedure can lead to a substantially improved prognosis. "Is it then ethical or fair to decide without the patient's knowledge what he should or should not know about his own life? Is it right to assess a personality, and its potential, without knowledge of its strengths and weaknesses, after a brief contact arranged for an entirely different purpose? The position is rather similar to knowing that an individual is going to have to perform a task requiring considerable fortitude and endurance. The individual is kept in ignorance of the true nature of the task on the grounds that it is best not to anticipate an unpleasant experience, so that the individual is shocked and unprepared for what then transpires" (Goldie, 1982).

Alternative treatments
Alternative treatments may not be proposed to the patient, who remains unaware of the options. Interestingly, a nurse who was practising in the United States of America, where there is a Patients' Bill of Rights ensuring that they have the right of self determination, chose to explain to a patient alternative methods of treatment available which a doctor had not, and was found guilty of professional misconduct — a decision against which

she is now appealing. Here an ethical argument arises; the nurse, acting as informer of the alternative treatment, presents an ethical dilemma involving her in the actual decision for the planned treatment whereas the doctor is more removed from the emotional aspect of the decision-making.

Where the information is given The circumstances in which information is presented are often overwhelming — the patient is usually in hospital, in unfamiliar surroundings with strangers around, being confronted with procedures to undergo and invasions of privacy. Often the information is given implying that the decision is required immediately and the patient does not appear to have an opportunity to discuss the proposals. Nurses are rarely present when surgeons or physicians explain the reasons for, and what is involved in surgical and medical procedures. This "right hand not knowing what the left hand is doing" syndrome confuses both nurses and patients and may have a disastrous impact on the patient's overall trust in the caring team. While it would be wrong to suggest many forms of consent are obtained without the patient being fully aware of his illness and its likely outcome, it would be equally wrong to pretend it does not happen.

"It is in situations such as these that a nurse is required to support her colleagues and assure the patient. Can the nurse be expected to support the decision that a patient is to have further surgery in the hope of curing what is known to all except the patient to be an incurable disease?" (Wells, 1982).

The values of effective communication between patient and carer seem easy to state but difficult to put into action. It involves a commitment to patients' rights to decide what happens to their own bodies. To uphold such views health professionals, especially doctors, must learn to become more communicative and less paternalistic and they must accept that informed consent is an essential part of the doctor-patient-nurse relationship and of proper patient care. The nurse's role as patient intermediary requires knowledge and a commitment to this concept of assisting patients in making an intelligent, educated decision; that is in ensuring patient autonomy.

As nurses we should not be regarded as a threat by our medical colleagues, but rather recognised as a source of support and information that has yet to be harnessed to improve the overall care for the patient.

References
Ashworth, P. (1984) Accounting for ethics. *Nursing Mirror,* **158,** 10, 34-6.
Barkes, P. (1979) Bioethics and informed consent in American health care delivery. *Journal of Advanced Nursing,* **4,** 23-38.
Besch, L. (1979) Informed consent: A patient's right. *Nursing Outlook,* January, 32-35.
Bucklin, R. (1975) Informed consent: past present and future. *Legal Medical Annual,* 203-214.
Ferguson, V. (1981) Informed consent: given the facts. *Nursing Mirror,* **155,** 35.
Goldie, L. (1982) The ethics of telling the patient. *Journal of Medical Ethics,* 8, 128-133.

Hanks, G. (1983) Management of symptoms in advanced cancer. *Postgraduate Update*, 1691-1702.

Hayward, J. (1973) Information – a prescription against pain. RCN, London.

Kennedy, I. (1980) Medical ethics are not separate from but part of other ethics. Reith Lecture, *The Listener*, 27 November.

MacDonald, M. and Mever, K. (1976) Medicolegal notes: informed consent. *The Mount Sinai Journal of Medicine*, **43,** 104-107.

Marks, M. A Patient's guide to Chemotherapy – Your Questions Answered. Royal Marsden Hospital Patient Guide series.

Martin, A.J. (1977) Consent to treatment. *Nursing Times*, **73,** 810-11.

Meisel, A. (1975) Informed consent – the rebuttal. *Journal of American Medical Association*, **234,** 6, 615.

Miller, L. (1980) Informed Consent. *Journal of American Medical Association*, **24,** 2661-2662.

Wells, R. (1979) Who, what and when to tell. *Nursing Mirror*, **75,** 22-3.

47

The ethics of brain death

Douglas Allan, RGN, RMN, RNT
Nurse Teacher in Continuing Education, South College of Nursing, Glasgow

Nothing in life has a greater finality than death, and nurses and other health care providers have had to learn to cope with dealing with it as part of their normal working practice. To many people outside the caring professions, death is a simple concept. Nurses will testify differently, having witnessed the different ways in which people can die. This chapter explores one of the rarer processes of death, that of brain stem death and all its ethical implications.

Brain stem death accounts for approximately 4,000 deaths per annum in the UK (less than one per cent of all deaths). Half of these occur as a result of head injury and another 30 per cent as the result of an intracranial vascular problem such as spontaneous haemorrhage (Jennett and Hessett, 1981). It is important to clarify terminology; brain death or cerebral death are terms often used, although a stricter description would be that of brain stem death. This is based on physiological reasoning and is outlined in the UK criteria, which sets out the practicalities of diagnosing brain stem death. However, all three terms appear to be readily interchanged in the literature; this is probably not that important provided that the reader has a sound understanding of the concept itself.

Historical perspective

Brain stem death is nothing new. The first description of this phenomenon was published in 1959 by Mollaret and Goulon in their classic work. Before this, attention was focused on the heart as a measuring stick for life; as long ago as 1740, a report determined that a sure sign of death was putrefaction (Jennett, 1981). Jennett continues by stating that the invention of the mechanical lung ventilator and its increasingly widespread use during two polio epidemics in 1952 and 1953, further complicated the situation.

In 1968 the World Medical Assembly declared that the point of death in various cells was not as important as the certainty of irreversibility (Gilder, 1968). During the same year the Ad Hoc Committee of the Harvard Medical School (1968) produced a set of criteria, using the term 'irreversible coma', which, in hindsight, was unfortunate as this led to confusion with the phenomenon of the vegetative state (Pallis, 1983). However, despite this, the report was hailed as a watershed in the attempt to clarify the situation.

The Harvard group was the first to state that its criteria was not the 'be all and end all' and that further modifications would take place as knowledge improved. Indeed, within 12 months of the issue of the report, the group acknowledged that the iso-electric electro-encephalogram was unnecessary, while retaining the opinion that it could constitute valuable supporting data (Beecher, 1969). Other aspects of the Harvard criteria remain an essential and indisputable part of present day criteria, such as the presence of apnoea and the notion of repeating the tests in their entirety to eliminate observer error.

In 1971 the notion of irreversible damage to the brain stem as the point of no return and the idea that a diagnosis could be based on clinical judgement was introduced by Mohandas and Chou. It was also at this stage that the existence of preconditions emerged. Twenty of the 25 patients in the study had sustained a head injury, a diagnosis found in at least half of the patients at present.

British criteria

After much deliberation and discussion among anaesthetists, neurologists, neurosurgeons and physiologists, the British criteria appeared in 1976 (Conference of Medical Royal Colleges and their Faculties, 1976). Following a further year of discussion, and in the absence of any adverse comment, copies of the guidelines were then distributed to hospital doctors for use in diagnosing brain death (Figure 1). (For details of these guidelines see Allan, 1987).

The UK guidelines in particular rely upon the presence of apnoea, an interval between testing, preconditions, the idea of irreversibility and a clinical diagnosis of brain stem death. Essentially, this is a combination of all the available data and was subsequently imitated in other parts of the world. Despite the publication of the Harvard criteria as long ago as 1968, it was not until 1981 that national guidelines were published in America (Report to the President's Commission, 1981), and it was possible to be declared dead in one state and not in another.

However, two years before this in the UK, a number of allegations were made in a Panorama television programme in October 1980. The programme, entitled Transplants – Are the Donors Really Dead?, focused on three particular issues. First, that brain death was a new concept introduced without prior consultation or discussion. Second, that it was created to satisfy organ transplantation demands and, finally, that the criteria were unreliable. The crux of the unreliability argument centred around the existence of two patients who had apparently survived, despite fulfilling the brain death criteria. This allegation was subsequently withdrawn (Paul, 1981). A relationship between the development of brain death criteria and organ transplantation was also proven not to exist. The brain death criteria had existed long before the ability to perform successful transplants and, indeed, if all organ transplants were stopped, it would still be necessary to diagnose patients

Diagnosis to be made by two doctors, one a Consultant and the other a Consultant or Senior Registrar.

Diagnosis should not be considered until at least 6 hours after the onset of Coma; 12-24 hours will be more usual.

Name .... Unit No ....

Pre-conditions Nature of irremediable brain damage		Time of event leading to coma
Dr A	....
Dr B	....
Do you consider that apnoeic coma is due to:	Dr A	Dr B
Depressant drugs		
Neuromuscular blocking (relaxant) drugs		
Hypothermia		
Metabolic or endocrine disturbances?		

Tests for absence of brain stem function		
Is there evidence of:	Dr A	Dr B
Pupil reaction to light		
Corneal reflex		
Eye movements with Cold Caloric Test		
Cranial Nerve Motor Responses		
Gag Reflex		
Respiratory movements on disconnection from Ventilator to allow adequate rise in $PaCo_2$?		

Date and time of first testing ....
Date and time of second testing ....

Dr A	**Dr B**
Signature	Signature ....
Status	Status ....

Figure 1. Criteria for diagnosis of brain death.

as clinically brain dead.

In the few months following the programme, much was written in both the general and medical press, debates took place and a mass of evidence emerged from various sources in the light of further experience.

In a small way, the Panorama programme did focus the general public's attention on the necessity of having brain death criteria, although at the time many individuals discarded their transplant cards.

Implications for nurses

Throughout the development of the brain death criteria, nurses have had little or no involvement in the formulation and performance of the criteria. Although not advocating that nurses are the appropriate people to diagnose patients as brain dead, it is unfortunate that they were not more closely involved during the early discussions in order that a nursing perspective could have been applied at the beginning.

Several fleeting references are made in the medical and nursing literature about the bad effect on the morale of nursing staff who are looking after brain-dead patients on a regular basis (Allan, 1984; Jennet, 1981; Pallis, 1983). Pallis (1983) in particular emphasises the damaging effect on the morale of highly trained nursing staff asked to clean the mouths or treat the pressure areas of patients who are already dead. He continues by recounting the plight of relatives who became emotional hostages to uncomprehending machines in the days of ventilating to asystole. Given the close relationship between the nurses and relatives of such patients, this must have had an enormous impact on the nurses.

Rudy (1982), commenting in an American nursing journal, states that in the concern for proper medical and legal determination of brain death, the very important role of nursing is neglected. She continues that it is imperative that nurses have a mechanism for making their feelings and views known. The same author outlines the additional difficulties faced by nursing staff where children or neonates are involved, and the particular problems posed by the family of the patient.

Nursing involvement with brain-dead patients can be considered under the following headings: physical care of the patient; psychological care of the patient and family; and psychological care of the nursing staff.

Physical care of the patient Physical nursing care of any critically ill patient will aim, initially, toward supporting and maintaining failing body systems. However, in some instances the priorities change. The goal in the nursing care of the brain-dead patient becomes one of facilitating a dignified death and, if organ transplantation is a possibility, the preservation of the remaining functioning body systems (Daly, 1982).

The nature of the patient's condition demands the use of critical care facilities and the highest possible standard of basic nursing care. The brain-dead patient is perhaps the ultimate example of total dependence upon nursing staff to deal with the physical needs of the patient as they arise. This implies a rigorous assessment of the patient's needs and meticulous application of effective nursing care, coupled with an ongoing evaluation process to deal with changing priorities. The nurse will need to assist in the tests for the absence of brain stem function.

Psychological care of the patient and his family   Any care plan must include the patient's family and significant others, and it is an emotionally traumatic and upsetting time for them. Many relatives show signs of the grieving process before the actual withdrawal of support from the patient. Daly (1982) suggests that it is helpful if the nurse is aware of the different stages of the grieving process and the ways in which these may be manifested in individuals, in order to enhance understanding of the needs of the relatives.

The patient is likely to be surrounded by technical machinery and it is imperative that the relatives sense that he or she is treated as a person and that the nurse demonstrates a humane, caring attitude in the performance of her care and interaction with the relatives. To reinforce this notion, the relatives are encouraged to touch the patient and there is no reason why they cannot perform simple nursing tasks. The nurse is usually the first person to make contact with the relatives and will certainly become their most consistent contact in the hospital.

It is important that the nurse is aware of the extent of the relative's knowledge with regard to the patient's condition so that any new information or reinforcement of existing information is carried out consistently. For example, a nurse could be present when the doctor speaks to relatives. To accommodate this, proper facilities must be provided whereby the family is afforded some privacy and time to make what are very personal major decisions. Involvement of others in the care of the relatives should be initiated, if appropriate. These may include a social worker or religious adviser.

Psychological care of the nursing staff   This aspect of caring for the brain-dead patient can be easily missed. Few nurses can fail to be affected in some way by their dealings with even one brain-dead patient. Several aspects are involved here, and this paper does not and cannot provide the answers to all the questions that are raised. With the close interaction which is inherent in any nurse–critically ill patient relationship, the nurse will often be the first person to notice the patient's deterioration. While undertaking routine nursing procedures, such as suctioning, the nurse may notice that the patient's gag reflex is weakened or absent or that the corneal reflex is weakened or absent, as would be observed during routine eye care.

Some nurses may have difficulties dealing with their own feelings and emotions in this situation. Rudy (1982) suggests that good communication between medical and nursing staff and peer support can help to alleviate or minimise these problems, but does not elaborate on how to achieve this. An understanding of the criteria and the medico-legal requirements would contribute to the avoidance of any possible misunderstandings, which might lead to difficulties for some nurses.

Difficulties do not end with the nurse directly responsible involved with the patient. This author can recall, as a charge nurse, wrestling with a quite separate set of problems. How to explain to a relative why the ECG monitor still has a 'heartbeat'? How to allow the mother of a brain-dead child to lift the child up in her arms when he is attached to a ventilator, monitoring machines and infusion pumps? What to do about the relative who insists on sitting at the bedside 24 hours a day, neglecting her family and her own health? How to allocate hard-pressed resources, both staff and equipment? Many readers can probably add other problems to the list.

This is undoubtedly an area of nursing practice which merits further attention. Some of the unanswered questions which demand closer examination might include:

- Can we identify the difficulties/problems/needs of nurses involved in caring for the brain-dead patient?

- What can we do to help?

- How can we help the ward manager deal with the managerial nursing problems?

Only with further research can we begin to address these issues.

References
Allan, D. (1987) Criteria for brain stem death. *The Professional Nurse,* **2,** 357-90.
Beecher, H.K. (1969) After the definition of irreversible coma. *New England Journal of Medicine,* **281,** 1070.
Conference of Medical Royal Colleges and their Faculties in the UK (1976) Diagnosis of brain death. *British Medical Journal,* **2,** 1187.
Daly, K. (1982) The diagnosis of brain death; an overview of the neurosurgical nursing repsonsibilities. *Journal of Neurosurgical Nursing,* **14,** 2, 85.
Gilder, S.S.B. (1968) Twenty-second World Medical Assembly. *British Medical Journal,* **3,** 493.
Jennett, W.B. (1981) Brain death, *British Journal of Anaesthesia,* **53,** 11, 1111.
Jennett, W.B. and Hessett, C. (1981) Brain death in Britain as reflected in renal donors. *British Medical Journal* **283,** 359.
Mohandas, A. and Chou, S.N. (1971) Brain death – a clinical and pathological study. *Journal of Neurosurgery,* **35,** 211.
Mollaret, P. and Goulon, M. (1959) Le coma depasse. *Revue Neurologique,* **101,** 3.
Pallis, C. (1982) From brain death to brain stem death. *British Mecical Journal,* **258,** 1487.
Pallis, C. (1983) ABC of Brain Stem Death. British Medical Association, London.
Paul, R. (1981) Survival after brain death: withdrawal of allegation. *The Lancet,* **1,** 677.
Report of the Ad Hoc Committee of the Harvard Medical School (1968) Examination of the definiton of irreversible coma. *Journal of the American Medical Association,* **205,** 85.
Report to the President's Commission (1981) Guidelines for the determination of brain death. *Journal of the American Medical Association,* **246,** 2184.
Rudy, E. (1982) Brain death. *Dimensions of Critical Care Nursing,* **1,** 3, 178.

Bibliography
Pallis, C. (1983) ABC of Brain Stem Death. British Medical Association, London.
A comprehensive series of articles from the *British Medical Journal* which examines brain death from historical, medical, ethical and legal standpoints. Does not contain any nursing aspects.
Rudy, E. (1982) Brain death. *Dimensions of Critical Care Nursing,* **1,** 3, 178.
One of the few articles available which examines for nurses the ethical and legal issues of brain death for nurses. Written for the American nurse, some parts of the paper are not applicable to British practice but it is still worth reading.

48

What are the legal implications of extended nursing roles?

Susannah Derrick, RGN

Senior Staff Nurse, Intensive Care Unit, St Mary's Hospital, London

Recent advances in medical technology have led to constant demands being made on both the knowledge and skills of nurses. This is highlighted in 'high tech' areas of nursing such as intensive care and renal units.

Nurses have a complex role in these areas. It requires not only competence in providing basic care, support and education to patient and family, but also a high level of theoretical knowledge and practical skill to understand and contribute to treatment. The role of the specialist nurse encompasses many procedures which have previously been considered within the medical domain, such as venepuncture and emergency defibrillation.

The legal issues

I would suggest that nurses working in these areas extend their role willingly. However, although they are trained for practice, they may not fully appreciate the legal issues surrounding it.

A research case study carried out using RGNs in an intensive/cardiac care unit as a sample population supports this suggestion and has provided factual information on the degree of knowledge and appreciation of the legal implications of the extended role held by this specific population (Derrick, 1987). The study also presents a reasonable overview of the RGN population as a whole, as it demonstrated the broad background and wide range of hospitals and health authorities in which the sample had previously worked.

What is an extended role?

An extended role can be described as one which is not included in basic training. They have developed for various reasons; the most obvious is development of new technology and treatment. However, economic factors can not be overlooked – nursing manpower may be cheaper than medical.

In the light of the change and extension of the nursing role the DHSS, medical and nursing professional organisations attempted to clarify the situation. The DHSS issued a circular in 1977 explaining the legal implications and training requirements (DHSS, 1977), and this was supported by a publication from the RCN and BMA (1978). These documents set out some clear guidelines for the management of extended roles for nurses, and are summarised by Rowden (1987.)

The guidelines stress the need for joint discussions, mutual trust and respect between professions and state that extension of role must be in the interests of patient care. An opinion often aired is that on a busy ward where staffing levels are low, skilled nurses should not be using precious time administering intravenous drugs.

The circular also states that 'Work which has hitherto been carried out by doctors ought therefore to be delegated to nurses only when:-
a) The nurse has been specifically and adequately trained for the performance of the new task and she agrees to undertake it;
b) this training has been recognised as satisfactory by the employing Authority;
c) the new task has been recognised by the professions and by the employing Authority as a task which may be properly delegated to a nurse;
d) the delegating doctor has been assured of the competence of the individual nurse concerned.'

It also states:- 'In order to be successful and safe such delegation should be in the context of a clearly defined policy . . . and it should be made known in writing to all staff who are likely to be involved.

These points should be considered very carefully and with particular reference to the Department of Health document, the Ministerial Group on Junior Doctors' hours (Department of Health, 1990). Reduction in the hours worked by junior doctors is a subject which rightly gains a great deal of support, and this document presents recommendations to achieve this. However, it is interesting to note one such recommendation in the document. II. Recommendations for Action No. 6 "the UK Health Departments should issue guidelines to health authorities and boards as follows" (d) "in consultation with the UKCC for Nursing, Midwifery and Health Visiting and the Royal Colleges of Nursing and Midwifery, on the need for reviews of local policies concerning activities which appropriately qualified nurses and midwives may reasonably undertake further to improve the quality of patient care. Where such local policies do not exist, arrangements should be made for them to be instituted."

Could this imply transfer of 'activities' or practices from a medical to a nursing responsibility?

It is important that nursing management and individual nurses are flexible to change and are able to respond to the needs of their patients in the light of increasing knowledge and advancing technology. But it is essential they understand the implications of the changes in practice.

Certification

A certificate of competence is issued for some extended role procedures. Unlike the administration of intravenous drugs (Breckenbridge, 1976) many procedures do not require certification in some authorities but do in others. Certification is not a legal requirement, but it does serve a worthwhile purpose.

Each individual nurse has a choice whether or not to extend her or his role. It can be generally accepted that any nurse choosing to work in specialised fields expects, and is willing to undertake an extended role, and with adequate training should be fully aware of the medical and nursing implications of her or his actions. Comment is rarely made, however, about the importance and need for training to enable nurses to appreciate the legal implications of their actions.

Law and the nurse

Accountability   "Each registered nurse, midwife and health visitor is accountable for his or her practice" (UKCC, 1984). Accountability means being answerable for work, decisions about work and being professionally responsible for the standard of practice. Nurses are first and foremost legally responsible for each and every nursing action undertaken or omitted, and must practise in accordance with the same standard of care of a reasonably prudent nurse practising under the same or similar circumstances. *Primary liability* is held by the individual nurse for her or his own actions.

It is possible for nurses to be persuaded or pressurised into carrying out treatment or procedures – extending their role – either to be helpful, to save time or 'to keep the peace', particularly when wards are busy or staffing levels are low. In such instances both medical and nursing staff should have the consequences of the unauthorised practise brought to their attention. Protecting one another from primary liability is a duty everyone should adopt, and be thanked for, albeit as an afterthought.

Greater awareness of legal issues surrounding nursing and the extension of the nursing role has developed in recent years. The number of study days and articles published on this subject has undoubtedly increased the level of interest and understanding.

In March 1989 the UKCC for for Nursing, Midwifery and Health Visiting published an Advisory Document 'Exercising Accountability'. It is designed to offer a framework to assist nurses, midwives and health visitors to consider ethical aspects of professional practise and is available free to all on the UKCC's professional register (UKCC, 1989).

Negligence   Negligence is divided into three main components (Rea, 1987):
● **The duty of care** The legal duty of care encompasses the professional, moral, ethical and sociological duties of care within which nursing operates. It is what the nurse is required to do under the terms of her

contract of employment. Deviation from this in any way is negligence.
- **The breach of the duty** This is the alleged wrongdoing.
- **The resultant damage** The damage to the patient must be the result of the breach of the duty of care.

The law relating to negligence principally seeks to identify conduct which does not reach an acceptable professional standard. If injury results from such conduct the possibility of an action for damages (compensation) arises. Liability to pay damages may be shouldered by the individual, covered by an insurance company or by membership of a professional organisation which offers legal liability insurance to its members.

Vicarious liability

In the DHSS circular (1977), and in law, it is made clear that any role extension *must* be approved officially by the employing authority. In the United Kingdom (Master-Servant Statutes) "the law takes the view that the master will accept responsibility for the actions of servants, where the servant is working in accordance with the policies agreed by master and servant" (Rowden, 1987). Within the NHS the employing authority is the master and the nurse the servant. It is normally accepted that the senior nurse will act on behalf of the authority.

The health authority will accept responsibility for the actions of nurses when they are working within policies agreed by both parties. It is suggested therefore that it may be good practice for nurses to be certificated for extended role procedures. In the extended role, a certificate not only facilitates education and the maintenance of a high standard of care but is proof of competence and of the authority's knowledge and agreement for the nurse to practise.

If the authority/employer is to accept legal liability for the action of the nurse/employee, it is necessary that the authority should know exactly the role being practised and agree to it. This is known as *vicarious liability* (sometimes called secondary liability). It is essential to confirm in writing any extension of role. It is too easy for confusion to arise where verbal agreements are concerned. How many times has a doctor been heard to say 'I will cover you'? Doctors are *not* permitted by their defence organisations to take responsibility for the actions of nurses. Documenting the extent and boundaries of an extended role may seem tedious and bureaucratic, but it is in the interests of practitioners and patients alike.

Ensuring knowledge

It is essential to ensure nurses have an appreciation and thorough understanding of the implications of the extension of the nursing role. With the ever increasing expectation that all nurses at all levels extend their role further, I would make the following recommendations:

- Individuals and management must be alerted to the need for more education.

- The teaching of the legal aspects of nursing should be incorporated into basic training and all nurses should be encouraged to question their own knowledge and safeguard their own practise.

- Incorporation of the legal implications in the criteria of certification for an extended role procedure would ensure awareness of the policy and requirements of the issuing health authority/employer.

- Attempts should be made to find time and finance to increase the number of study days, teaching sessions, workshops and discussions available.

Each registered nurse, midwife and health visitor is accountable for his or her practice. It is every nurse's individual responsibility to understand the legal implications underlying that accountability. Do you?

References

Department of Health (1990) *Heads of Agreement. Ministerial Group on Junior Doctor's Hours.* December. DoH, London.

Derrick, S.M. (1987) Unpublished case study on nurses' appreciation of the legal implications of taking an extended role.

DHSS (1977) *The extending role of the clinical nurse – legal implications and training requirements.* DHSS, London.

RCN/BMA (1978) *The Duties and Position of the Nurse.* RCN, London.

Rea, K. (1987) Negligence. *Nursing,* **3,** 576.

UKCC (1984) *Code of Professional Conduct for the Nurse, Midwife and Health Visitor.* UKCC, London.

UKCC (1989) *Exercising Accountability.* UKCC, London.

49

Balancing public concern and patients' rights in HIV testing

Ann Shuttleworth, BA
Editor, Professional Nurse

The issue of HIV testing gained further controversy recently with the news that doctors are being asked to take blood for tests from patients who have not given informed consent. The British Medical Association said insurance companies have been asking doctors to take the blood from people who have applied for life insurance. The doctors are then asked to send the samples to a laboratory who will inform the insurance company of the result. The first indication people have that they are HIV positive could be the refusal of their application for insurance.

The BMA argue that the standard letter issued to applicants, briefly outlining the test with an attached consent form does not constitute informed consent. They insist counselling is essential before a test is given and then after for the result to be followed up correctly. This view is shared by the DHSS (1986).

Implications for nurses
The whole issue of HIV testing has wide implications for nurses, who often take the blood samples. If they do so without the full consent of the patient, they could find themselves defending civil actions for damages or criminal actions on charges of battery. If they knowingly collude with a doctor in taking such a specimen they may face charges of aiding and abetting an assault, while they also risk being struck off their professional register if they mislead patients about the reason for taking blood samples.

In a circular on professional conduct, the UKCC emphasise that nurses must especially heed the first two clauses of their Code of Professional Conduct with respect to people with or suspected of having HIV infection. These state that they must always act in such a way as to promote and safeguard the wellbeing and interests of patients, and ensure that no action or omission on their part or within their sphere of influence is detrimental to the condition or safety of patients.

Sherrard and Gatt (1987), defining informed consent, say that it must be genuine, and not obtained by misrepresentation, fraud, deceit or duress. Surely the prospect of not being allowed life insurance, and therefore a mortgage, could be construed as duress? The law may interpret a test taken in such a situation as being taken without informed consent.

More generally, practitioners taking blood for HIV tests must take account of the patient's 'right of bodily integrity' – the right to determine what is to be done with his or her own body. Sherrard and Gatt say the far reaching implications of a positive result for the patient would probably make implied consent insufficient from a legal point of view. It is not good enough to take a blood sample 'to run a few tests' and assume the patient realises an HIV test will be among them, and consents to this. The patient must explicitly consent to an HIV test. Obviously nurses should beware of taking blood for HIV tests without the explicit consent of the patient. But does anyone benefit from HIV testing anyway – apart from the insurance companies?

Those responsible for planning and allocating services for AIDS sufferers would certainly be grateful for more information on how many people are HIV positive and therefore likely to contract AIDS. Such information is currently in short supply. Nor is there much information on how far HIV infection has spread into the heterosexual community.

The more people who have HIV tests, the more information will be available on the epidemiology of the virus. This would enable services to be more efficiently planned before a situation arises, rather than when it has reached crisis proportions. This is assuming such action would really be taken, which is by no means certain.

Who should be tested?

While mandatory testing of the entire population is logistically impractical and undesirable from the aspect of individual rights, the voluntary testing of certain groups may be beneficial. Pregnant women are one important group, for two reasons. Pregnancy has been shown to make HIV positive women more likely to develop AIDS because the functioning of mother's immune system is lowered so that her body does not reject the foetus (ACHCEW, 1988). This is thought to give the HIV virus more chance to gain ascendancy. Half of HIV positive mothers can also be expected to pass on HIV to their children either during pregnancy or at birth. Testing would give them the option of having an abortion.

Pregnant women could also be epidemiologically extremely valuable. Brain (1988) said that midwives and antenatal women would be unwise to oppose the routine screening of all pregnant women if they are the only group who would give a clue to the spread of the disease into the heterosexual community. She recommended that testing be voluntary and that the women know its full implications. She also expressed concern at reports that a group of antenatal women had been tested without their consent.

The Government is to decide whether or not pregnant women should be tested anonymously – and whether this should be with or without their consent – when it receives a report on surveillance and monitoring for the Expert Advisory Group. However, Britain's Chief Medical Officers recently refused to support a call for such anonymous screening without the women's consent. They were criticised by Black et al (RSM, 1988), who said anonymous testing would be easy to administer, using blood left over from that taken for routine tests, and would provide a sensitive index of the rate at which the disease is entering the heterosexual community. Women could be told their results if they wished, the rest of the samples would be sent to a central laboratory.

The question of who should be tested and under what circumstances is an emotive one which many nurses will feel strongly about. They have their safety and that of patients and colleagues to consider but must also protect their patients' rights, which may be compromised in the quest for information.

Testing certain groups would not only provide epidemiological information and give pregnant women the chance to have an abortion, say Masters, Johnson and Kolodny (1988). Infected people who were unaware of their status could be identified and counselled to modify their behaviour and avoid infecting others.

As well as pregnant women, they recommend testing all people admitted to hospital between the ages of 15 and 60. Again, the epidemiological information would be valuable. The results would also ensure that staff were aware of the hazard of contact with biological fluid from seropositive patients, and that immunocompromised people were not put at unnecessary risk by exposure to contagious illnesses.

How reliable are the tests?

However, there are other factors in the debate about HIV testing. While the tests currently used are highly reliable compared with many other routine medical tests, some errors are made.

The main test used is the enzyme-linked immunosorbent assay (ELISA), which works by mixing serum with protein pieces of HIV in the presence of chemical reagents. These cause a colour reaction if the HIV antibody is present. ELISA is relatively cheap to administer, and under ideal conditions will detect 98-99 per cent of samples correctly. However, high sensitivity means it occasionally registers false positive results, especially in people who have had numerous blood transfusions and women who have had numerous pegnancies.

The effect of a false positive test on a person could be almost as catastrophic as a true positive. They will suffer the same stigmatisation and emotional trauma as if they were infected, and from a practical point of view, are unlikely to be able to get life insurance or a mortgage among other things. While they may not have the same health problems as a seropositive person, the stress of believing themselves to be infected would be likely to have a detrimental effect on their health. ELISA also shows a small percentage of false negative readings.

To guard against a high number of false positive test results, readings are only considered positive if they are consistent with a repeated ELISA and confirmed by a more specific test like the Western blot. This test is carried out only on samples which have given positive readings with ELISA, because it is much more expensive and requires a higher degree of technical skill to administer. This means false negative readings are not retested. The two tests give a high degree of accuracy, but they are not infallible, or free of the possibility of human error.

Compulsory testing

Compulsory testing of either the whole population or certain groups, usually those who are at high risk of infection, is a subject raised from time to time. At present, however, the question is really academic. The purpose of such screening would be to discover all those who are infected with HIV, and presumably to take steps to ensure that they do not spread the infection. The time lapse between infection with HIV and the body producing the antibodies to the virus can be anything from two months to over a year, so even screening the entire population would not give an accurate picture of who was infected. Until a test is devised which isolates the virus itself, rather than the antibodies, the compulsory testing lobby is unlikely to get very far. If such a test does become available, however, nurses may have to defend their patients' right to bodily integrity from more sustained and vociferous campaigns.

The arguments about HIV testing are bound to continue, but common sense on the part of health care professionals can do much to protect both those afraid of infection with HIV and those already infected. For example, nursing care should not change if a person is diagnosed seropositive – body fluids from seronegative patients may contain other biohazards and should be treated as potentially hazardous. This weakens the argument for compulsory testing – why bother if the same precautions are necessary for seronegative and seropositive people?

The case for voluntary testing, either anonymously or otherwise, is probably the strongest. The information such a programme, properly conducted, could yield would be invaluable if it were used to plan services and public education programmes, and full patient confidentiality were retained. If it were simply used to whip up hysteria against minority groups, however, it would be worse than useless. In such a case it would merely deflect attention from the real issue of how to care for people with AIDS effectively and prevent other people from infection. It would discourage people from going for the test, and make the already catastrophic personal situation of being HIV positive much worse. Any testing programme must be carefully conducted.

How nurses can help

By remaining calm and giving effective education to those who need it nurses can help people take reasonable steps to protect themselves from infection and overcome any unreasonable fears they may have. Hopefully they will also be able to ensure that HIV testing is never used in a negative way against those who are infected with the virus.

Nurses have a huge part to play in protecting both their patients' health and their rights. The medical establishment has expressed its voice in the public debate – albeit often in a contradictory fashion. Nurses are often at the 'coal face' in these issues. It is time the nursing profession made itself heard as well.

References
ACHEW (1988) AIDS and HIV Infection (Health News Briefing). Association of Community Health Councils for England and Wales, London.
Brain, M. (1988) President's address to the 1988 RCM annual conference.
DHSS (1983) AIDS. Booklet 3. DHSS, London.
Masters, H., Johnson, V.E., Kolodny, R.C. (1988) Crisis – Heterosexual Behaviour in the Age of AIDS. Grafton, London.
RSM (1988) Anonymous testing for HIV. *The AIDS Letter*, **1**, 5, 7.
Sherrard, M. and Gatt, I. (1987) Human immunodeficiency (HIV) virus antibody testing. *British Medical Journal*, **295**, 911-2.
UKCC (1987) AIDS – testing, treatment and care. Circular PC/87/02. UKCC, London.

50

When right and wrong are a matter of opinion: the ethics of organ transplantation

Heidi J. Satterthwaite, RGN
Cardiothoracic Nurse, formerly with QARANC

The ethics of any topic can easily become the subject of heated debate. Individuals become roused to defend their opinions and feelings, and the debates are to be found on television and in newspapers, classrooms, pubs and bus queues, as people strive to find an answer to their differing opinions. While there is probably no right answer in most cases, certain facts will be accepted, and compromises reached. These compromises do not stop the debates, but they do allow 'life to go on'.

"Ethics is critical in the sense explained, its subject matter is human conduct and character, not as natural facts with a history and causal connection with other facts, but as possessing value in view of a standard or ideal." The Scope of Ethics.
Encyclopaedia of Religion and Ethics (1979, Clark, Edinburgh).

The difficulty with ethical debates is that you cannot say that one is right and another wrong, it is often a matter of personal opinion, and it is the difficulty in accepting another's view along with your own that causes the conflict. One of the most recent debates is that of heart and lung transplants. Initially these were highly publicised, but now are accepted as routine. The ethical arguments, however, continue unabated.

"Thirty years ago only rarely did experienced physicians have any difficulty in deciding whether or not a person was dead and if there was the slightest doubt this was solved by postponing the decision for an hour or two. A few people did have a fear of being buried alive, Hans Christian Anderson had a note by his bedside 'I only seem to be dead'. Today some are aftraid that they may be eviscerated before they are dead" (Papworth, 1981).

Kidney transplants have been accepted for many years with few objections, although the recent 'kidneys for sale' case has brought them back into the limelight. The difference with heart transplants is the deeper emotions evoked.

New technology
The advanced technology which has allowed the development of heart and lung transplantation has also given us improved methods of ventilation and system support which in some circumstances may enable

a person to be kept alive indefinitely. The need for a new definition of death was obvious – and one which could not be said to be aiding the surgeons in their search for donors. While ethical issues continue to be debated, those working in controversial areas still need rules and guidelines for their work, regardless of their own feelings.

Diagnosis of death by lack of brain stem function is now recognised in this country. Some States in America will still only equate heart and respiratory cessation to death. Diagnosis of brain stem death is governed by criteria set by the Transplant Advisory Panel, the working party of the Royal College of Physicians and the working party of the Royal College of Surgeons, and has been approved by the Conference of Medical Royal College and their Faculties in the UK. Their criteria are accepted as being sufficient to distinguish between those patients who may have even a partial recovery and those in whom no such possibility exists.

A diagnosis of brain stem death can only be considered when the patient is deeply comatose with no possibility that it may be drug induced, primary hypothermia or metabolic and endocrine disturbances. Spontaneous respiration must be inadequate or have ceased altogether and there must be no doubt that the condition is irreversible. This decision must be made by two doctors, individually and on separate occasions, and these doctors must not be connected to a transplant team. According to the code of practice drawn up by a working party on behalf of the Health Department of Great Britain and Northern Ireland in 1978 "If a patient carries a signed donor card or has otherwise recorded his wishes, there is no legal requirement to establish lack of objection on the part of relatives . . ." However, relatives' wishes are always followed.

Great Britain has an opting-in system where people must express a wish to donate organs. Other countries, France, Belgium, Sweden and Norway have adopted an opting-out system where "a person's organs may be removed for transplantation as soon as he is pronounced dead unless he has left specific instructions to the contrary." Many people here feel an opting out system would make more organs available for transplantation and the issue is currently the subject of debate (Farfor, 1977).

The process of death

The circumstances under which death is pronounced and death rites begin are an area full of human concern . . . "from the earliest archeological records of modern man – in fact as far back as Neanderthal Man – the evidence of funeral rites indicates that various rituals have been associated with death. Even a person of the lowest social status was assured of being treated with dignity in death and not as a mere carcass. Arnold Toynbee (1968) states that this 'respect for the dead may conceivably be inborn in us'," (Shanley, 1982).

Now, with medical advances, "death has become dissected, cut into bits by a series of little steps which finally make it impossible to know which step was the real death. All the little silent deaths have replaced and erased the great dramatic act of dying and have deprived the individual of the dignity that through the ages has been an integral part of death" (Shanley, 1982). While irreversible brain stem death forms a legal criteria, ethical nursing care must recognise more general perceptions of a sleeping relative. A young donor's mother says of her daughter "leaving her for the last time, supported by machines, but looking just like our own sleeping Katie was the most wrenching experience of our lives" (Coolican, 1987). For many, death implies a departure of the soul – unseen, unscientific, but deeply felt.

People's uncertainty about death and what it really means to them leads many not to carry organ donor cards, and for many, heart transplantation has intensified their feelings of doubt. The heart is an organ tied up with many emotions and sentiments, and these must be overcome before the idea of receiving someone else's heart or of donating a heart can be fully accepted. People are classified in society as being 'hard hearted', 'soft hearted', having 'hearts of stone' or ultimately, 'having no heart'. Given a choice, would you choose a heart from someone who was known as being hard hearted or soft hearted? It is difficult to disassociate these feelings and to view the heart as a biological pump. However, many relatives may be helped to cope with a sudden, unexpected death if a part of their relative has saved someone else's life. It makes the death seem less pointless.

It is easy to see that relatives have to sort out many emotions before coming to a decision. Nurses looking after these patients may find the situation equally difficult – they must help the relatives through this period as well as cope with their own feelings on the subject.

Having looked afer a young boy being maintained on a ventilator while waiting for his organs to be harvested, one nurse said "knowing he was declared dead, but having to act as if he were not, made those the most difficult hours I have ever worked" (Sandro, 1980). The problem seems to be that although nurses are aware of the diagnosis of brain stem death, and may have been present while the tests are carried out, many will still define death as the cessation of respiration and heart beat.

A survey in America showed that six out of 10 nurses felt it was ethically acceptable to maintain a patient on a ventilator to enable harvesting of the organs. Most of these nurses did specify that it was only acceptable for a few hours, and that prolonging dying for organ use was not acceptable. This still leaves four out of 10 nurses feeling it is unethical to maintain a patient to enable organ harvesting. These nurses felt there is never an acceptable excuse for prolonging a family's suffering and that organs could be obtained without heroic measures (Sandroff, 1980).

Nurses must be prepared to help the family through the process of organ donation, and it is undoubtedly easier if units have a policy for this. Although intellectually the family are aware the patient is dead, emotional understanding is another matter, and they will need reinforcement of the explanation of brain death. Once the decision has been made to donate, it is important that the family know the organs are being kept in the best possible condition and will all be used. Many relatives will attach their acceptance of the death on the knowledge that organs have been successfully used.

Nurses have the most important role to play with the family at this time. It is to nurses they will turn with their questions. If the area has a transplant coordinator, she or he can offer much support and help to both the family and nursing staff.

Patients awaiting organs

For nurses in many intensive care units, the question is how much medical support should be given to patients awaiting heart and lung transplantation. Nurses are often asked their opinion at case conferences. A few years ago, only the patients with the best chances of survival were considered, and one potential recipient said "waiting for the test results was like waiting for a death sentence. I knew if I did not qualify as a good transplant prospect, I would not be accepted into Stanford's programme" (Jelkmann, 1982).

With further experience and increasing knowledge, the decision is no longer so easy. Many of the patients requiring maximal support, such as intra-aortic balloon pumping, or even extra-corporeal membrane oxygenation, may do equally well postoperatively as a patient who has not required this level of intervention. The increasing survival of these patients may mean units will have to rethink their selection policies.

As in the case of relatives of prospective donors, the nurse's role in caring for a patient awaiting a heart transplant is supportive. If the patient needs a lot of medical support, the family has to cope with the possibility of imminent death, as well as the eternal hope that a donor is found in time. The see-sawing of emotions may lead to depression, euphoria and occasionally hysteria, all of which nurses must be able to deal with. Hardest to come to terms with is not having an answer for questions such as 'when?' and 'how long left?'.

If the patient does die, the relatives often find it difficult to accept a heart has not been found in time, and here again nurses must give support. Although the patient has undoubtedly needed much nursing, nursing staff must also ensure relatives were involved in the patient's care, and understood what was happening.

Following on from the debate about how much treatment should be given is one of cost. How much money should be spent on one patient? Is it actually possible to say 'this patient is costing us too much, treatment must stop'. Those against transplants argue that the cost of one heart transplant can pay for 20 hip replacements and thus improve the quality and length of life for more people. However, it is highly unlikely money saved would be allocated to hip replacements, and as the technology exists to give someone a new heart, how can you deny them?

Figures have been produced which show that heart transplants can actually save the country money. The cost of treating an invalided patient and paying benefits is greater than that of performing a heart transplant and giving the associated follow-up (Habernam, 1980). The cost of treating a patient is probably rarely realised at the time – only when the administrators do the accounts are costs highlighted and by then it is too late. However, in the present economical climate it is future patients who will suffer as wards and facilities are withdrawn.

Many other issues are involved in heart and lung transplantation: should donors' families have a say in who the recipient is? Should there be incentives to donate and therefore create a market? Who shall decide who will and who won't be treated? Are we 'playing God'? Who should approach the relatives about donation? How much persuasion should be used? The questions are endless and there are no real answers. What is ethically acceptable today may not be tomorrow.

Super nurses?

Nurses involved in both donor and recipient heart and lung patient care should perhaps be trained as 'super-nurses'. They need all their nursing skills and compassion to care for the patients and relatives, as they are perhaps the mainstay of their sanity during this period. Nurses should, therefore, take part in ethical debates and decisions. It is they who often have to carry out the decisions made.

An issue of the *Nursing Times* (December, 1987) reported a knee transplant in a lady in New Jersey. One has to wonder if we are approaching a time where a person with multisystem failure will be able to have a new heart, lungs, liver, kidney, and legs, a face lift, skin grafts and new eyes – colour of their choosing. Where will it end? How do we control it? Will Frankenstein become a reality? Who knows? However, someone donating a heart to someone who will otherwise die is giving the gift of life, and what greater gift can there be?

References
Bayles, M.D. (1980) The value of life – by who's standard. *American Journal of Nursing*, **89,** 12, 226–30.
Coolican, M.B. (1987) Katie's legacy. *American Journal of Nursing*, **87,** 4, 483–85.
DHSS (1979) The Removal of Cadeveric Organs for Transplantation. A Code of Practice. HMSO, London.
Farfor, A. (1977) Letter from . . . Paris. *British Medical Journal*, **1,** 497–98.
Haberam, S. (19800) Putting a price on life. *Health and Social Service Journal*, **2,** 877–79.
In Brief (1987) *Nursing Times*, **83,** 48, 7.
Jelkmann. C.H.M. (9182) My heart transplant: a second chance to live. *AORN Journal*, **36,** 53–56.
Keogh, A. (1987) Transplantation and organ donation. *Nursing 16*, **3,** 16, 590–92.
Kimball, L.)1982) Organ donation: one family's story. *AORN Journal*, **36,** 1, 50–52.
Knight, B. (1976) Law and ethics in transplantation. *The Practitioner*, **216,** 471–74.
Papworth, M. (1981) The definition of death. *World Medicine*, 12 December, 72–76.

Roach, S. (1986) Reflections on the ethics of organ donation and retrieval. *Dimensions*, **63**, 7, 34.

Sandroff, R. (1980) Is it right? *Registered Nurse*, 24–27.

Shanley, E. (1982) The medicalisation of dying – 1, 2 & 3, *Nursing Times*, **78**, 1360–62; 1403–05; 1449–50.

Wight, C. (1987) Concerns of the family. *Nursing Times*, **82**, 20, 53.

51

Euthanasia: the way to a peaceful end?

Peter Ellis, BSc (Hons), RGN,
Staff Nurse, Guy's Hospital, London

How many times has an elderly suffering patient said, "If I were an animal you'd put me down" – and how many times have you replied, "Now then dear you don't really mean that", as you scuttle off knowing full well they do mean it. Most nurses probably experience similar situations a number of times in their careers. Euthanasia, though, is illegal and, as a subject of discussion, taboo.

Why is this? Is this stance logical in the light of an ever increasing elderly population, advances in medical technology and increasing freedoms for the individual? Who has the right to choose if a person should live or die? Who can judge if the length of life is more important than its quality, or indeed the quality of death? The simple answer would be 'the patient of course!', except for the fact that death is perhaps the most emotive of all subjects.

There is an important distinction to be drawn between involuntary and non-voluntary euthanasia. Involuntary euthanasia is when the decision to shorten a person's life is made by others, despite the fact that he or she is able to be involved in the decision making; ie, is conscious and coherent. Non-voluntary euthanasia involves the decision being made for the individual as he or she is unable to make the decision, due to being unconscious, mentally incapacitated or too young.

Definitions of euthanasia

Literally translated from the Greek, euthanasia means 'good death'. It is only in recent years that it has come to mean "the deliberate killing of someone by a fatal intervention" (Whitefield, 1987).

Goldberg defines the various types of euthanasia as:

Active euthanasia The purposeful shortening of human life through active or direct assistance, with or without medical assistance.

Passive euthanasia Withdrawal or renunciation of life-prolonging measures with or without medical assistance.

Voluntary euthanasia The freely given consent of the individual to his death, after he has been fully informed.

Involuntary euthanasia Purposeful shortening of an individual's life without the individual's consent (Darbyshire, 1987).

There is a further category, non-voluntary euthanasia, when a life is taken when it is impossible to ask the person's consent (Melia, 1988), as in the case of a comatose person, or an infant.

A moral distinction

Active euthanasia is illegal in the UK, even if it is voluntary. The BMA (1988) supports this, referring to the practice of active euthanasia as "killing the patient". On the other hand, the report accepts the practice of passive euthanasia as "morally acceptable".

In criticising the view that there is a moral distinction between 'allowing to die' – as in passive euthanasia – and actively ending a life, it can be argued that in law, and in practice, what counts is intent (Wright, 1988; Nowell-Smith, 1989). Whether we either allow the patient to die, or become actively involved in his or her death, the outcome is the same – the death of the patient – and in both cases there is an element of intent.

There is an argument sanctioned by the Catholic church called the argument of 'double effect'. "This distinguishes between what we do, and what we intend the outcome to be" (Melia, 1988), meaning that if we give opiates to a terminally ill patient we can say 'It's for pain relief', even though we know the opiates may suppress that patient's respiration and lead to premature death.

Beauchamp and Childress (1983) state that the principle of double effect involves four conditions:

1. That the action in itself should be 'good' or at least morally 'indifferent'.

2. The action should be undertaken purely in order to achieve the 'good' effect, and that while the 'bad' effect is foreseen and is 'allowed', it is not intended.

3. That the two effects should arise as the result of the same action, the 'bad' effect cannot be allowed if it occurs as part of the means to achieving the 'good' effect.

4. The 'good' and 'bad' effects should be relatively equally balanced.

It appears from this definition, therefore, that the death of a patient (the 'bad' effect) as a result of administration of a large dose of opiates is viewed as acceptable, as the primary intention of the care giver would be to control the patient's pain and distress (the 'good' effect). This argument, while it does not answer the questions surrounding the issue of the administration of large doses of opiates to people who are terminally ill, goes a long way towards helping us cope with this dilemma at a personal level.

One way of helping medical staff make the decision to stop treatment is to carry what is commonly known as a 'living will', but what the Voluntary Euthanasia Society (VES) call an 'advance declaration'. These forms do not ask attending doctors or healthcare professionals to do anything illegal, but state that the bearer does not wish to be kept alive should there be "no reasonable prospect of my recovery from physical illness or impairment expected to cause me severe distress or render me incapable of rational existence" (VES, 1989). It is not mandatory for doctors in the UK to execute the advance declaration, but it may prove helpful should members of the healthcare team find themselves in the position of having to make a life and death decision for a patient who is unconscious, or otherwise incapable of voicing their opinion.

Sanctity of life

There are those who would argue that the sanctity of life is of paramount importance when considering euthanasia. They believe that life should be sustained at all costs, and for them there is no quantity/quality dilemma. This view is probably best explained in the words of Dr Tendler, "... human life is of infinite value. This in turn means that a piece of infinity is also infinity, and a person who has minutes to live is of no less value than a person who has 60 years to live..." (Kuhse, 1989).

Tendler, however, misses the point: value often has more to do with quality than it does quantity. No-one who advocates euthanasia does so on the grounds that one life is worth less than another, the reality, in fact, is exactly the opposite. Kennedy (1991) describes euthanasia as the "last act of compassion and love". Brewer (1988) cites the case of an elderly dying patient who reproached the staff at the hospice where she was dying with the words "You wouldn't let it happen to a dog". This elderly lady was judging between the quality and quantity of her life, as well she might, and she had come down in favour of quality – there are many such documented cases, and even more undocumented.

In Holland about 10 per cent of deaths are by active euthanasia, or 'mercy killing' as its practitioners prefer to call it (*Viewpoint '90*, 1990). This accounts for 2,000-6,000 deaths a year (Darbyshire, 1987), which are bound by strict guidelines laid down in law (Table 1). While euthanasia is not actually legal in Holland, prosecutions do not occur if the death has been handled according to law (Ridder, 1989).

There is much argument that legislation in favour of active euthanasia would be open to considerable abuse. This, according to Dr John Keown, of Leicester University, appears to have been the case in Holland: he says, "There is...disturbing evidence that patients in Holland are being killed without their request and even sometimes against their will" (*Viewpoint '90*, 1990).

- The patient should be suffering from a terminal illness.
- The patient (and only the patient) should ask for the euthanasia – he or she should not be coerced into it – requests need to be consistent, and preferably in writing.
- The doctor who is asked should consult with another doctor whom he or she doesn't know.
- The doctor should inform the public prosecutor prior to euthanasia, but should not name the patient.
- The next of kin should be informed of the wish.
- The euthanasia needs to be reported to the coroner after it has occurred.

Table 1. Main guidelines governing the practice of active euthanasia in Holland

If we had legislation for active euthanasia in the UK, where would we eventually draw the line? At elderly people? Those suffering from dementia? Those with disabilities? (Whitefield, 1987). This has been called the 'slippery slope' argument, and is often reputed to be a reaction to the Nazi holocaust more than to any solid evidence (Ellis, 1990). A working party for the Institute of Medical Ethics (1990) does not see the argument as a real threat: "Such a moral slide seems improbable... disapproval of involuntary termination of patients' lives is strongly entrenched in the concepts of most doctors and laymen. Furthermore, despite the denials of the BMA report, we know that many doctors have assisted and still assist the deaths of occasional patients in their own homes. These rare acts have been accepted as desirable without any consequent moral decline."

Another major argument says patients will have difficulty in trusting doctors and nurses if they feel these people, whom they expect to strive to 'save life', are also involved in the deaths of other patients (Wright, 1988). This is unlikely, as public opinion appears to be mostly in favour of legislation legalising euthanasia (Waller, 1986; Humphry and Wickett, 1986; VES, 1989). Despite public opinion, however, Roland Boyes' Private Member's Bill to legalise euthanasia failed at its first reading in the House of Commons in 1990.

Although it remains illegal in this country, there is a consensus of opinion that active euthanasia does occur here (Walker, 1988; Nowell-Smith, 1987). Dr Pieter Admiral, a leading Dutch euthanasiast is quoted as saying: "I am sure that they are doing this in England but dare not talk about it. I am sure that in most countries, good doctors are helping people to die peacefully" (Turton, 1987).

The law

The law in England and Wales (with only minor differences of wording in Scotland) does not recognise euthanasia as 'mercy killing'. Anyone found to be aiding, counselling or arranging the suicide of another, as specified by the 1957 Homicide Act, faces a charge of murder. Nicholas Purnell, chairman of the Bar Council, says:"Mercy killings are another example where the law has to look at whether or not the evidence shows a deliberate intention to take life. It doesn't look at motive; it doesn't look at consequence; it doesn't look at the reasons why people may be driven to make very unhappy decisions. If the evidence shows that it was a deliberate act, then murder or attempted murder will be the only offences that can be charged in those circumstances" (*Viewpoint 90*, 1990).

The mandatory sentence for murder since 1957 has been life imprisonment – that for attempted murder, however, remains at the discretion of the judge. This anomaly can have serious consequences for any successful euthanasiast. Nicola and Andrew Thompson were lucky that a medical team was able to reverse the morphine overdose they had administered to their dying mother in July 1990: they only faced a charge of attempted murder. They were equally lucky to come before a judge as compassionate as Mr Justice Tudor Evans who explained his decision to give them no more than a conditional discharge with the words: "I am sure that it was the deep attachment and love that you both had for your mother that led you to act as you did" (*Times*, 1990).

Andrew Thompson later explained the reasons for his action thus: "I didn't want her to suffer anymore, it was the only thing that kept me going. I loved my mum so much...it wasn't easy...she'd had enough. No-one else seemed to be able to do anything, therefore there didn't seem to be any choice...We are talking about someone who was existing in a rotting carcass...It was a moral issue...allowing her to die slowly was an injustice, when she asked me to kill her, then I had the right" (*Viewpoint 90*, 1990).

Thompson states that it was his mother's wish that her suffering should end. Did she have the right, if not to take her own life, then to ask that somebody do it for her? In a society committed to personal autonomy and the freedom of the individual, she was unable to exercise this freedom (and indeed was legally disbarred from doing so).

Nurse involvement

Darbyshire (1987) argues that nurses all too often stop thinking about ethics because "others make the critical decisions and orders have to be obeyed". These 'others' are usually doctors, whom nurses allow to make the most vital of all decisions: 'not for resuscitation'; 'terminate life support'; 'ordinary interventions only'. Why is this, and what is a medical decision? Benjamin and Curtis (1986) define two types of medical decision. First there are those based upon the superior training of the doctor, called 'medical decisions in the technical sense', and include such things as drug regimens and appropriate types of surgery. Second there are 'medical decisions in the contextual sense' which are based on morals, values and beliefs. While medical knowledge may affect these decisions, they do not depend on any technical expertise.

If we accept this distinction, in medical decisions in the contextual sense the feelings of the nurse are as valid as those of the doctor. More important than any 'clinical' decision, however, are the beliefs, values and wishes of the patient about whose life the decisions are being made.

As nurses, we often stress that we are the patient's advocate. Should we not, therefore, take the time to find out what he or she wants and do our best to represent those wishes. If this means opposing the decisions of our medical colleagues, we must learn to do so. It would be unrealistic to suggest active sabotage of medical decisions, but we should not be afraid to make our feelings, and those of our patients, known – indeed the UKCC Code of Conduct states that nurses: "in the practice of professional accountability shall: take account of the customs, values and spiritual beliefs of patients/clients."

In undertaking to do this nurses will increase their standing as members of the healthcare team, and improve on the reality of the team approach wherever they work. To do this effectively, we need a common consensus about what is acceptable in individual cases, so we can represent our feelings and, more importantly, those of our patients. When medical decisions in the contextual sense are being made, it should be remembered that nurses have as much right to resist do not resuscitate orders as they do to promote them, and the same can be said of any withdrawal of treatment decision. Nurses need to stand up for whatever they feel is right for individual patients, whether that is to draw back from further treatment or to continue to try to save them.

Nurses' feelings about euthanasia

There has been little research on nurses' feelings about euthanasia; it is an emotive subject, and one with which researchers may feel uncomfortable. What we do know, however, is that about 72 per cent of the general population are in favour of active voluntary euthanasia, but what nurses feel remains debatable.

Lovett (1988), in a study of nurses working in psychiatric, elderly and elderly mentally ill rehabilitation wards, found 51 per cent felt people have the right to end their own life when they choose; 29 per cent were in favour of aiding those who are incapable of acting, while only 16 per cent felt they could become actively involved. Nurses who worked with elderly people were more in favour of the individual's 'right to die' – probably because they saw their patients as capable of making this decision for themselves, whereas nurses working with psychiatric and elderly mentally ill people did not. These findings are supported by those of Stewart and Rai (1989), who showed that nurses felt more comfortable with euthanasia if the patient involved was elderly.

Three quarters of nurses in a *Nursing Times* survey (1988) felt there is a moral difference between passive and active euthanasia. This appears to endorse the BMA's report of 1988 which labelled active euthanasia as 'killing the patient', and passive euthanasia as a 'non-treatment decision'.

There appears to be a general agreement that individuals should have the right to choose how and when they die, especially when suffering from terminal illness. What should be done, therefore, about the issue of active euthanasia? Would we be 'playing God' if we were to implement such a policy? Do we not 'play God' when we use modern technology to sustain – or even restore – life which under 'normal' circumstances would have ended?

Where does all this lead us? Surely we need strictly policed legislation in favour of voluntary euthanasia, so that we, as nurses, can deliver in death the dignified care we strive hard to deliver to our patients in life.

References
Beauchamp, T. and Childress, J. (1983) Principles of Biomedical Ethics (2nd Edn). Oxford University Press, Oxford.
Benjamin, M. and Curtis, J. (1986) Ethics in Nursing (2nd Edn). OUP, Oxford.
Brewer, C. (1988) An option on death. *Nursing Times*, **84**, 11, 22.
British Medical Association (1988) Euthanasia. BMA, London.
Darbyshire, P. (1987) Whose life? Whose decision? *Nursing Times*, **83**, 45, 26-29.
Ellis, P. (1990) A baby's right to die. *Nursing Standard*, **5**, 9, 51.
Humphry, D. and Wickett, A. (1986) The Right to Die: Understanding Euthanasia. The Bodley Head, London.
Institute of Medical Ethics Working Party (1990) Viewpoint: Assisted death. *The Lancet*, **336**, 610-13.
Kennedy, L. (1991) Euthanasia: Lecture presented at King's College London as part of the lent season of Public Lectures for the Centre of Medical Ethics and Law.
Kuhse, H. and Singer, P. (1989) The quality/quantity of life distinction and its moral importance for nurses. *International Journal of Nursing Studies*, **26**, 3, 203-12.
Lovett, L. (1988) A comparative attitudinal study of nurses working in geriatrics, psycho-geriatrics and psychiatric rehabilitation. Unpublished work: Liverpool University.
Melia, K. (1988) An easy death? *Nursing Times*, **84**, 8, 46-48.
Nowell-Smith, P. (1989) Euthanasia and the doctors – a rejection of the BMA's report. *Journal of Medical Ethics*, **15**, 3, 124-28.*Nursing Times* (1988) Euthanasia what you think? *Nursing Times*, **84**, 33, 38-39.
Ridder, C. (1989) A model for euthanasia. *Nursing Standard*, **3**, 48, 35-37.
Stewart, K. and Rai, G. (1989) A matter of life and death. *Nursing Times*, **85**, 35, 27.
Turton, P. (1987) The death debate. *Nursing Times*, **83**, 45, 31.
Victor, P. (1990) Brother and sister go free after trying to kill dying mother. *The Times*, 14 November.
Viewpoint '90 (1990) Let Me Die. Granada Television.
Voluntary Euthanasia Society (1989) The Last Right. VES, London.
Walker, I. (1988) Killing for kindness. *New Society*, **83**, 13.
Waller, S. (1986) Trends in public acceptance of euthanasia worldwide. *Euthanasia Review*, **1**, 1, 13-47.
Whitefield, S. (1987) Going gently into that good night. *Nursing Times*, **83**, 45, 30.
Wright, S. (1988) The power over death. *Nursing Standard*, **2**, 11, 22.

Further information
The Voluntary Euthanasia Society, 13 Prince of Wales Terrace, London W8 5PG.
Tel: 071-937 7770.

Product Appraisal

52

Resources review: product appraisal

Brenda Pottie, SRN, SCN, DN (Lond)
Senior Nurse, Specialist Research, East Surrey Health Authority

The nurses' involvement with purchasing decisions

In many purchasing decisions, the nurse on the ward or in the community has an important role. She uses many items of equipment and supplies every day, and also has the most detailed knowledge of the needs of the individual patient.

There has been, and often still is, a very large gap between the contracting supplies officer and the nurse on the ward, in the department, or in the community. This can widen if, for example, a company representative shows nurses products that are not available to them because there is a regional contracting system for purchase which excludes these products on grounds of cost or unsuitability. To be involved with decision-making at ward and regional levels nurses must be aware of the cost and be systematic in their appraisal of products. This information must then

PRODUCT APPRAISAL FORM

ITEM .... DURABLE ☐ DISPOSABLE ☐

MANUFACTURER/BRAND ....

Placement of contract for purchase of this item is being considered. If you have been using this product for not less than 3 months would you please assist the Supplies Department by completing this form.

When completed please return to ....

Name and Address of Unit ....

Type of Nursing e.g. "General" ....

Please tick the appropriate reply to these statements and questions	STRONGLY AGREE	AGREE	DISAGREE	STRONGLY DISAGREE	COMMENTS
1. This product is easy to use					
2. The quality is about right					
3. There are no major disadvantages					
4. It is suitable for the job					

5. Would you like this product to be available for ordering? YES ☐ NO ☐

6. If you know of an alternative product which is equally acceptable or better please give details

NAME ....

DESIGNATION ....

DATE ....

Figure 1. Product appraisal form.

be circulated to the appropriate people, and used effectively in reaching purchase decisions.

A system for product appraisal

A product appraisal system was devised by Doreen Norton by which to obtain basic facts about products in use (Norton, 1982). In such a survey, the nurses using the item are asked to complete a product appraisal form

PRODUCT APPRAISAL RESULTS   Ref. No. ....

ITEM ....   Date ....

MANUFACTURER/BRAND ....

Number P.A. Forms completed ....

Question 1-4:   4 × .... = ... (100%)

ANALYSIS OF RESULTS	A	B	Y	Z
	Strongly Agree	Agree	Disagree	Strongly Disagree
1. Product easy to use				
2. Quality about right				
3. No major disadvantages				
4. Suitable for the job				
TOTALS				

Total of **A + B** (favourable) .... (...... %)
Total of **Y + Z** (unfavourable).......... (...... %)

COMMON COMPLAINTS: in order of frequency of mention, with approximate number making comment.

	Number
....	
....	
....	
....	
....	
....	
....	
....	
....	
....	
....	

5. Would like product available for ordering
   number .... percentage ....

ACTION TAKEN

Figure 2. Product appraisal result form.

(Figure 1), having had experience of using a product for three months. The opinion of nurses in different specialties can be included in the survey. The forms are then collated onto the product appraisal result form (Figure 2) for analysis and for use in decision making by the appropriate person or department.

This information gathered from the completed forms does not in itself constitute a rigorously researched evaluation of the product, but it does give a practical survey of the opinions of nurses and should reveal which products are suitable for purchase. The survey may indicate that further evaluation should be carried out.

This simple system can be used successfully in conjunction with a monitoring and costing exercise, for example examining three different types of wipe or cleaning tissue for incontinent patients.

Different manufacturers' products 1, 2, and 3 were each used for one week on one ward, over a period of three consecutive weeks. The product appraisal forms were completed by all nurses working on the ward during the trial and the results were collated onto the product appraisal result form. The results were as follows:

Product 1: $A + B = 75\%$ $Y + Z = 25\%$
Product 2: $A + B = 25\%$ $Y + Z = 75\%$
Product 3: $A + B = 100\%$

This information was then forwarded to the contracting officer with the recommendation that **Product 3** should be selected for the regional contract (Smith; Unpublished Report).

A system for evaluation

More detailed evaluation of products may be required, and this will take more planning and research than the simple example just given.

To evaluate means "To determine significance or worth of usage by careful appraisal and study" (Webster, 1977). This means that there must be a commitment by staff, and in many circumstances patients, if the evaluation is to take place and be of value. A protocol must be written first to establish the criteria and the plan for the research. The process of product evaluation will be discussed in the following chapter.

Conclusion

Nurses have a vital role to play in appraising and evaluating resources, but the necessary research must be done in a systematic way and be carefully planned and properly documented. If the need for this discipline is recognized prior to an evaluation, this will surely stop the use of so-called "trials", in which one or two products are used with only one patient and then one product either praised or rejected. Incorrect decisions are often made as a result of inadequate or insufficiently documented factual information.

Nurses are increasingly involved with the decisions made on purchase. Ward budgeting is used in some hospitals and is a system that is likely to become more widely adopted in the future. One of the results of this system is that the ward sister or charge nurse may now be accountable for sizeable budgets for ward-based purchases. We owe it to our patients, our employers, our colleagues, and ourselves to make the best decisions.

References

Norton, D. (1982) What's in Store. Nursing Times, 1221.
Websters Dictionary (1977) Cassells, London.

53
Resources review: product evaluation

Brenda Pottle, SRN, SCM, DN (Lond)
Senior Nurse, Specialist Research, East Surrey Health Authority

Ward budgeting is a system that is used now in some hospitals and it is likely to be more widely adopted in the future. As a result, ward sisters may be accountable for sizeable budgets and they need to know how to make the best decisions on ward-based purchases of equipment and supplies.

A system for evaluation

In the previous chapter, the nurse's involvement with purchasing decisions was discussed and it was stressed that to be involved with decision making at ward and regional levels nurses must be aware of the costs and be systematic in their appraisal of products.

A simple system for product appraisal was illustrated which can provide a practical survey of nurses' opinions and reveal which products are suitable for purchase, but sometimes a more rigorous and detailed evaluation of products may be required, and this will take more planning and research.

To evaluate means "To determine significance or worth of usage by careful appraisal and study" (Webster, 1977). This means that there must be a commitment by staff, and in many circumstances patients, if the evaluation is to take place and be of value. A protocol must be written first to establish the criteria and the plan for the research.

Protocol for product evaluation

Purpose There may be a number of reasons for undertaking product evaluation. A new product may have become available and an existing product in use over a number of years may not now be the best choice. Suitability of a product for a particular group of patients may be questioned. A comparison of products may be required and the cost-effectiveness of each may need to be evaluated.

Products to be used All products to be included in the evaluation must be listed; details are taken from the manufacturer's specifications and literature.

Costs   These should be carefully defined and VAT included where applicable. The unit cost if a bulk purchase on a regional contract is made should also be known. If the product is not available on prescription, evaluation of it with patients in the community should be questioned, and the value of assessing these products considered carefully.

Literature search   Has anyone been down this path before? If so, what did their research cover and what were the results? Should those findings be tested again, or new methods employed?

Criteria to be tested   The manufacturer's literature can be used to draw up some of the questions that may be asked in finding out if it is suitable for the patient and the nurse to use. For example, a bandage to be evaluated has in its manufacturer's literature (Johnson and Johnson, 1984):
"Easy to apply and remove
Stick only to themselves
Easy for home and ward use
Aid compliance
Do not stick to hair or skin

Less discomfort and skin trauma
Tears easily to length without scissors
Conforms even on awkward sites
Extremely comfortable
Highly absorbent and permeable
Kind to skin
Fewer complications and fewer changes
Can be worn in water
Radiolucent"
   These statements can be used to draw up a questionnaire to assess the practical use of this product. Other criteria may include suitability for different groups of patients (such as children or the elderly) or the effectiveness of use by untrained personnel, who could include relatives.

Method of evaluation   The method used in the research must be planned out in detail. This should include the following:
Length of time in days, weeks, or months
Staff to be consulted
Numbers of patients and locations in hospital and/or community
Ethical issues
Instructions for using the products (company representatives could be involved here)
Design of the forms and questionnaires: Should these be piloted?
Monitoring the use of detailed forms. Is someone able to give the time personally to monitor the evaluation? Time and staff must be available to collate the results.

The research With this planned out in detail, the forms and questionnaires devised (and if necessary piloted), and all the staff fully briefed, the information gathering can begin.

Results Once the forms and questionnaires are collected, it takes time to collate the results. If a computer is available time can be saved, but monitoring forms and questionnaires must be designed before the research with full knowledge of the computer's potential in order to make best use of this resource. The limitations of the research must also be clearly identified (for example it may only be appropriate for one group of patients, or one setting for care). The problems encountered while undertaking the research should also be reported.

Report This needs to have all the details of the evaluation, limitations, problems encountered, costs, results, conclusions, and recommendations in a clear, typed format. Before writing the report, consideration must be given to its future use. It may be circulated to other nurses, administrators, or supplies officers only, or it may be made more widely available to the manufacturers or even for publication.

Reports are best written as soon as possible after the research is completed so that the most up-to-date information is made available to colleagues. Imposing a deadline for the completion of the report may help with this. The report must be circulated to appropriate colleagues, including the nurses involved with the evaluation and the budget holder.

Conclusion
Incorrect decisions on purchasing are often made as a result of inadequate or insufficiently documented factual information. Nurses have a vital role to play in appraising and evaluating resources, and the necessary research must be done in a systematic way, with careful planning and proper documentation. Recognition of the need for such discipline prior to an evaluation should avoid the use of so-called "trials", when one or two products are used with only one patient and then one product is praised or rejected on this basis.

References
Johnson and Johnson Ltd (1984) New Secure and Secure Forte Literature.
Norton, D. (1982) What's in Store. *Nursing Times*, 1221.
Websters Dictionary (1977) Cassells, London.

54

Measuring product performance

Doreen Norton, OBE, MSc, SRM, FRCN

Retired; formerly Nursing Research Liaison Officer, South West Thames RHA and Professor of Gerontological Nursing, Case Western Reserve University, Cleveland, Ohio

Evaluation means measuring performance against prescribed criteria. The first step to conducting a reliable trial of a product is writing the prescription for the performance, as these criteria are the basis for planning the data-collecting form or questionnaire to be used in the trial. 'Measuring' means the information sought and obtained must be capable of interpretation in numerical form.

This article offers guidance on these aspects of product performance trials. It is written in terms of a single product but the same principles apply when two or more of the same kind are subjected to comparative

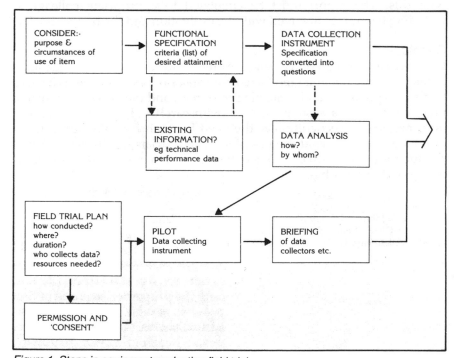

Figure 1. Steps in equipment evaluation field trial.

evaluation of performance. Any field trial must be systematically planned (Figure 1) and based on scientific principles.

Criteria prescription

What is the purpose of the product and the general circumstances of its use? Write a concise statement answering these two questions (Figure 2). This is not always easy, but worthwhile because it focuses the mind and throws up issues which can easily be missed through familiarity with the nursing tasks involved in using such an item.

a) Roughly list all the functions and properties which, ideally, are desired of the product in fulfilment of its purpose and in the circumstances of its use. Note any information supplied by the manufacturer, particularly technical specifications, and adjust the list accordingly.

Figure 2. Criteria specifications.

ITEM: Disposable theatre cap.
PURPOSE: To keep hair enclosed for (a) hygenic reasons and (b) uninhibited vision and movement.
MAIN SITUATIONS OF USE: Operating theatres and intensive care units.

REQUIREMENTS	EXPLANATION AND CONSTRAINTS
MATERIAL 1. Shall be reasonably non-generating of static electricity.	(i) Cap worn in the presence of anaesthetic gases.
2. Shall allow ventilation.	(ii) Operating theatres have a temperature of 18-24°C and humidity of 40-50%; therefore the head covering must not impede heat evaporation from the scalp nor generate its own heat.
3. Shall remain intact when handled (donning of cap) and throughout use.	(iii) Must not disintegrate, stretch or contract under conditions of heat and humidity (ii).
4. Shall be non-irritating to skin.	(iv) Length of time in contact with skin (v) and environmental conditions (ii) increase risk of skin irritation.
THE CAP 5. Should be reasonably light in weight and softly flexible.	(v) Cap may be worn up to eight hours and therefore should not give awareness of weight or rigidity in the interests of comfort.
6. Shall be easy to put on.	(vi) —
. . .etc. . .	. . .etc. . .

This example of prescribed criteria was developed as an exercise with a group of nurses from East Surrey Health Authority in 1982.

b) Now examine each entry critically, with a view to revising the list by deletions and modifications. Extract and record separately, for example, any factor which would require to be tested other than in the field trial, such as a bacterial test in a laboratory. Bear in mind throughout that demands made of the product must be realistic and that each stated requirement will later involve framing questions to ascertain if, and to what extent it is met in performance of the product.

c) Assemble the remaining entries into some form of order, eg grouping of related factors or an appropriate logical sequence.

d) Against each entry, record into which of three categories it falls — essential (it shall), desirable (should), permissible (may). The terms in brackets will apply when finalising the wording of the criteria.

e) Prepare for the revised list by dividing a large sheet of paper into two sections, one headed **Requirements** and the other **Explanation and Constraints.** Now comes the brain-teasing part — not to be rushed! It is advisable to study the example (Figure 2) at this stage.

f) Make each entry under 'Requirements' a precise statement in terms of functional performance. (Do not specify design or materials — express only the properties required of them.) Try to make the statements in the positive, ie what the product must, should or may do, rather than what it must not do. (The 'must nots' should become apparent under the other section heading). Under 'Explanation and constraints' record information which clarifies the entry opposite. Indeed, it is advisable to work through such information and assemble any extrinsic facts necessary before attempting to finalise the wording of the statement of Requirements.

Data collecting instrument

Whatever the plan decided for conduct of the trial, the criteria have to be converted into some form of questioning of observers about the product's performance under working conditions.

The kind of questioning varies with the nature of the requirement; it can be a direct question or a statement for agreement/disagreement. In either, a 'yes/no' type of answering may be appropriate for some factors but for others allowance usually has to be made in the data collecting instrument for recording degrees of the product's compliance with the requirement. An even number of degrees (say, four or six) is preferable to an uneven number (say, three or five) as this allows for a balance of degrees towards satisfactory and unsatisfactory and avoids the less helpful 'middle of the road' reply. The more degrees there are the more refined the information obtained but it is often necessary to strike a compromise between the amount and sophistication of information sought and the resources available for collecting and analysing the data.

Scoring of points

To achieve measurement of a product's performance, a weighted value of points is allocated to the optional replies to a question. Maximum points are given for total compliance with the requirement (completely satisfactory) to nil for no compliance (completely unsatisfactory). The number of intervals between depends on the number of degrees of compliance allowed for, eg four degrees will be in the order of 3,2,1,0 in value, but in any event the points' 'weighting' must be proportionately equal in their graduation steps.

Measurable analysis

The sum of the maximum points obtainable to all questions gives the 'ideal' performance score. The points scored by the product are then totalled and this figure calculated as a percentage of the 'ideal' score.

Example: Ideal score 58; obtained score 38.

$$\frac{3800}{58} = 65.5 \text{ per cent compliance with the criteria.}$$

If the product is a disposable or requires treatment before being used again (such as laundering) it may be decided to record observations at each incident of use rather than to collect data at the end of the trial period. In this case, the formula for analysis is to multiply the 'ideal' score by the number of times the item was used and the total of the obtained scores calculated as a percentage.

Example: Ideal score 58 x 110 incidents of use = 6380 max.
Obtained score total = 4125.

$$\frac{412500}{6380} = 64.6 \text{ per cent compliance with the criteria.}$$

Refinement of results   Irrespective of when data are collected, a refinement of results can be obtained if desirable. Namely, by isolating those requirements earlier identified as essential (shall) and applying the same procedure to their respective total of maximum points possible and the obtained score. It may be decided that the product is unacceptable if it fails to satisfy any one of these requirements or achieves less than, say, 90 per cent, in respect of these, however well it rated overall.

Comparative evaluations   When two or more products of the same kind (and used in the same way) are to receive a field trial to determine the most suitable, the principle is the same as for a single product. That is, the performance of each is measured against the prescribed criteria (and not simply compared with each other) and rated accordingly. All, however, must be subjected to the same trial conditions and, preferably, using the same observers.

It was mentioned at the outset that reliable information is the key to products being designed suitable for purpose and acceptable in the work situation. Manufacturers are starved of such information, and weaknesses in the design of products can be generally attributed to the failure of health care professionals to produce user-specifications. A performance criteria drawn-up for trial purposes and a user-specification are one and the same, so performance criteria made known to manufacturers can influence future design for the better. In any event, a full report of a product trial (including details of the methods) should always be sent to the manufacturer concerned.

References
Buckles, A.M. (1980) How should we dispose of our used needles and syringes? *Nursing Times*, **76**, 34, Journal of Infection Control Nursing, ICNA, 5–11.
An evaluation of four different types of containers for the disposal of sharps which serves as a good example of a comparative type of field trial using product performance measurement.
Norton, D. (1978) Equipment fit for purpose. *Nursing Times*, **74**, 19, Occasional Papers, 73–76.
Describes in detail the principles of specifying and evaluating equipment and for conducting field trials.

55

A tube to suit all NG needs? Evaluation of fine bore nasogastric tubes

Helen Fawcett, RGN
Nutrition Nurse Specialist, The Royal London Hospital, Whitechapel

Claire Yeoman, BSc, SRD
Former Chief Dietitian, The Royal London Hospital, Whitechapel

Fine bore nasogastric (NG) tubes are now widely used in hospitals and by patients at home for the administration of commercially made feeds. These tubes have replaced the wide bore Ryles tubes which were traditionally used, but which caused patient discomfort, oesophagitis and gastric reflux due to their size. Being made of PVC, Ryles tubes could also only be used for a week before they hardened and often cracked. Ryles tubes are, however, indicated where gastric emptying is impaired, and should be reserved for postoperative aspiration and gastric lavage only.

A wide selection of fine bore NG tubes are available on the market and these vary in quality and cost from 80 pence to £11.00 (retail price at the end of 1990). To ensure the tubes chosen are best suited to patient needs, nurses need to know the properties of each and to establish a criteria for selection. To be cost-effective, tubes must be long-lasting, comfortable *in situ* and well secured with adhesive tape to avoid slippage. The NNS in conjunction with ward and endoscopy staff and dietitians at the Royal London Hospital organised a trial to determine which tubes best fulfilled the criteria for nasogastric administration of feed. This chapter charts the progress of the trial and records the results.

The trial first established the criteria fine bore NG tubes must meet to achieve effective administration of commercially made feeds. The criteria identified by discussion between NNS, ward nurses and dietitians to ensure nursing care best fulfils patient needs is listed below:

- All tubes must conform to British Standards.

- Nasogastric tubes must be no greater than FG size eight to prevent nasal trauma and oesophageal discomfort.

- Tubes must be compatible with the feeding equipment used on the ward to avoid both leakage and unnecessary use and expense of different connections and adaptors.

- Tubes must be easy to pass and to aspirate. Confirmation of position by aspiration and then testing with litmus paper, avoids the need for post-insertion X-ray.

- Tubes should be soft and, preferably, made from polyurethane to prevent cracking after prolonged use - polyurethane tubes can be left *in situ* for three months.

- Radio-opaque tubes enable X-rays to be taken clarifying the tube position, if required.

- Wide internal diameter is required to prevent blockage of NG tubes.

- A cap situated at the proximal end of the nasogastric tube to prevent contamination and blockage.

- Tubes must be comfortable for the patient, and, where appropriate, it should be easy for fluids to be swallowed around them.

- Tubes must be cost-effective to avoid overspending on the nutritional support budget.

Study sample

Six fine bore NG tubes which fulfilled the necessary criteria and were widely and easily available were chosen for the trial. These were:

- Fresenius 'Freka' (CH8).
- Merck 'Silk' (CH6).
- Abbott 'Flexiflow' (CH6).
- Cow and Gate 'Flocare' (CH8).
- Viomedex 'Swallow' (CH7/8).
- Portex tubing (cut to the required size) with adaptor (used in the endoscopy unit) (CH6).

Table 1 lists the characteristics of each tube; 10 tubes of each type were tested. They were randomly distributed among patients on the wards and in the endoscopy unit. A good representative sample of patients (60) requiring nutritional support was used; indications for placement included anorexia (17 patients); CA oesophagus (16 patients); orofacial and ENT surgery (9 patients); neurological disorders such as scleroderma and cerebral problems (10 patients) and inability to swallow - CVA and unconscious patients (8 patients). There was random selection of patients although those having endoscopically placed tubes had portex tubes.

A questionnaire was issued with each tube used in the trial, and nurses were required to complete and return it to the nutrition nurse specialist (NNS). The questionnaires asked nurses to record specific advantages and disadvantages of the tubes, and the results were collated to provide a rating for the equipment used.

Name of tube	1990 price (retail)	Material and size	Internal and external diameter	Distal end shape	Proximal end (cap etc)	Radio-opaque	Tube length	Comments
Fresenius' 'Freka' tube	£4.15	Polyurethane CH8	Ext. 2.8mm Int. 2.1mm	Two, large round side holes	A fitted cap compatible with feeding equipment	Yes	120 cm	Soft, flexible tube, well designed introducer, Easy to pass. Easy to aspirate. Securing tape in patient and 'cigar' connection. Needs a cigar shaped connection for flushing with syringes.
Merck 'Silk' tube	£11.00	Polyurethane CH6	Ext. 2.18mm Int. 1.37mm	Scooped spoon end	Fitted cap not compatible with feed equipment without connection	Yes	92 cm	Very soft and flexible. Easy to pass and particularly suitable when tube passage is diffcilt ie, ENT patients. Expensive in comparison to other tube. Needs male/male connection for feeding equipment. Securing tape in packet.
Abbott 'Flexiflow' (now with-drawn from sale)	£2.95	Polymeric PVC CH6	Ext. 2.0mm Int. 1.0mm with two	Round closed end with feed side holes	No cap compatible equipment	Yes	85 cm	No cap. Easy to pass. Tendency to block. Proximal end sometimes cracks.
Viomedex 'Swallow' tube	£5.46	Polyurethane 7/8FG	Ext. 2.5mm Int. 1.7mm	Round closed end. Two large outlet holes	Cap compatible with feed equipment	Yes	80 cm	Slightly stiff tube. Good size outlet holes. Difficult to aspirate due to poor seal on connection. Well packaged with a tray for water and a glove.
Cow & Gate 'Flocare' tube	£3.70	Polyurethane 8FG	Ext. diameter measurements not avaialble Int. 1.5mm	Open ended. Small side holes	No cap. Compatible with feed equipment	Yes	110 cm	No cap. End sometimes kinks as tube is passed.
Portex tubing (with adaptor)		Size 6FG	Ext. 2.0mm Int. 1.0mm	Open ended. No side holes	No cap. Requires adaptor to connect to tube.	Yes	As required cut to size	Cheap. Difficult to aspirate. Tendency to block.

Table 1. Characteristics of each tube.

The study

The tubes were passed by the NNS or qualified nursing staff in accordance with hospital policy, and marked with indelible ink at the nasal exit site so that any slippage could be recorded. All patients on the trial received pump assisted feeding of commercially made feeds, and where there was any risk of perforating the oesophagus (for example, patients with cancer, oesophageal varicies or stricture), tubes were placed by a gastroenterologist in the endoscopy unit. Patients were studied for ten days, and if their tube was changed during the trial, the same type was used.

The questionnaires identified the main nursing requirements for NG administration, and nurses were asked to record the progress of individual patients. Questions included:

- Which type of NG tube was used?

- Was intubation easy or difficult?

- Did any blockages occur? If so, why?

- Was the tube compatible with the feeding equipment?

- Was the tube comfortable (a rating score of 1-5 was given)?

- Were any specific problems encountered with the tube ?

- Why was the tube was removed?

The staff were confident the answers would provide a clear understanding of which fine bore NG tubes best met patients' needs.

Results of the survey

The questionnaire highlighted the main problems affecting the management of patients receiving NG feeding. Tube blockage relating to the size of the internal diameter of the tube was cited as a common problem (14 occurrences). Wider internal tube diameter was shown to reduce the incidence of blockages; Portex tubes (internal diameter 1.0mm), for example, saw most blockages (six) and Fresenius tubes (internal diameter 2.1mm) least (none). Difficulty also occurred in passage of some tubes due to swallowing difficulties, tubes kinking (Cow and Gate two kinked), and tube slippage due to poor adhesive taping (13 occurrences). Incompatible connections with the feed equipment caused delay and extra expense where new connections had to be found, and tubes which could be easily removed by patients were noted as a cause for concern (this happened four times during the trial). The full list of results is given in Table 2.

Tube	Number of tubes	Days in studies	Blockages	Slippages	Removed by patient
Fresenius	10	14	0	1	0
Merk	10	14	2	2	0
Abbott	10	14	3	2	1
Viomdexe	10	14	0	2	2
Cow & Gate	10	14	3	3	1
Portex	10	14	6	3	0

Table 2. Results of the questionnaires.

The results of the questionnaire prove that the design of NG tube is important for the effective management of patients requiring nutritional support. Blockage is always a potential problem, and tubes with wide internal diameters were shown to reduce the risk. Nasogastric tubes require a secure adhesive to prevent slippage, and this was achieved by 'Freka' (Fresenius) and 'Silk' (Merck) tubes. Both tubes were shown in the trial to provide the most effective all-round administration, fulfilling the criteria set in the trial to find a tube which best fulfilled patients' needs.

Bibliography

Taylor, S.J. (1988) A guide to nasogastric feeding equipment. *Professional Nurse*, 4, 2, 91-94.
Neohane, P.P. *et al* (1983) Limitations and drawbacks of 'fine bore' nasogastric tubes. *Clinical Nutrition*, 2, 85-86.
Hobbs, P. (1989) Enteral feeds. *Nursing Times*, 85, 9, 71-73.
Pritchard, A. (Ed.) The Royal Marsden Hospital manual of clinical nursing procedures, (2nd edition).

Acknowledgements

The authors wish to thank the ward nursing staff; the endoscopy unit nursing staff; Dr P. Swain and Dr N. van Someren (for placement of NG tubes in the Endoscopy Unit).

56

Achieving a competitive edge: an assessment of the cost effectiveness of Clinitron therapy

Trevor Patchett, BA, AHSM, Grad IPM
Healthcare Partner, Price Waterhouse

The trend towards greater productivity in terms of patient throughput continues to be strong in the NHS, even in the face of a tightening financial situation. Developments in medical technology, changes in treatment patterns and the decline in the number of available beds have all contributed to this situation, while the introduction of the internal market has also added to this pressure. Purchasers are looking to obtain maximum quantity and quality of service from their available resources and the concept of competition between providers is starting to emerge.

As part of the process of becoming competitive, hospitals must pay attention to their variable costs and the length of stay, which can be seen as an element of productivity. The approximate relative proportions of fixed and variable costs for inpatient work are illustrated in Figure 1, showing the possible impact a reduction in length of stay might have.

Hospital management may therefore find it expedient to look again at the available technology which can help their cause. They will also need to look at their existing and potential investments in technology and how this can be offset against improvements in productivity, as well as the impact on unit costs and quality. As part of this process, hospitals will also need to look at the impact, on both quality of care and productivity, of a variety of medical equipment products currently available in the market place. This chapter describes research undertaken by Price Waterhouse as to the potential contribution of Clinitron therapy.

Clinitron therapy
Clinitron therapy was developed to help meet the needs of a wide range of critically ill patients. The Clinitron Air Fluidised Therapy unit consists of a tank of glass microspheres which are fluidised by the upward flow of warm filtered air, and offers particular benefits in wound healing, temperature control, exudate management and infection control.

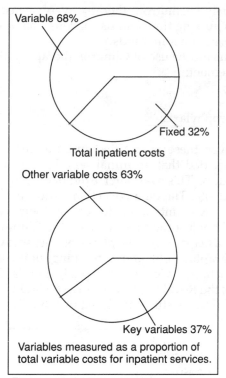

Total inpatient costs

Variables measured as a proportion of
total variable costs for inpatient services.

Figure 1. Variables and inpatient costs.

The unit is used by hospitals for a daily rental charge of £60 plus a one-off installation charge of £95. The service, from SSI Medical Services Ltd, includes advice from one of their nurse advisors on how to derive the best possible benefit from Clinitron therapy throughout the period of treatment, with special emphasis on wound care and technical support from the SSI technicians who are responsible for installation, main-tenance, repair and decontamination of the units between patients.

The primary objective of the study was to determine whether treatment involving Clinitron therapy was demonstrably more cost-effective, overall, than that given to similar patients using other methods such as turning them twice hourly or using other support surfaces. It was agreed at the outset that a large-scale randomised clinical trial would be neither feasible nor appropriate, nor would it be acceptable to consider denying patients Clinitron therapy if clinicians considered it an appropriate regimen, simply for the purposes of a study. Such an approach would be unethical and in direct contradiction of the MRCP guidelines on therapeutic research. It was therefore agreed to conduct a study comparing actual Clinitron patients with a control group.

A number of patients being treated using Clinitron therapy were studied in three hospitals, while staff in two other hospitals who were experienced in using Clinitron therapy were asked to assess what resources, such as nursing time and use of consumables were used when treating patients with other methods.

The main reasons for the use of Clinitron therapy in the study were:
- nursing management;
- tissue friability;
- pain;
- pressure sore prophylaxis;
- immobility.

In order to cover these specialties and the reasons for using the product, it was decided that an initial sample of 10 patients would be studied on two sites. This was later extended to include two further patients on a third site. The data collection period for patients receiving Clinitron therapy was intended to cover their complete hospital inpatient stay and not just the time spent on the Clinitron unit. Hospitals who agreed to participate in this phase of the study represented the north/south geographic split and a teaching/non-teaching split; they were North Manchester General Hospital, King's College Hospital, Ashford Hospital, the Royal Liverpool Hospital and Guy's Hospital. The specialties involved in the study are listed in Table 1.

- Intensive care;
- surgical/medical;
- plastic surgery;
- oncology;
- trauma/orthopaedics.

Table 1. Specialties involved in the study.

The researched control group was set at a sample size of 20 patients, of whom 10 were drawn from the SSI database of previous patients, and detailed patient profiles were drawn up to represent their clinical histories. The other 10 were based on the patients studied using Clinitron therapy. The rationale for the two sets of profiles was to try to establish consistency of data collection. Again, two hospitals participated in this phase of the study and replicated the teaching/non-teaching and north/south splits.

The key variables on which data was collected during the study were:
- direct nursing time;
- consumables: drugs, dressings, disposables;
- linen;
- length of stay (admission-discharge);
- paramedical time;
- outcome.

Figure 1 shows the relative proportions of the nursing, linen, drugs and dressings variables, measured against the total variable costs.

At the outset, it was difficult to determine how long the study would continue in terms of elapsed time, as there was no control over the incidence of patients who would be suitable for treatment by Clinitron therapy following our criteria for the study nor any control on their ultimate length of stay. In fact, the data collection spread over a period of 12 months from September 1988 to August 1989.

The study was conducted by our trained nursing consultants with assistance from SSI nurse advisors.

Conclusions

From this study, which has not concentrated on the improvement in quality of care which is described in other studies (see bibliography), the major determinates of whether Clinitron therapy can be justified in terms of cost-effectiveness are:
- reduction in the length of stay, and
- reduction in required nursing time per day.

The reduction in length of stay, as shown by our study, correlates with some of the work undertaken in America, for which literature was reviewed. The primary cause of this reduction was the promotion of wound healing which is intrinsic to the Clinitron therapy concept, and which has been validated on numerous occasions. One of the largest studies was conducted at Johns Hopkins Hospital by Allman *et al* (1986), while Hibbs (1988) bears witness to the role of Clinitron therapy in the treatment of pressure sores in the UK.

Similarly, the reduction in nursing time and cost for patients treated using Clinitron therapy is validated by other trials in the US whose literature was also reviewed.

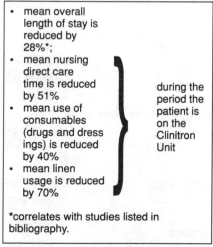

- mean overall length of stay is reduced by 28%*;
- mean nursing direct care time is reduced by 51%
- mean use of consumables (drugs and dressings) is reduced by 40%
- mean linen usage is reduced by 70%

during the period the patient is on the Clinitron Unit

*correlates with studies listed in bibliography.

Table 2. Key benefits of Clinitron on cost-effectiveness.

The results

It must be recognised from the outset that the study is based on a small sample of patients. The net effect of these factors do not detract from the overall conclusions but suggest the results should be treated as indicative rather than absolute.

The key benefits of Clinitron therapy's cost-effectiveness are shown in Table 2. If, therefore, a patient treatment costs £5,000 for a 25 day length of stay:

Total cost £5,000	= £200 per day
Length of stay 25 days	
Fixed cost (32 per cent)	= £ 64per day
Variable cost (68 per cent)	= £136 per day

If the patient were put on a Clinitron unit for 10 days within this overall length of stay, the potential reduction in variable cost from the results of the study would be:

(10 x £136) x 37 per cent   = £500 (approx).

The overall reduction in cost, taking into account the potential effect on length of stay would be:

25 days x 28 per cent   = 7 days reduction in length of stay.

Therefore new length of stay   = 25 - 7
          = 18 days.

Total treatment cost   = 18 x £200 per day
          = £3,600

Less variable cost savings while patient is on Clinitron therapy
          = £3,600 - £500
          = £3,100

Compared to previous cost,
therefore reduction: = £5,000
          = £5,000 - £3,100
          = £1,900

Deduct cost of renting Clinitron therapy service
          = (10 x £60 per day) + £95 installation fee
          = £695

Overall potential net saving   = £1,900 - £695
          = £1,205 per case

A competitive advantage

The use of Clinitron therapy can be viewed as having two kinds of benefit: clinical and cost. This article is concerned solely with the latter.

In order to take maximum advantage of the reduction in variable costs and the overall length of stay, it is clear that patients will have to be targeted carefully, with clinicians making judgements about possible length of stay and likely outcome. It will also require hospitals to have a good understanding of the level of their variable costs, particularly the direct nursing care time per patient. This information is becoming more readily available from the implementation of nursing workload systems as part of the resource management initiative currently in practice in many hospitals. Figure 2 illustrates the results of this study set in the context of the likely mix of contracts immediately post April 1991 and for the following three years.

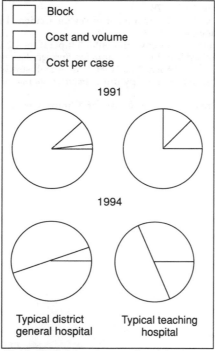

Figure 2. *Estimated proportions of cases by contract type.*

Managers will be able to develop a framework for targeting the application of the Clinitron product and any others which can be shown to have a similar impact on costs, in order to maximise their competitive advantage, assuming the product continues to be used in a similar way. This will be, perhaps, most important in the cost per case and cost and volume contract areas, but will demand the use of detailed cost, outcome and case mix data together with some fairly sophisticated forecasting.

References
Altman R.M. *et al* (1986) Pressure sores among hospital patients. *Annals of Internal Medicine*, **108**, 337-352.
Hibbs, J. (1988) Prevention Plan for Patients at Risk from Developing Pressure Sores. Policy for the Management of Pressure Sores. Pressure Area Care for the City and Hackney Health Authority.

Bibliography
Cooker, K.E.(1979) The intermittent air fluidised bed and the neurologically impaired patient. *J. Neurosurg. Nsing*, **11**, 1.
Dolezal, R. *et al* (1985) The use of Clinitron therapy unit in the immediate postoperative case of pressure ulcers. *Anals of Plastic Surgery*, **14**, 1
Hanson, J.E. (1985) Air fluidised therapy brings relief for decubitus ulcers. *Am. Health Care Association Journal*, Nov.
Jones, G.A. *et al* (1985) Demonstration of reduction in postoperative body protein breakdown using the Clinitron Fluidised Bed with an ambient temperature of 32ºc. *British Journal of Surgery*, **72**, 574-78.
Miles, J.M., Thompson, G.R. (1987) Treatment of severe accidental hypothermia using the Clinitron bed. *Anaesthesia*, **42**, 415-18.
Ryan, D.W. (1983) The influence of environmental temperature (32°C) on catabolism using the Clinitron air subsidised bed. *Intensive Medicine, Springer Ventag*, **9**, 279-81.
Vesley, D., Hankinson, S.E., Lauer, J.L. (1986) Microbial survival and dissemination associated with an air-fluidised therapy unit. *American Journal of Infection Control*, **14**, 1, 35-40

The above list illustrates the clinical use of Clinitron in a range of patients and conditions.

57

How are you supporting your patients? A review of pressure relieving equipment

Carol Dealey, SRN, RCNT

Clinical Nurse Specialist, Tissue Viability, Moseley Hall Hospital and Queen Elizabeth Hospital, Birmingham

In recent years, pressure sores have 'come out of the closet'. Nurses are no longer automatically given the blame when they occur (Anthony, 1989), and as a result, there is much more interest in their management and prevention. There have also been cases of litigation over the development of pressure sores: Livesley and Simpson (1989) state that lack of adequate equipment to provide pressure relief is negligence in the eyes of the law. It is the responsibility of health authorities to provide reasonable facilities for their patients (Tingle, 1990) so it is nurses' responsibility to alert management to the needs of their patients.

The most common places for pressure sores are the sacrum, buttocks and heels (Locket, 1983). They may arise from lying or sitting for long periods on hard surfaces, such as trolleys, operating tables, X-ray tables, worn out mattresses and inappropriate chairs. Nothing lasts forever and all hospitals need to establish regular review and replacement programmes. Where there is no such policy, nurses can instigate a review of equipment, producing evidence of the need for change.

The Department of Health recommends standard hospital mattresses have a life-span of four years. It should be remembered that the covers only remain water resistant if cleaned with soap and water, and that spraying with alcohol damages them. All mattresses should be at least 130mm in depth - the foam in shallower mattresses has been found to collapse after a short time, and once this has happened, the patient is resting on the metal bed base.

To ensure mattresses are replaced at the appropriate time, nurses can instigate a check and replacement programme. Mattresses can be checked by placing both hands on the centre and pressing down. If the metal base can be felt, the mattress needs replacing. All mattresses should be tested annually, and their check date should then be marked on them. As new mattresses arrive, they should also be marked with the date they come into use.

Pressure relief

There is a huge range of pressure relief equipment available, ranging from highly sophisticated beds to heel pads, and this can be confusing when trying to determine what to use and when. Hibbs (1988) has suggested the requirements for a district general hospital. Ward-based nurses may wish to calculate the requirements for their wards, and this can be done by taking a weekly audit of all the patients. On a set day each week, all patients are assessed using a risk assessment scoring system such as Norton (1975) or Waterlow (1985). Those patients with pressure sores are indicated, as is any pressure relieving equipment being used. According to their score, all patients can be identified as falling into no risk, low, medium or high risk categories: the Waterlow score lends itself nicely to this. Over a period of time, a pattern will emerge indicating the average numbers of patients in each category and, thus, the requirements of the ward. Ideally there should be an adequate supply of equipment so that each patient has what is suitable to his or her needs. Table 1 gives appropriate suggestions, which are discussed in more detail in the text.

Low-risk patients
• Sheepskins
• Hollow core fibre pads
• Bead overlays
• Foam overlays
• Gel pads

Medium-risk patients
• Foam overlays
• Foam replacement mattresses
• Combination foam/water mattresses
• Combination foam/gel mattresses
• Alternating air pads
• Water beds
• Double layer alternating air pads

High-risk patients
• Double layer alternating air pads
• Air floatation pads
• Dynamic air floatation mattress
• Air wave mattress
• Low air loss bed
• Air fluidised bed

Table 1. The range of pressure relieving

Low-risk patients
The standard hospital mattress can be used in conjunction with various overlays.

Sheepskins   Probably readily available in most areas, sheepskins have several limitations. They do not provide pressure relief, although they do prevent friction, and while they absorb moisture, such as perspiration, some patients find them too hot. Many sheepskins become lumpy after frequent laundering, and this can actually cause pressure problems.

Hollow core fibre pads   These are also widely used, and many frail and emaciated patients find they provide great comfort. The recent development of vapour-permeable (VP), water resistant covers has made them easier to use with incontinent patients. They can also reduce the frequency of washing, as the cover can easily be washed between patients. A major problem with these mattresses is that many hospital laundries reduce their life-span by washing them at too high a temperature. Some mattresses have the fibre in individual bolsters inside an outer cover. This can be useful in the community, as several bolsters can be washed together in an ordinary washing machine.

Bead overlays   These are made with beads of polystyrene, which help to spread the pressure, and although they are quite thin, they can be amazingly comfortable. Bead overlays are best used with lighter weight patients, as very heavy patients can squash the beads. VP water resistant covers are available.

Foam overlays   These have recently become popular, probably since the provision of VP water resistant covers. An overlay should be between 70-100mm in depth, and most are partly cut through in cube or egg crate shapes, which provides additional pressure relief. While many patients find these overlays comfortable, they raise the height of the bed, which can be a particular problem in fixed height beds, as it can make it difficult for the patient to get in and out of bed.

Gel pads   These help to disperse pressure because of their density. They can be used on trolleys, X-ray tables and operating tables, as they are not radio-opaque. The major disadvantage is that they are rather heavy and cumbersome to move about.

Medium-risk patients
It is possible to use some of the support systems in this category as a replacement mattress. Others may be used on top of a standard mattress.

Foam overlays   May also be suitable for medium-risk patients providing they are at least 100mm in depth.

Foam replacement mattresses   These are being used to replace standard mattresses in some areas. They are made of different densities of foam put together in such a way as to provide extra pressure relief. Usually fairly firm, they are very popular in orthopaedic and spinal injury units. The expected life-span is double that of standard mattresses (Lowthian, 1989), which can be a useful selling point to management.

Combination foam/water mattresses   Made up of cells of water set in a foam surround, these may also have a foam layer over the cells. Some are deep enough to be a replacement mattress, and they provide the advantages of water floatation without the disadvantages found with water beds. However, some patients feel 'sea sick' on them or find it more difficult to move. They are inappropriate for patients being rehabilitated as it is difficult to sit on the edge of the bed and push up to standing, and are best used for light patients who are bedfast.

Combination gel/foam mattresses   Similar to the above, these are quite heavy to move around as the gel cell remains intact, unlike the water cell, which can be emptied.

Alternating air pads   Commonly referred to as ripple mattresses. The original small-cell ripple mattress was unreliable and actually caused pressure problems, but the types now commonly used either have bubble shaped cells or large horizontal cells. The motor causes the cells to alternately inflate and deflate. Care is needed to avoid pucturing the cells, and this equipment should be regularly maintained to avoid breakdown.

Water beds   These provide true floatation and pressure relief, but there are several disadvantages in their use. The beds are extremely heavy and must be placed where the floor will carry the weight. This is often near a wall and may cause the patient to feel isolated. It is also not very easy moving patients on a water bed. Some beds are lower than standard beds which puts added strain on the nurses' backs. They are no longer widely used.

Double layer alternating air pads   Usually in the form of two layers of alternating air cells. The two layers may work in unison or the bottom layer may be static. A maintenance programme needs to be established for these mattresses.

High-risk patients
Equipment appropriate for these types of patients is of the more sophisticated variety, although some of the support systems from the previous group, such as the double layer alternating air pads, may still be appropriate.

Air floatation pads   Designed so that the patient lies 'in' them rather than 'on' them, these are made up of interconnecting cells which are pumped up with air. The pads should not be pumped up too hard, or the pressures will be high. For some patients these pads are an excellent form of pressure relief, but others may find the rubber from which they are made too hot for comfort.

Dynamic air floatation mattress These have figure-of-eight shaped cells which alternately inflate and deflate. The pressures are automatically adjusted according to the weight and position of the patient, and the motor can also be set on static mode, when the pressures remain constant throughout the cells. These mattresses are useful for a range of patients.

Air wave mattress Made up of two layers of air cells which work together as one; the cells work in a sequence of inflation, partial deflation and deflation. The motor is able to regulate the amount of pressure in the cells according to the weight of the patient. An appropriate support system for those patients who cannot be turned.

Low air loss beds These have a mattress composed of a series of air sacs which lie on edge crossways across the bed. The pressures in the sacs can be adjusted either individually or according to the position on the bed, for example, the pressures for the sacs under the patient's buttocks can be set to be different to those under the chest. The bed can be put in a variety of positions by means of electrical controls, which may be used by patients, giving them some control over their immediate environment. These beds can be particularly useful for very heavy patients who are difficult to move or those with contractures who have limited range of positions.

Air fluidised bed Composed of a large tank which is filled with silicone coated beads. The motor causes the beads to aggitate, producing a fluidising effect. The pressures created are lower than capillary pressure and so do not cause ischaemia by capillary closure, while body fluids such as sweat pass from around the patient's skin into the beads and sink to a sieve at the bottom of the tank. These beds are extremely heavy, and should only be used where the floor can carry the weight. They are mainly used in ITU and burns units for critically ill patients.

Seating

For many excellent reasons, patients are 'mobilised' as soon as possible. Unfortuately, this often results in them being left in chairs for long periods, and often, little or no attention is paid to pressure relief on the grounds that the patient is now 'up'. At this stage in their recovery, many patients lack energy and the desire to move about, and are still likely to be at risk of pressure sore development - considerable pressure may be exerted over the ischial tuberosities when seated. Lowry (1989) considered the principles of good seating.

In the hospital setting it is difficult to cater for the many differing needs of patients. Hospital armchairs often fail to promote good posture, but allow the patient to sit in a slumped position. Not only is the patient likely to slide down the chair, increasing the risk of shearing, but it is also more difficult to rise to standing from this position.

Another fairly common sight is that of a patient sitting with legs dangling a few inches from the floor. There is no way this patient can easily help him- or herself to stand, and this may slow down the process of rehabilitation. Finding suitable chairs for tall men can also be a problem, as the seat may not be deep enough, front to back, as well as the chair being too low.

---

1. Instigate a mattress checking and replacement programme in your ward/unit. Encourage management support by warning of the dangers of litigation!

2. Identify all at-risk patients by means of a risk assessment score and then instigate a plan of care. Remember, once the risk has been identified the responsible nurse is accountable for any lack of care.

3. Ensure that turning regimes include regular pressure relief for patients when sitting out of bed.

4. Liaise with the physiotherapist to identify chairs which provide good posture.

5. Weekly audits can be used to identify the average degree of dependency in a patient population as well as the numbers of pressure sores. This provides objective evidence for the equipment requirements for the area and is a useful bargaining tool.

6. Establish contact with local charity, who will often help with the purchase of equipment.

7. Set up teaching programmes for staff and patients to improve understanding in the causes and prevention of pressure sores. Include the medical staff so they understand their responsibilities.

8. Continue to evaluate the progress being made. This provides encouragement and possible justification for further expenditure.

Table 2. Guidelines for preventing pressure sores.

Apart from the fact that many chairs are generally inappropriate, little attention has been paid to developing maintenance or replacement programmes. One hospital survey (Dealey *et al*, 1990) showed that many armchairs were in need of repair and/or the foam in the seat cushions had collapsed. Many hospitals are writing standards of care for their patients, and it should be possible, within the structure component, to cover armchair maintenance programmes as well as mattress checking.

Another aspect of seating which is often neglected is that of wheelchairs, which are extremely important for moving patients from place to place as well as increasing the mobility of those with disabilities. Wheelchairs are often used without a cushion, allowing the canvas base to exert extremely high pressure. Rithalia (1989) stressed the importance of wheelchair cushions, having found mean pressures of 226.1mm/Hg when testing the base alone. Such high pressures would cause sores in a very short time, and time can pass almost unnoticed as a patient waits for an X-ray, a test or to be seen in casualty or outpatients.

Other forms of pressure relief

Unfortunately not all nurses have easy access to adequate pressure relieving equipment, so other strategies need to be employed. The most widely used is a regular regime for turning patients, and this should be extended to standing or lifting patients when they are sitting out of bed. Preston (1988) highlighted the advantages of using the 30 degree tilt position to reduce pressure even on a standard mattress, while judicious placing of pillows or padding can help protect bony prominences such as heels or elbows. Regular checking of all pressure areas can identify other vulnerable spots.

It is easy to feel intimidated by the huge range of equipment regularly advertised in the nursing press, and by the cost of many items. However several simple aims can be set which will improve the quality of patient care and help to reduce the suffering caused by pressure sores. Table 2 gives guidelines for practice. Although pressure sores may not be seen as a 'glamorous' topic, it is a rewarding one. It can also become addictive - you have been warned!

References

Anthony, D. (1989) The pressure sore debate. *Nursing Times* , **85**, 26,74.

Dealey, C., Eden, L., Earwacker, T. (1990) Are your patients sitting comfortably? *Care of the Elderly*, in press.

Hibbs, P. (1988) Action against pressure sores. *Nursing Times* , **84**, 13, 68-73.

Livesley, B. and Simpson, G. (1989) Hard cost of soft sores. *Health Service Journal*, **99**, 5138, 231.

Locket, B. (1983) Prevalence and Incidence. Pressure Sore Disease. Symposium at Royal Hospital and Home for Incurables, London.

Lowry, M. (1989) Are you sitting comfortably? *Professional Nurse*, **5**, 3, 162-64.

Lowthian, P. (1989) Pressure sore prevention. *Nursing*, **3**, 34, 17-23.

Norton, D., McLaren, R., Exton-Smith, A. N. (1975) An Investigation of Geriatric Nursing Problems in Hospital. Churchill Livingstone, Edinburgh.

Preston, K.W. (1988) Positioning for comfort and pressure relief: The 30 degree alternative. *Care - Science and Practice*, **6**, 4, 116-19.

Rithalia, S.V.S. (1989) Comparison of pressure distribution in wheelchair cushions. *Care - Science and Practice*, **7**, 4, 87-92.

Tingle, J. (1990) The important case of Bull. *Nursing Standard*, **4**, 37, 54-55.

Waterlow, J. (1985) A risk assessment card. *Nursing Times*, **81**, 48, 49-55.

Index